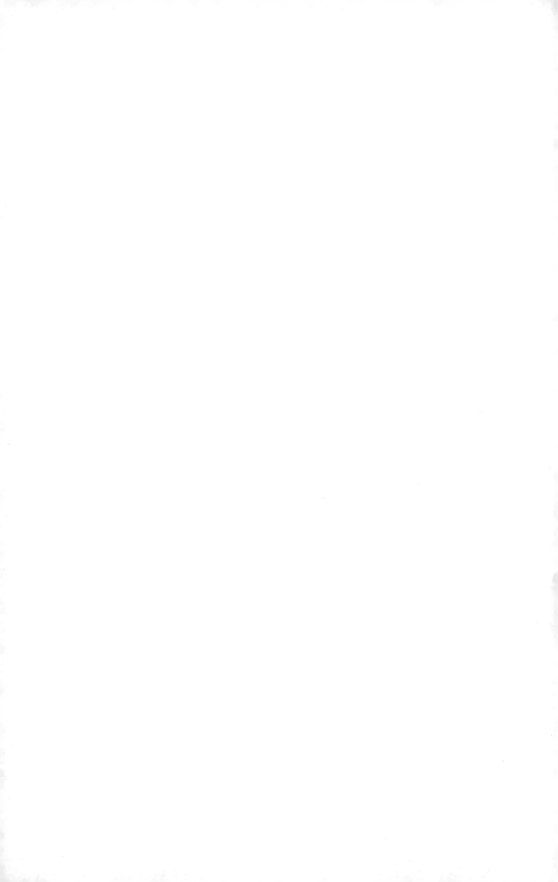

HANDBOOK OF FAMILY THERAPY TRAINING AND SUPERVISION

THE GUILFORD FAMILY THERAPY SERIES
Alan S. Gurman, *Editor*

Casebook of Marital Therapy
Alan S. Gurman, *Editor*

Families and Other Systems: The Macrosystemic Context of Family Therapy
John Schwartzman, *Editor*

The Military Family: Dynamics and Treatment
Florence W. Kaslow and Richard I. Ridenour, *Editors*

Marriage and Divorce: A Contemporary Perspective
Carol C. Nadelson and Derek C. Polonsky, *Editors*

Family Care of Schizophrenia: A Problem-Solving Approach to the Treatment of Mental Illness
Ian R. H. Falloon, Jeffrey L. Boyd, and Christine W. McGill

The Process of Change
Peggy Papp

Family Therapy: Principles of Strategic Practice
Allon Bross, *Editor*

Aesthetics of Change
Bradford P. Keeney

Family Therapy in Schizophrenia
William R. McFarlane, *Editor*

Mastering Resistance: A Practical Guide to Family Therapy
Carol M. Anderson and Susan Stewart

Family Therapy and Family Medicine: Toward the Primary Care of Families
William J. Doherty and Macaran A. Baird

Ethnicity and Family Therapy
Monica McGoldrick, John K. Pearce, and Joseph Giordano, *Editors*

Patterns of Brief Family Therapy: An Ecosystemic Approach
Steve de Shazer

The Family Therapy of Drug Abuse and Addiction
M. Duncan Stanton, Thomas C. Todd, and Associates

From Psyche to System: The Evolving Therapy of Carl Whitaker
John R. Neill and David P. Kniskern, *Editors*

Normal Family Processes
Froma Walsh, *Editor*

Helping Couples Change: A Social Learning Approach to Marital Therapy
Richard B. Stuart

HANDBOOK OF FAMILY THERAPY TRAINING AND SUPERVISION

Edited by
HOWARD A. LIDDLE
University of California, San Francisco

DOUGLAS C. BREUNLIN
RICHARD C. SCHWARTZ
Institute for Juvenile Research, Chicago

THE GUILFORD PRESS
New York London

© 1988 The Guilford Press
A Division of Guilford Publications, Inc.
72 Spring Street, New York, N.Y. 10012

Printed in the United States of America

Last digit is print number: 9 8 7 6 5 4

Library of Congress Cataloging-in-Publication Data

Handbook of family therapy training and supervision / [edited by] Howard A. Liddle, Douglas C. Breunlin, Richard C. Schwartz.
    p. cm. — (The Guilford family therapy series)
    Includes bibliographies and index.
    ISBN 0-89862-073-2
    1. Family psychotherapy—Study and teaching—Supervision.
I. Liddle, Howard A. II. Breunlin, Douglas C. III. Schwartz, Richard C. IV. Series.
   [DNLM: WM 18 H236]
RC488.5.H334 1988
616.89′ 156′071—dc 19   87-24848
                                        CIP

To Our Parents and Families:
Loving and Superb Teachers All

Contributors

James F. Alexander, PhD, University of Utah, Salt Lake City, Utah

Donald R. Bardill, PhD, Florida State University School of Social Work, Tallahassee, Florida

Mary Jo Barrett, MSW, Midwest Family Resource Associates, Chicago, Illinois

Michael Berger, PhD, Atlanta Institute for Family Studies, Atlanta, Georgia

Douglas C. Breunlin, MSSA, Institute for Juvenile Research, Chicago, Illinois

Betty Carter, MSW, The Family Institute of Westchester, Mt. Vernon, New York

Gianfranco Cecchin, MD, Centro Milanese di Terapia della Famiglia, Milan, Italy

Rocco A. Cimmarusti, MSW, Center for Family Development, Chicago, Illinois

Jorge Colapinto, Lic., Wynnewood, Pennsylvania

Lee Combrinck-Graham, MD, Institute for Juvenile Research, Chicago, Illinois

Gail S. Davidson, MEd, Private Practice, Princeton, New Jersey, and Yardley, Pennsylvania; Seton Hall University, South Orange, New Jersey

Celia Jaes Falicov, PhD, La Jolla Marital and Family Institute, La Jolla, California

Richard Fisch, MD, Brief Therapy Center, The Mental Research Institute, Palo Alto, California

Alan S. Gurman, PhD, University of Wisconsin Medical School, Madison, Wisconsin

Leonard J. Haas, PhD, University of Utah, Salt Lake City, Utah

Jay Haley, The Family Therapy Institute of Washington, D.C., Rockville, Maryland

Fredda Herz, PhD, The Family Institute of Westchester, Mt. Vernon, New York

Betty M. Karrer, MA, Institute for Juvenile Research, Chicago, Illinois

David P. Kniskern, PsyD, University of Cincinnati College of Medicine, Cincinnati, Ohio

Maureen Leahey, RN, PhD, Holy Cross Hospital, Calgary, Alberta, Canada

Howard A. Liddle, EdD, University of California, San Francisco, California

Cloé Madanes, Lic., The Family Therapy Institute of Washington, D.C., Rockville, Maryland

C. Haydee Mas, PhD, University of Utah, Salt Lake City, Utah

Judith Mazza, PhD, Center for Problem Solving, Bethesda, Maryland

Dennis E. McGuire, MA, Carthage College, Kenosha, Wisconsin

William C. Nichols, EdD, Tallahassee, Florida

Daniel V. Papero, PhD, Georgetown University Family Center, Washington, D.C.

Sergio Pirrotta, EdM, LCSW, Mental Health and Retardation Services, Inc., Lawrence, Massachusetts

Donald C. Ransom, PhD, University of California, San Francisco, California

Benjamin E. Saunders, PhD, Medical University of South Carolina, Charleston, South Carolina

Richard C. Schwartz, PhD, Institute for Juvenile Research, Chicago, Illinois

Douglas H. Sprenkle, PhD, Purdue University, West Lafayette, Indiana

Lorraine M. Wright, RN, PhD, University of Calgary, Calgary, Alberta, Canada

Acknowledgments

The vision and appearance of this book are owed in large measure to three sources of support for our work as teachers of family therapy: the wide variety of settings that funded, housed, and nurtured our training efforts over the last 14 years; our colleagues and fellow trainers; and the many students who challenged us to teach and supervise with precision, humanity, and compassion.

The following list represents those settings in which we conducted or were involved in major training programs: Adolescents and Families Project (funded by the National Institute of Drug Abuse) of the Department of Family and Community Medicine, University of California, San Francisco, California; Department of Pediatrics and Family Practice, Cook County Hospital, Chicago, Illinois; Dupage County Health Department, Wheaton, Illinois; Department of Psychiatry, Eastern Pennsylvania Psychiatric Institute, Philadelphia, Pennsylvania; Family Institute, Cardiff, Wales; Family Practice Residency Program of San Francisco General Hospital, San Francisco, California; Family Systems Program, Institute for Juvenile Research, Chicago, Illinois; Marriage Guidance Council of New South Wales, Australia; Mental Research Institute, Palo Alto, California; Purdue University, West Lafayette, Indiana; and the Department of Counseling Psychology, Temple University, Philadelphia, Pennsylvania. Many other settings, unfortunately too numerous to mention, also provided important opportunities to train and supervise clinicians in family therapy.

The dedication, support, and challenges of our teachers and the professional stimulation of collaboration with colleagues and fellow trainers contributed mightily to this book. We are particularly thankful to Toni Bernotas, Betty Bosdell, Brian Cade, Rocco Cimmarusti, Terry Colling, John Constantine, Max Cornwell, Celia Falicov, Earl Goodman, Jay Haley, Gordon Hart, Bonnie Henkels, Betty Karrer, Phil Kingston, Agnes Lattimer, Sue Mackey, Salvador Minuchin, Jamshed Morenas, Don Murphy, Joel Richman, Anthony Richtsmeier, George Saba, Philippa Seligman, Jim Smith, Doug Sprenkle, Bernice Tucker, Sue Walrond-Skinner, and Marianne Walters.

Finally, many talented students have shared with us their excitement, skepticism, and curiosity about family therapy, as well as their clinical work with families. We have enjoyed and learned from participating in and observing their emergence as family therapists and in many instances, as talented trainers.

We also thank those who assisted in the preparation of the manuscript, particularly Nikki Settles, Joann Godbold, and Linda Kellett for professional typing and the Family Systems Program Women's Group for reviewing manuscripts.

We pay special thanks to Seymour Weingarten, of The Guilford Press, for his continued support; to Alan Gurman, the Family Therapy Series Editor, for constructive guidance; and, most important, to our contributors, whose translation of their expertise to the printed page made this a volume in which we take great pride.

Howard A. Liddle
Douglas C. Breunlin
Richard C. Schwartz

Preface

The intent of this book is to provide a comprehensive examination of family therapy training and supervision, an area of the family therapy field with a rich diversity of ideas and practices. In this volume, we have attempted to organize this breadth and variation of content and thinking into six sections. Section One orients the reader, offers a macrolevel, grand tour of the vast terrain of family therapy training and supervision, and identifies many of the content areas addressed more fully in the chapters.

SECTION TWO

"Family Therapy Models: Approaches to Training," explores, within the various models of family therapy, how differences in theories of therapy reflect differences in training practices. Leaders of several family therapy models describe their training approach. Particular attention is given to the connections between the therapy and training models, as well as to the assumptions, methods, content, notions about trainee change and development, and context of each training approach.

   The differences in clinical practices among various models of family therapy have been addressed repeatedly in the literature, but the similarities and differences among the training and supervision practices of various models of family therapy have rarely been scrutinized (see McDaniel, Weber, & McKeever, 1983). In this section, the training philosophy and methods of seven different models of family therapy are described by prominent trainers from each model.

   In Chapter 2 Colapinto describes the spatial, jigsaw puzzle view of families that structuralists hold; details the structural training philosophy, which parallels the approach to therapy; and outlines the practices of the extern program at the Philadelphia Child Guidance Clinic. He offers sound advice regarding the practice of live and videotaped supervision, and, in a final section, clearly illustrates typical training problems and their solutions. Throughout his chapter, Colapinto interweaves the principles of structural therapy into the training and supervision context.

   The Milan Team's radical departure from other family therapy models has had a powerful impact on the field. These differences in theory are both subtle and complex and, fortunately, Pirrotta and Cecchin have organized Chapter 3 so that tenets like epistemology, circularity, relativity, and neutrality are understandable and provide a context for the evolution of their training methods. Since the Milan Team's clinical practices are so different from those of other therapies, one expects the same to be true of their training methods. As detailed by Pirrotta and Cecchin, their training process is, indeed, unusual, and consistent with their systemic world view. The authors conclude with feedback from current and former students on their experiences and on problems with this approach to training.

In Chapter 4 Papero provides a concise but comprehensive review of Bowen theory, which, he states, is "the product of an effort to see the human from a broad perspective," and thus is a philosophy of life rather than just a framework for understanding family interaction. Papero fully discusses the central concept of differentiation of self and identifies six other concepts that form the conceptual core of Bowen theory. In the second half of the chapter, Papero outlines the training process at the Georgetown Family Center, which he describes as "a dialogue between engaged minds." The most important goals of this program are for trainees to understand the concept of differentiation and to become more differentiated themselves. Papero describes in rich detail how these goals are achieved through lecture/discussion and supervision.

The hallmarks of the brief therapy approach of the Mental Research Institute (MRI) are its simplicity and brevity. In Chapter 5, Fisch's description of the nonpathological and non-normative theory behind this approach is, of course, brief and simple. Fisch succinctly explains the more-of-the-same-attempted-solution sequence that is the cornerstone of the MRI model. The training at the MRI that he describes is designed to teach the techniques and theory in the most pragmatic and efficient manner possible. Fisch's description of the problems trainees have in remaining true to the brief therapy model indicates that, while the approach is simple, it is not necessarily easy to learn. Thus, the training issues covered in this chapter are very important.

In Chapter 6, Mazza presents a strategic approach to raining derived from the work of Jay Haley and Cloé Madanes. Unlike the other theories discussed in this section, the theory of strategic family therapy is not outlined in a separate section of the chapter; instead, it is embedded among the many illustrations of training situations that Mazza provides. These examples highlight the strategic trainer's use of the same indirect, hypnotically derived techniques to change trainees that the strategic therapist uses to change families. In addition, in a unique section, Mazza describes eight types of trainees that strategic trainers are likely to encounter and gives strategies for dealing with each type.

For the most part, the models covered thus far in this section have spurned psychodynamic concepts and training paradigms. Nichols, in contrast, presents a model of family therapy in Chapter 7 that retains an appreciation of the unconscious, insight, and historical processes in individuals and incorporates the newer systems perspectives on family interaction. Nichols presents a model for training and educating therapists that is consistent with this integrative clinical approach. His approach to training is long-term and gradual, involving a solid conceptual foundation as a prerequisite to clinical experience, and it is relatively nondirective in its emphasis on allowing trainees to develop their own ideas and style.

In Chapter 8, Haas, Alexander, and Mas describe a university-based model called Functional Family Therapy that incorporates aspects of the Structural and Strategic models described above as well as the concepts and rigor of behavioral approaches. In their graduate school context, the authors are faced with a different set of issues and opportunities; consequently, their training practices, and the Functional Family Therapy model itself, reflect the adaptations they have made to these differences. Their training process, like their model, is based on well-articulated and specific phases.

SECTION THREE

In "Pragmatics of Supervision," the editors and some of our associates reflect on the conceptual, behavioral, and technical aspects of family therapy supervision. These contributions are intended to be detail- and skill-focused explorations of various aspects of the mechanics of supervising family therapists.

Family therapy supervision has emerged as a subspeciality within the field of family therapy, possessing its own body of knowledge and extensive literature. (It is beyond the scope of this volume to review this literature, but a comprehensive, categorized set of references is provided in the Appendix. Additionally, Liddle [in press] offers a comparative analysis and critique of this literature in the second edition of the *Handbook of Family Therapy* [Gurman & Kniskern, in press].) This section includes five chapters devoted to particularly relevant topics in contemporary family therapy supervision.

In a national survey of family therapy trainers representing the full range of training sites, respondents expressed a desire for the development of clear models of family therapy training and supervision (Saba & Liddle, 1986). Responding to this finding, in Chapter 9 Liddle develops a series of practically presented conceptual overlays or action-suggesting maps that can guide the supervisor's work. The isomorphic nature of training and therapy, key variables in the training system's formation, and the stages of training are the major overlays offered in this evolving model of systemic supervision.

The new technology of live and videotape supervision, as well as the emphasis on changing the trainee's world view rather than just teaching skills, has placed a great deal of strain and importance on the trainer–trainee relationship. In Chapter 10, with these pressures taken as a starting point, Schwartz provides practical advice for maintaining a good working supervisory relationship. He includes guidelines for creating a workable and mutually satisfactory frame for the training, for handling a range of difficulties in the trainer–trainee relationship, and for helping trainees focus on the family and on their overall and session plans rather than on their trainer's opinion of them. Threaded throughout the chapter are suggestions for negotiating the delicate relationship balance among encouraging trainee autonomy and insuring trainee learning and help for the family in treatment.

Live supervision can be an effective, efficient training tool. It is, however, an intricately complex endeavor containing the possibility of numerous technical and interpersonal difficulties. In Chapter 11, Schwartz, Liddle, and Breunlin present illustrations of the most common of the problems faced by supervisors using live supervision and offer practical suggestions for either avoiding or untangling them. Two processes inherent in live supervision are emphasized: the tendency toward trainee robotization and the tendency for sequences of interaction to be mirrored at all levels of the training system.

Videotape supervision has gained widespread acceptance as an effective method of family therapy supervision, but surprisingly little has been written about it. In Chapter 12, Breunlin, Karrer, McGuire, and Cimmarusti address this gap in the literature by offering a model of videotape supervision. They compare videotape supervision based on three theories: psychodynamic, first-order cybernetics, and second-order cybernetics. The authors choose second-order cybernetics to organize their model. This framework connects the internal, distinction-drawing processes of the therapist with the interactive process these distinctions elicit. Videotape supervision is defined as a process whereby the tape material is used by the supervisor to help therapists refine their ability to draw distinctions and hence work more effectively with interactive process. A protocol for videotape supervision is proposed with a set of guidelines for effective implementation and control of negative effects.

As family therapy increases in popularity, greater numbers of family therapists will seek to become supervisors. In Chapter 13, Breunlin, Liddle, and Schwartz propose that becoming a supervisor can be seen as another stage in the never-ending process of one's development, as well as a step that entails the acquisition of new skills and professional identity. They believe that becoming a supervisor requires practice under the guidance of an experienced supervisor. They describe training programs where this *live supervision of supervision* occurs simultaneously with supervision of therapy. To manage this program's complexity, the authors attend closely to complementary sets of training objectives for therapist and supervisor. These objectives are categorized as systemic thinking, technical skills, and professional identity. Actualization of training objectives is orchestrated through additional training formats involving appropriate combinations of therapists and supervisors over the course of the training year.

SECTION FOUR

"Contexts for Training," describes the many forms that family therapy training assumes according to the setting in which it occurs. The issues and unique challenges posed by a broad spectrum of training contexts are detailed by authors representing a variety of professional disciplines and settings.

In this volume, seven chapters address the following settings: degree-granting programs in marriage and family therapy, free-standing institutes, psychiatry, nursing, family medicine, academic psychology, and social work.

In Chapter 14, Sprenkle describes training in programs that offer academic degrees in marriage and family therapy. He provides compelling arguments for the importance of such programs to the field of family therapy. Sprenkle traces the development of degree-granting programs, examines their context, and describes how training prepares students to view themselves as entering the profession of family therapy.

Using their experience from the Family Institute of Westchester, in Chapter 15, Herz and Carter analyze the life cycle of a free-standing institute. Such institutes, which often began with a group of colleagues seeking opportunities to work together, have survived through their ability to manage successfully a series of organizational and fiscal crises. The authors describe the evolution of an integrated set of training objectives and describe marketing strategies to attract students.

In Chapter 16, Combrinck-Graham addresses family therapy training in psychiatry. She argues that psychiatrists, who operate at all levels of a biopsychosocial continuum, should be taught an ecosystemic epistemology to enable them to understand the recursiveness among levels of that continuum and to be equipped to intervene at any of the levels. She describes a "systemic" residency that possesses many opportunities for learning ecosystemic thinking and describes family therapy training per se as but one aspect of that training. Included in her analysis are a discussion of the problems associated with offering a systemic residency within a medical setting and suggestions for addressing those problems.

Wright and Leahey, in Chapter 17, describe family therapy training in nursing. They distinguish between bachelor and graduate level programs and argue that generic training in family nursing is appropriate for the former while specialist training in family therapy should be reserved for the latter. They describe the trend toward family therapy in nursing and offer suggestions about training programs including training objectives, supervision methods, and training facilities. They also include an interesting section that details the contributions nursing can make to family therapy.

In Chapter 18, by posing and answering a set of questions relevant to the topic, Ransom tackles family therapy training in family practice settings. What results is a thorough discussion of the place of family therapy within family medicine. Ransom discusses the personal and professional pitfalls, obstacles, surprises, and breakthroughs family therapists can expect and provides a glimpse at future trends that suggest an increase in collaboration between family therapists and family physicians. Ransom offers useful suggestions to help family therapists adapt their training efforts to the context of family practice.

In Chapter 19, Berger tackles the status of family therapy training in academic psychology. He identifies five areas within psychology in which connections with family therapy theory and practice might easily be made. These include social psychology, child development, ecological and community psychology, clinical child psychology, and behavior therapy. He uses the Georgia State psychology program as a model for introducing family therapy into academic psychology, an effort that he believes should be handled strategically. Berger concludes by offering content areas, such as research and developmental theory, where psychology has much to offer family therapy.

Bardill and Saunders begin their discussion of family therapy training in social work in Chapter 20 by tracing the long history of social work's involvement with families. This history reveals many systemically oriented social workers involved with families long before family therapy became a movement in the 1950s. The authors present survey findings suggesting that great interest in family therapy currently exists in schools of social work, but argue that philosophic squabbles between the "people changers" and "social changers" and trends toward a generalist approach in social work education still limit the availability of quality family therapy training. They propose a curriculum for master's level family therapy education in social work that meets the accrediting requirements for both social work and the American Association of Marriage and Family Therapy.

SECTION FIVE

Section Five, "Special Issues," supplies a sampling of salient issues and topics that keep training and supervision an exciting, and sometimes controversial, area of family therapy. The contributors' identification and development of content domains such as cultural sensitivity, research and evaluation, and meta-analyses of training and supervision not only illustrate current trends but also highlight areas that require further conceptual specification and guidelines for implementation. Volumes could be filled with special issues, but, because of limited space we decided to include five chapters.

In Chapter 21 Falicov presents a framework that integrates culture into family therapy training. Her cultural perspective uses an ecosystemic view that draws upon Bronfenbrenner's model of ecosystems and is designed to help trainees make culture relevant to therapy in the following ways: first, to assess a family's ecological fit at all levels of an ecosystem; second, to determine an index of ecological stress based on the family's dissonance within the ecosystem; third, to choose appropriate goals and interventions; and fourth, to assess and use the degree of cultural consonance-dissonance between the family and therapist. Falicov shows how important family therapy concepts such as organization and development can be used with a cultural perspective in mind. Key aspects of her training approach are the integration of a cultural perspective with other training objectives, interviews with nonclinical families, and experiential exercises.

A consistent theme in Haley's writing on training, and one that runs through this book, is the parallel nature of clinical practice and supervision. In Chapter 22, Haley uses this principle to predict the consequences of different types of supervision for both clients and trainees. He criticizes supervision models that focus on the personality of the trainee because the trainee will in turn focus on the personality of the clients rather than on how they can change. Similarly, he takes issue with supervisors who focus on family dynamics rather than on the requisite skills for helping people. Haley also discusses the degree to which trainees need to be made aware of why they are directed by their supervisors to make interventions. In sum, this chapter presents both Haley's personal overview of the world of supervision and a theoretical rationale that complements the strategic supervisory techniques described by Mazza in Chapter 6.

In reviewing the state of family therapy research and providing guidelines for future research endeavors, Kniskern and Gurman have updated their earlier (1979) survey of research on family therapy training in Chapter 23. They highlight two recent projects that "break methodological ground and provide models for future investigators" interested in evaluating training. Finally they offer a comprehensive list of researchable questions that remain unaddressed in the area of training.

Is therapy art or science? Most of the chapters in this book emphasize the latter, but in Chapter 24 Madanes considers family therapy as a form of popular art and entertainment and draws parallels from other forms of entertainment such as drama, television, and rock music. Likening the supervisor to a playwright "who has been given the task of entertaining by writing for each family and therapist a script," Madanes humorously shows how the techniques of family therapy such as circular questioning, enactment, reframing, directives, ordeals, and use of metaphors become ingredients for constructing a therapeutic drama. Madanes's paper, while playful at one level, calls attention to the influence our larger culture has on the practice of therapy and training.

In Chapter 25, Liddle, Davidson, and Barrett present the results of in-depth interviews with 85 family therapy trainees regarding their experience of being supervised. These trainees, from various contexts and different levels of experience, offer a wide range of frankly-expressed opinions and observations on specific topics such as the value of during-session phone calls and consultations, preferences regarding trainer style, and the qualities of a good training group. The authors conclude with suggestions to trainees on how to get the most out of the live supervision experience.

CONCLUSION

The book concludes with a discussion of the future of family therapy, followed by an appendix, in which Liddle and Breunlin have compiled and organized the family therapy training and supervision literature. Their outline of over 400 articles, chapters, and books on training and supervision permits efficient location of salient references in a wide variety of content areas, disciplines, and sources.

REFERENCES

Gurman, A., & Kniskern, D. (Eds.). (in press). *Handbook of family therapy* (2nd ed.). New York: Brunner/Mazel.

Kniskern, D., & Gurman, A. (1979). Research on training in marriage and family therapy: Status, issues, and direction. *Journal of Marital and Family Therapy, 5*(3), 83–94.

Liddle, H. A. (1988). Family therapy training and supervision: A critical review and analysis. In A. Gurman & D. Kniskern (Eds.), *Handbook of family therapy* (2nd ed.). New York: Brunner/Mazel.

McDaniel, S., Weber, T., & McKeever, J. (1983). Multiple theoretical approaches to supervision: Choices in family therapy training. *Family Process, 22*, 491–500.

Saba, G., & Liddle, H. A. (1986). Perceptions of professional needs, practice patterns, and critical issues facing family therapy trainers and supervisors. *American Journal of Family Therapy, 14*, 109–122.

Contents

HANDBOOK OF
FAMILY THERAPY TRAINING
AND SUPERVISION

SECTION ONE

OVERVIEW

1

Family Therapy Training and Supervision: An Introduction

HOWARD A. LIDDLE
University of California, San Francisco

DOUGLAS C. BREUNLIN
RICHARD C. SCHWARTZ
Institute for Juvenile Research, Chicago

A contextual perspective has been the hallmark of family therapy, and, not surprisingly, it is also a useful framework for understanding the area of training and supervision, one of family therapy's most active and rapidly expanding subsystems. Early in the history and development of the family therapy field, training was a fairly homogeneous concept, modest in scope and influence and characterized by the clinical wizardry of "the Great Originals" (Hoffman, 1983) rather than by clearly articulated curricula and objectives. This is no longer the case. In the last decade, we have witnessed exponential growth in family therapy training and supervision, which now have their own body of knowledge, publications, conferences, and experts (Liddle, in press, b). This growing interest in training and supervision has resulted in a specialty within the family therapy field that is more sophisticated and varied in its mission, content, and methods than ever before.

The contemporary context of training is characterized by a tremendous heterogeneity of backgrounds, biases, intentions, and objectives. For example, training is operationalized in different ways depending on whether the goal is to expose students to a family approach or to prepare postdegree clinicians to work with families. The context in which training occurs also influences the processes and outcomes of training and supervision (e.g., Framo, 1976; Haley, 1975; Liddle, 1978). Training that occurs within settings that define family therapy as a profession is different from training that takes place within established professional disciplines, such as psychology, social work, nursing, pastoral counseling, and psychiatry. Additionally, the training site's financial stability and means of support, stage of development, embeddedness or lack thereof in the community, plans and prospects for the future, and physical facilities influence the nature of the training provided.

The characteristics of those conducting the training as well as those who are being trained also codetermine the definition and translation of family therapy training. Previous clinical training in family therapy and in other models, as well as formal instruction in supervision and the personal characteristics and interpersonal styles of trainers and trainees all interact to define and shape the training. Also, as both the locales of family therapy training and the variety of professionals designating themselves, or being designated, as family therapy trainers or supervisors have increased, the content, too, has expanded and become more complex. Family therapy training may cover one therapeutic approach or several distinct models, or can assume an integrative form that

3

attempts to blend principles, rules, and methods of therapeutic operation into a single comprehensive model. The definition of family therapy training, therefore, depends on the stated purpose of the specific training, the training site, the amount of time devoted to the training, whether it is for actual clinical work with families or for exposure to family systems thinking, and how these factors synergistically interact to create the teaching and learning process called training.

SHIFTING VISIBILITY AND STATUS

Why is training and supervision becoming a more prominent fixture in the family therapy field? Also, what accounts for its increase in stature and attention? The skills of training and supervision, once taken for granted, are less likely to be unarticulated and underappreciated today, partly because of an increased awareness of the difficulty and complexity of the training task. In a survey of supervisors, we found that family therapy teachers wanted superordinate frameworks to guide their work, and they believed that their previous clinical training had inadequately prepared them for the duties and identity of a family therapy supervisor (Saba & Liddle, 1986). Further, the mystique and charisma of the family therapy pioneers have given way to a developing technology of therapy, and, by inference at least, if there can be a technology of therapy, there can be a corresponding technology of training. Clinical models are being defined more systematically, often along integrative lines, and, not surprisingly, so are the developing training models. The clinical models are part of a changing zeitgeist that increasingly demands demonstration of accountability to funding-related health care systems. Similarly, the manner in which these more externally scrutinized clinical models are taught and implemented is also subject to a lens of evaluative inquiry.

This growing recognition of the difficulty and complexity of training is contrary to the often unstated but operative notion that training is merely something one *does*—a straightforward extension of therapeutic skills. Although making the transition from therapist to supervisor requires a significant leap in thinking, skills and professional role identity, it is often taken for granted. Agencies frequently promote clinicians into supervisory positions without sufficient preparation; and while teachers of therapists would not consider screening clinicians without some assessment of their abilities (e.g., conceptual and perceptual skills), those responsible for designating and selecting supervisors often do not exercise equal care.

Today the training and supervision subsystem has become vital to the family therapy field because it transmits the field's values, body of knowledge, professional roles, and skills to new clinicians. Training and supervision are also primary vehicles through which a field evolves. They prepare future generations to be the representatives and developers of the field's viewpoint, with the hope that they will move beyond their mentors in conceptual, therapeutic, and professional development.

THE CONTEMPORARY SCENE OF TRAINING
AND SUPERVISION

As we have mentioned previously, family therapy training is developing rapidly: workshops and training institutes abound, inroads have been made into the traditional academic institutions in a variety of disciplines, and advances in the development of a technology for teaching the complex behavioral skills of family therapy are evident (see Everett, 1980; Kaslow et al., 1977; Liddle, 1988b, for comprehensive reviews of the literature).

Live and video supervision and, within certain models, the role of the group behind the mirror are primary examples of these gains. On the conceptual front, work on the specification and practical implications of the isomorphic nature of training and therapy has appeared and serves as an organizing schema for trainers. Finally, as we have said, family therapy trainers have long been concerned with and sensitive to the contextual aspects of training, and the literature illustrates the difficulties of conducting family therapy and training in a variety of settings (e.g., Malone, 1974; Meyerstein, 1977; Shapiro, 1975, 1979; Stanton, 1975; Sugarman, 1984). The increasing interest in family therapy training has generated the excitement that often characterizes a growing field. Yet it has also resulted in uncertainty, a lack of standards and guidelines, and a lack of consensus on how best to train and supervise.

Current Trends and Developments

In recent years, presentations and workshops on training and supervision have dramatically increased at the annual meetings of the American Association for Marriage and Family Therapy (AAMFT) and the American Family Therapy Association (AFTA). Additionally, training has become a more serious area of focus within these and other professional organizations. The AAMFT, through its Commission on Accreditation, has been accrediting training programs since 1978. Also within AAMFT, the Commission on Supervision, in addition to setting standards for and approving new supervisors within its parent organization, has been increasingly concerned with setting standards for the practice of supervision in marriage and family therapy.

On a related professional front, the American Psychological Association has established a Division of Family Psychology, which has its active Training and Education Committee designed to influence doctoral education in psychology in family systems therapy. The Division's *Journal of Family Psychology* has taken its place in the scholarly community of organized psychology as the primary representative of the family systems paradigm (Liddle, 1987a, 1987b).

The role of free-standing institutes relative to teaching family therapy in traditional institutions such as academic departments within universities remains to be defined, although work has begun in this regard, with models of collaboration being proposed (Lebow, 1987).

Content Needs

What are the content themes in training and supervision? Which areas can help this corner of the field to become more sophisticated? Several themes have been identified and are beginning to influence how therapists are trained to work with families. First, the impact of the women's movement and feminist thinking has been felt in the family therapy field. In training and supervision, various authors are addressing gender-related concerns about power, hierarchy, discrimination, and sex-role–stereotyped thinking

(Caust, Libow, & Raskin, 1981; Goldner, 1987; Hare-Mustin, 1987; Libow, 1985; Libow, Raskin, & Caust, 1982; Okun, 1983; Wheeler, Avis, Miller, & Chaney, 1985). Second, the family life cycle has also become a valuable content overlay in the training of family therapists (Liddle, in press), and has emerged as a developing content domain that can inform a therapist's work in positive and powerful ways (Breunlin, 1988; Falicov, 1988; Liddle & Saba, 1983). Third, work in the area of cross-cultural issues and ethnic differences has advanced considerably: several people have offered concrete guidelines for how this new sensitivity can help a therapist's work (Falicov, Chapter 21, this volume; Saba, Karrer, & Hardy, in press). Fourth, the notion of stages in therapy (Breunlin, 1987), in training (Liddle & Saba, 1983, Chapter 10), and in therapist development (Schwartz, 1981) is evolving and also has important implications for training and supervision (Liddle, in press). Theory development specific to training has proceeded slowly; thus far, it has been limited to ideas about the isomorphism between therapy and training.

Several other content domains that need further elaboration have also been recognized. For example, ethical and legal issues in training family therapists represent a fairly new content area, with only a few papers available (Cormier & Bernard, 1982; Margolin, 1982; Piercy & Sprenkle, 1983); also, in the research realm, although it is certainly not a problem peculiar to family therapy, practitioner utilization of relevant research findings is a vexing concern for clinicians and researchers alike (Andreozzi & Levant, 1985; Cohen, Sargent & Sechrest, 1986; Hazelrigg, Cooper, & Borduin, 1987; Morrow-Bradley & Elliot, 1986).

Despite many advances in the area of training and supervision methods, the evaluation of these methods, especially as they exist and are attempted by supervisors of various experience levels and across multiple contexts, remains a fertile area for further work. Additionally, the issue of the personality of the therapist and related matters of therapist and supervisor development will certainly receive growing attention and focus in the years ahead.

FAMILY THERAPY TRAINING AND SUPERVISION: A CRITICAL REAPPRAISAL

Why is it necessary and appropriate to examine critically the complex mission of family therapy training and supervision? A straightforward rationale could be cast in terms of developmental readiness: the field is now ready to withstand and undertake such inquiry. The clinical area of the field is beginning to look critically and realistically at its methods and at many elemental, cherished assumptions. The research arena is improving, with an increase in the number and quality of family-oriented studies and a growing concern with the establishment of an empirical base to the field. On the political and policymaking fronts, there is a clear mindfulness of both the needs and the challenges involved in attempts to influence social service delivery and policy institutions. Within the context of health and mental health care delivery systems, we are increasingly becoming aware of the need for long-term realistic (Ryder, 1987), if not modest, plans in this regard.

As we venture into the new and uncharted realm "beyond family therapy," trainers will conceive of their mission and role in appropriately expanded ways; in the process, they will challenge the boundaries, roles, and definitions of family therapy training and supervision (Liddle, 1985b)—and, indeed, of family therapy itself (Liddle, 1985a). This new generation of trainers will have a greater comprehension of (and options regarding) the politics of family therapy, partly out of choice and partly out of necessity. If political (e.g., economic and gender) factors are ignored or not centrally embedded in their philosophy and methods, trainers risk training and treatment failure. Successful trainers will need to be ever more cognizant of contextual factors in the construction and implementation of training programs.

Another major issue facing contemporary training and supervision is identical to that facing the clinical area of the field. That is, how can family therapy training and curricula be adapted to and designed for the wide variety of settings in which training is now offered? How can the idiosyncrasies of any context be taken into account in designing and implementing a training model, given its strengths, limitations, and politics?

The matter of how the current and future generations of trainers should be trained is in need of clear guidelines and additional thinking. Issues concerning the skills and body of knowledge required to produce competent trainers, indeed a definition of what constitutes effective training, remain to be substantively addressed. Professional identity and affiliation issues are also in need of inquiry and specification. Family therapy training and supervision can be seen as a barometer of change as well as a context in which change can contribute to and influence the broader field of family therapy. Creativity, innovation, and commitment to evaluation and research in the training and supervision area can thus have obvious generative influences on the clinical, research, theoretical, and political domains of the family therapy field.

Finally, as the mission, methods, and scope of training are being reexamined, difficult questions arise. To what extent should trainers be concerned with the preparation of their trainees as family therapy advocates, representatives of a viewpoint and way of working that is not widely accepted as legitimate or even helpful? Are we, as some have suggested, training therapists with insufficient attention to the settings and communities in which they will work? Should trainers not only teach a set of skills or content to trainees, but also prepare them (conceptually and practically) for the potential difficulties that arise in the implementation of family therapy?

SUMMARY

Just as the models of family therapy are, unsurprisingly, isomorphically represented in their corresponding training models and methods, so the development of the clinical realm of family therapy can serve as a metaphor for the development of the training and supervision area. Within family therapy, training and supervision have become increasingly visible and important, well defined, and sophisticated. The importance of training is reflected by a questioning of the appropriate role of trainers and the need to *train* supervisors and teachers of therapy. There has been a heightened sensitivity to context in the maturation of the training and supervision area. An expanding awareness of the limitation of our training settings, the political fallout of our training mission, the consequences of having therapists work in a particular work setting, and the need to change established institutional structures (e.g., child protective services, Aid to Families with Dependent Children, juvenile court) are examples of the contextualization of training and supervision.

In summary, then, progress has been seen in the noteworthy emergence of technology (e.g., live and videotaped supervision), curricular development in the form of learning objectives, the rise of free-standing institutes, and a widening appreciation of the need to train supervisors. Accountability, sometimes externally imposed, has taken hold in the clinical and therapy domains; along with it has come the establishment of standards and beginning guidelines for the practice of training and supervision. Along with workshops, often masquerading as training, have evolved the more conservative but perhaps longer lasting degree-granting and postdegree programs and the introduction of family systems ideas in traditional academic departments such as psychology, social work, and psychiatry. Special content areas and activities—including evaluation and research, feminism, cultural factors, epistemology (i.e., conceptual issues and theory development), and the family life cycle—have begun to inform and contour the training area in recent years. Also, there has been a macro-level reexamination of training and supervision; this welcome and long-term process has, at this stage, generated significant questions but few convincing answers. This book proposes some steps toward such answers.

References

Andreozzi, L. L. (Vol. Ed.), & Levant, R. F. (Consulting Ed.). (1985). *Integrating research and clinical practice.* Rockville, MD: Aspen.

Breunlin, D. C. (1985). *Stages: Patterns of change over time.* Rockville, MD: Aspen.

Breunlin, D. C. (1988). Oscillation theory and family development. In C. Falicov (Ed.), *Family transitions: Continuity and change across the family life cycle.* New York: Guilford Press.

Caust, B., Libow, J., & Raskin, P. (1981). Challenges and promises of training women as family systems therapists. *Family Process, 20,* 439–448.

Cohen, L., Sargent, M., & Sechrest, L. (1986). Use of psychotherapy research by professional psychologists. *American Pscyhologist, 41,* 198–206.

Cormier, L., & Bernard, J. (1982). Ethical and legal responsibilities of clinical supervisors. *Personnel and Guidance Journal, 60*(80), 486–490.

Everett, C. A. (1980). Supervision of marriage and family therapy. In A. Hess (Ed.), *Psychotherapy and supervision.* New York: Wiley-Interscience.

Falicov, C. (Ed.). (1988). *Family transitions: Continuity and change across the family life cycle.* New York: Guilford Press.

Falicov, C. (1988). Learning to think culturally. Chapter 21, this volume.

Framo, J. I. (1976). Chronicle of a struggle to establish a family unit within a community mental health center. In P. Guerin (Ed.), *Family therapy: Theory and practice.* New York: Gardner Press.

Goldner, V. (1987). Instrumentalism, feminism, and the limits of family therapy. *Journal of Family Psychology, 1*(1), 109–116.

Haley, J. (1975). Why a mental health clinic should avoid doing family therapy. *Journal of Marriage and Family Counseling, 1,* 3–12.

Hare-Mustin, R. (1987). The problem of gender in family therapy theory. *Family Process, 26,* 15–27.

Hazelrigg, M. D., Cooper, H. M., & Borduin, C. M. (1987). Evaluating the effectiveness of family therapies: An integrative review and analysis. *Psychological Bulletin, 101,* 428–442.

Hoffman, L. (1983). *Foundations of family therapy.* New York: Basic Books.

Kaslow, F. W., et al. (Eds.). (1977). *Supervision, consultation and staff training in the helping professions.* San Francisco: Jossey-Bass.

Lebow, J. L. (1987). Developing a personal integration in family therapy: Principles for model construction and practice. *Journal of Marital and Family Therapy, 13,* 1–14.

Libow, J. A. (1985). Training family therapists as feminists. In M. Ault-Riche (Ed.), *Women and family therapy*. Rockville, MD: Aspen.

Libow, J., Raskin, P. A., & Caust, B. (1982). Feminist and family systems therapy: Are they irreconcilable? *American Journal of Family Therapy, 10*(3), 3–12.

Liddle, H. (1978). The emotional and political hazards of teaching and learning family therapy. *Family Therapy, 5*, 1–12.

Liddle, H. A. (1985a). Beyond family therapy: Challenging the boundaries, roles, and mission of a field. *Journal of Strategic and Systemic Therapies, 4*(2), 4–14.

Liddle, H. A. (1985b). Redefining the mission of family therapy training. *Journal of Psychotherapy and the Family, 1*(4), 109–124.

Liddle, H. A. (1987a). Editor's Introduction I: Family psychology: The journal, the field. *Journal of Family Psychology, 1*(1), 5–22.

Liddle, H. A. (1987b). Editor's Introduction II: Family psychology: Tasks of an emerging (and emerged) discipline. *Journal of Family Pscyhology, 1*(2), 149–167.

Liddle, H. A. (1988a). Integrating developmental thinking and the family life cycle paradigm into training. In C. Falicov (Ed.), *Family transitions: Continuity and change across the life cycle*. New York: Guilford Press.

Liddle, H. A. (1988b). Training implications of the family development paradigm. In C. Falicov (Ed.), *Family transitions: Continuity and change across the family life cycle*. New York: Guilford Press.

Liddle, H. A. (in press). Family therapy training and supervision: A critical review and analysis. In A. Gurman & D. Kniskern (Eds.), *Handbook of family therapy* (2nd ed.). New York: Guilford Press.

Liddle, H. A., & Saba, G. (1983). Clinical implications of the family life cycle: Some cautionary guidelines. In H. A. Liddle (Ed.), *Clinical implications of the family life cycle*. Rockville, MD: Aspen.

Liddle, H. A., & Saba, G. (1984). The isomorphic nature of training and therapy: Epistemologic foundations for a structural-strategic family therapy. In J. Schwartzman (Ed.), *Families and other systems*. New York: Guilford Press.

Malone, C. (1974). Observations on the role of family therapy in child psychiatry training. *Journal of the American Academy of Child Psychiatry, 13*, 437–458.

Margolin, C. (1982). Ethical and legal considerations in marital and family therapy. *American Psychologist, 37*, 788–801.

Meyerstein, K. (1977). Family therapy training for paraprofessionals in a community mental health center. *Family Process, 16*, 477–494.

Morrow-Bradley, C., & Elliott, R. (1986). Utilization of psychotherapy research by practicing psychotherapists. *American Psychologist, 41*, 188–197.

Okun, B. F. (1983). Gender issues of family systems therapists. In B. Okun & S. T. Gladdings (Eds.), *Issues in training marriage and family therapists*. Ann Arbor, MI: ERIC/CAPS.

Piercy, F., & Sprenkle, D. (1983). Ethical, legal and professional issues in family therapy: A graduate level course. *Journal of Marital and Family Therapy, 9*(4), 393–401.

Ryder, R. (1987). *The realistic therapist*. Newbury Park, CA: Sage.

Saba, G. W., Karrer, B., & Hardy, K. (Eds.). (in press). *Minorities and family therapy*. New York: Haworth.

Saba, G. W., & Liddle, H. A. (1986). Perceptions of professional needs, practice patterns, and critical issues facing family therapy trainers and supervisors. *American Journal of Family Therapy, 14*, 109–122.

Schwartz, R. C. (1981). The pre-session worksheet as an adjunct to training. *American Journal of Family Therapy, 9*(3), 89–90.

Shapiro, R. (1975). Problems in teaching family therapy. *Professional Psychology, 6*, 41–44.

Shapiro, R. (1979). The problematic position of family therapy in professional training. *Professional Psychology, 10*, 876–879.

Stanton, M. (1975). Psychology and family therapy. *Professional Psychology, 6*, 45–49.

Sugarman, S. (1984). Integrating family therapy training into psychiatric residency programs: Policy issues and alternatives. *Family Process, 23*, 23–32.

Wheeler, D., Avis, J. M., Miller, L. A., & Chaney, S. (1985). Rethinking family therapy education and supervision: A feminist model. *Journal of Psychotherapy and the Family, 1*(4), 53–72.

SECTION TWO

FAMILY THERAPY MODELS:
APPROACHES TO TRAINING

Introduction

The field of family therapy encompasses a remarkably wide range of disparate and often contradictory approaches to clinical practice. The seven chapters in this section demonstrate that the training practices and principles of the various models of family therapy are no less disparate and contradictory. These differences are less perplexing, however, if one considers the isomorphic nature of theory, clinical practice, and training; that is, that the training practices of any single model will necessarily reflect the therapeutic approach and theory of which it is a part.

With the isomorphism between training and therapy in mind, we asked each author to summarize their model's basic assumptions and clinical methods in their chapter's first section, then to describe their training methods and their rationale for using those methods. Thus, after reading the summary of a model's clinical assumptions, the reader could try to predict the chapter's content on training practices and philosophy. To facilitate such an exercise, some salient variables of a model's theory that will be reflected in its clinical and training practices are presented below.

1. Patients and/or trainees need to learn a "big picture" epistemology.	vs.	Trainees and/or patients need only learn as much theory as it takes to be effective in therapy or life.
2. The verbal content of therapy sessions is of primary importance.	vs.	The verbal or nonverbal process (sequences or interaction) is of primary importance.
3. Patients and/or trainees need to undergo major changes in personality.	vs.	Patients and/or trainees need only learn a set of skills or frames regarding their task or problem.
4. Understanding or insight precedes changes in behavior in patients and/or trainees.	vs.	Understanding follows or occurs concurrent to changes in behavior.
5. Relationships, whether trainer–trainee, therapist–family, or within-family, should be open and egalitarian.	vs.	Relationships should be hierarchically organized and/or may be, if necessary, manipulative or indirect.
6. Lasting change cannot be accomplished quickly.	vs.	Lasting change can be accomplished quickly.

In short, we believe that the positions that a model takes on these and other variables will influence much of the model's clinical and training practices. To illustrate this process we will examine the relative importance and use of live supervision among the seven models. The structural (Colapinto), functional (Haas *et al.*) and both the strategic (Fisch and Mazza) models all rely heavily on live supervision (i.e., shaping a trainee's skills by observing and intervening directly into the trainee's session from behind a one-way mirror). The Bowen (Papero) and psychodynamic (Nichols) models eschew this training modality, while the systemic Milan model (Pirrotta & Cecchin) uses live observation primarily to focus on the family's process rather than on the trainee's skills.

These differences make sense in light of the structural and strategic models' greater emphasis on changing present interactional sequences, on hierarchical training and therapy relationships, on the possibility of relatively short-term change, and their de-emphasis of the need for major personality or theoretical reorganization. All of these positions point toward the need for a direct and efficient method of changing in-session interactions and therapist behaviors; hence the genesis of a method like live supervision.

The structural model diverges from both strategic models, however, on one variable in its application of live supervision. Both strategic models believe that patients' under-standing of their problems follows changes in their behavior, and is not always necessary to maintain changes. Similarly, both strategic models focus on changing their trainees' interactional sequences with families rather than giving trainees broad understanding of what they are to do through extensive lectures on theory. As Fisch states, "we assume that learning a new approach to treatment, both conceptually and technically, best comes about by doing that treatment. . . ." Mazza agrees: "Generally, the therapist's insight will most naturally follow other changes and would not be a direct result of the supervisor's evaluation." Indeed, Mazza's chapter is filled with indirect strategies to get trainees to change their behavior without their full awareness and without a direct request from the trainer.

In contrast, the structural position is that theory and technique (understanding and behavior) can and should occur simultaneously. This position is reflected clinically in prompting families to change within the context of therapist-created "workable realities." Colapinto relates that when structural therapists first began training students, they held the assumption that insight follows behavior. These trainers eventually discovered, however, that with a technique-focused approach to training, "spontaneous theoretical integration was the exception rather than the rule." The present structural position argues for the concurrent teaching of technique and theory. Colapinto states that, "The conceptual understanding of the model and the practical operations in the therapy room need to be taught simultaneously and as an integral paradigm." In sum, live supervision is the centerpiece of the structural training model. In practice, this includes extensive pre- and postsession discussion of both technique and theory, as well as teaching the group behind the mirror during the session.

The Bowen and psychodynamic models assume very different and critical postures toward live supervision: they deemphasize technique and, instead, teach trainees to acquire a comprehensive theory of life that organizes their therapy behaviors. Papero explains that a "clear understanding of theory seems to be of greater assistance in the long run than specific techniques." Thus, just as a major part of the therapist's responsi-bility in this approach is to teach patients about the "functioning of emotional systems," the primary role of the Bowen trainer is to teach trainees the Bowen model's concepts and principles. Implicit in this training philosophy is the assumption that understanding precedes, guides, and is necessary for competent therapist behavior. That is, as trainees (or patients) gain greater understanding of the functioning of emotional systems, they will become more differentiated from those systems. This freedom then enables therapists to understand more fully and help the families they see in therapy.

Nichols expresses another objection to live supervision. While he believes it can produce rapid change initially in trainee behavior, Nichols has found that a year or so after the training, "the student had tended to either rebel against the stance taken by the supervisor or to slavishly follow the mentor's actions." He therefore is concerned that live supervision, while seemingly effective in the short run, can stifle the trainee's long-term growth and autonomy.

Hierarchy in the trainer–trainee relationship is another dimension that illustrates distinctions among the training models. Papero's chapter highlights the Bowen model's desire to avoid the hierarchical, expert-versus-novice relationship that is often a part of live supervision. In contrast, the structural and both strategic models advocate a hierarchical organization in both therapy and training, and so have little problem with this aspect of live supervision. For example, Colapinto makes the point that in structural training the supervisor is explicitly the expert who must correct "errors" in the trainee's thinking and action, and that trainees are not autonomous until training is over.

However, among the models that accept and utilize hierarchically structured live supervision, there are different emphases in how this training mode is implemented. Differences in theory can account for these contrasting emphases. For example, structural family therapy gives verbal and nonverbal process within a therapy session paramount importance, while the M.R.I. strategic model (Fisch) attaches "little or no importance" to nonverbal events; instead, this model emphasizes verbal interaction and the generation of between-session tasks. This difference in theory translates into very different styles of live supervision. The structural trainer actively tries to shift the process of the session by challenging the trainee to "use himself or herself" more effectively through phone calls or consultations behind the mirror. On the other hand, rather than calling in to change in-session process, the M.R.I. trainer phones in either to ask the trainee to obtain or clarify information from the family, or to help the trainee correctly word a task's rationale or directive. Indeed, the M.R.I. group's reliance on verbal interaction alone is highlighted by their use of audiotape rather than videotape for supervision.

The Milan model represents a unique situation regarding live supervision. Its position on the six variables listed above is, overall, more similar to those of the models that eschew live supervision (Bowen or psychodynamic) than to the structural or strategic positions. The Milan model focuses on helping trainees learn a "big picture" epistemology rather than on techniques, and they avoid authority–hierarchical arrangements in favor of a "group mind" approach. The Milan theorists are, however, interested in the process as well as the verbal content of sessions; indeed, they believe that through the process of relatively few sessions, lasting change in a family may be achieved. Thus, for the Milan school, observing and participating as a team in therapy sessions is a primary training tool, although the trainer does not focus on the trainee's performance of verbal or nonverbal technique, as is the conventional focus of live supervision.

This range of positions on live supervision, presented against the backdrop of each model's basic assumptions, illustrates the extreme disparity that exists on this training modality. Other training variables could have been employed for this cross-model comparison (e.g., trainee–trainee relationship, screening for certain trainee characteristics, use of videotape supervision, amount of didactic versus experiential training), but this diversity would have held, given the isomorphic nature of therapy and training models and the lack of consensus in the field. This section is intended to help the reader view the training practices advocated in each of its chapters in the context of each model's assumptions. Each training practice can best be evaluated in terms of how well it achieves the goals of its corresponding therapy model; and by its degree of theoretical and practical fit relative to the therapy model's assumptions.

2

Teaching the Structural Way

JORGE COLAPINTO[1]
Wynnewood, Pennsylvania

On finishing one year of training in structural family therapy, a group of fun-loving practitioners produced a spoof videotape that they titled "The Structural Way." In a comic fashion, the piece demonstrated the trainees' understanding of a fundamental tenet in their teachers' philosophy: that structural family therapy should be learned, not as an assortment of efficient techniques, but rather as a disciplined way of looking at families in pain, at the intricacies of change, and at the role of the therapist.

What, however, is, the "structural way"? The adjective "structural" is usually employed to identify the approach originally developed by Salvador Minuchin at the Philadelphia Child Guidance Clinic. Today, however, a good number of family therapists invoke it to describe their practice—in some cases without much justification—while many others are producing excellent structural work that they do not label as such. Pinpointing the "real" structuralists is difficult by the absence of a formal model that would define the essential features of structural family therapy. Minuchin's own theoretical writings, while abundant and inspiring, display noticeable variations in emphases and are not without inconsistency—probably the result of an open-minded interest in what other thinkers had to say about his own clinical work. The influence of Jay Haley can be detected through the pages of the classic *Families and Family Therapy* (Minuchin, 1974), and many clinicians and even taxonomists of family therapy would not acknowledge any substantial differences between the two masters. There have been attempts to systematize the essential tenets of the structural model (e.g., Aponte & VanDeusen, 1981; Colapinto, 1982; Nichols, 1984; Umbarger, 1983), but none of these renditions can be regarded as the "official" version.

THE STRUCTURAL PARADIGM

It could certainly be argued that there is no such thing as "the structural way," but only the inimitable style of Salvador Minuchin, an idiosyncratic expression of genius that manifests itself anew each time and does not allow for formalization. Indeed, the master himself, worried that his creation might be turned into dogma by others, has all but disowned anything resembling a comprehensive model of therapy that can be taught and learned (Minuchin, 1982). The contrary position reflected in these pages is that there exists a core system of perspectives on families, change, and therapy that directs the structuralist's work in the therapeutic arena and sets the "structural way" apart from other approaches. Such a paradigmatic core can be primarily distilled from certain redundancies in Salvador Minuchin's clinical operations and in his case discussions, more than from his theoretical presentations—where the search for dialogue with other thinkers has occasionally blurred the shape and boundaries of the structural paradigm.

A Structural View of Families

Family therapists of all persuasions look beyond the apparent behavior of family members in search of some kind of pattern that will introduce a unifying meaning into what would otherwise be a confused bundle of unrelated observations. But they are not all searching for the *same* kind of pattern (Scheflen, 1978). Some pursue clues to the distribution of power; others, styles of conflict resolution; still a third group, redundancies in the sequence of speakers. The list could continue almost indefinitely.

The structural way is one among many methods of putting together the richly complex manifestations of family life. Although generically speaking it conceptualizes the family as other systemic approaches do—as a system in evolution that constantly regulates its own functioning—it features a distinctive focus on concepts that describe *space* configurations: closeness/distance, inclusion/exclusion, fluid/rigid boundaries, hierarchical arrangements. The key notion of complementarity is used by the structuralist to denote not an escalation of differences (Bateson, 1972), but a fit among matching parts of a whole. Visually, the relational patterns that the structuralist "sees" can be better described by maps and jigsaw puzzle–like figures than by circular series of arrows.

From the structural point of view, symptomatic behavior is a piece that fits into a dysfunctional organization. An adolescent's anorexia may be related to a mutual invasion of the patient's and her parents' territories; a school phobia may reveal excessive proximity between mother and son; a runaway may signal a "leaky" structure. Structural configurations are deemed functional or not according to how well or how badly they serve the developmental needs of the family and its members. In a dysfunctional family, development has been replaced by inertia. Stuck in a rigid arrangement, such a family cannot solve its problems and continue growing. For example, following mother's death a father and a daughter maintain the same distance that they had kept when mother was alive; the girl becomes a truant, mother is not there to make sure that she attends school, and the vacuum in parental functions is filled neither by the father nor by the relatives who are now mediating between him and the girl.

Thus, unlike other systemic approaches that focus on the *function of the symptom* ("Joey's temper tantrums distract his parents from their marital conflict"), the structural view focuses on the *organizational flaw* ("The couple's avoidance of conflict is crippling their parenting of Joey").

A Structural View of Therapeutic Change

Breaking away from such an organizational impasse requires the mobilization of resources that the family already possesses in latent fashion and which are often apparent in a different context; the widower of our example was a competent professional who could display leadership in his job but not in relation to his adolescent daughter. Systemic change, in the structural view, equals an increase in the complexity of the structure—an increment in the availability of alternative ways of transacting. The function of the therapist is to create a context for the family to experience those alternative patterns as accessible (father does have an influence on daughter), possible (neither father nor daughter will collapse while dealing with each other), and necessary (daughter is in for trouble if she and father abdicate their relationship). This definition of the therapist's role explains the structuralist's preference for changing transactions in the therapy room, where he or she can punctuate sequences of behavior and literally create a different experience.

What the structural therapist is trying to *build* through his or her restructuring efforts is more important than what he or she is trying to *uncover.* If father becomes paralyzed when his truant daughter blames him for her mother's death, identifying the accuser–defendant pattern that renders him impotent is only a preliminary step toward the promotion of a more functional father–daughter relationship. This health-oriented search for the "missing pattern" is a characteristic mark of the structural approach: the survey of differing views about the nature of the problem, the gathering of information on family background and history, and other diagnostic operations are guided by the need to assess the system's resources and weaknesses in preparation for a reorganization.

The structural therapist does not emphasize the pursuit of individual change or the prescription of specific solutions. Instead, he or she tries to modify, enrich, and make flexible the family structure. The goal is to help the family discover patterns that are missing and that will, when developed, provide the scenario for the solution of individual problems. The family (like a recovered ecosystem) is the healer, while the therapist's job is to recruit individual resources for the project and to provide a context that can defeat inertia. Unlike other systemic approaches that prescribe for the therapist the role of an invariably neutral commentator, the structural view requires therapists to become protagonists as well. The creation of healing scenarios and the mobilization of individual resources demand the therapist's active involvement as well as a broad perspective. In helping a father to find better ways of relating to his children, the structural therapist may ressemble a coach—mostly straightforward, in principle benevolent, sometimes impatient, rarely neutral. In undoing a rigid triangle in a psychosomatic family, he or she will enter into selective alliances, and will alternately unbalance, support, and push. Rather than cautiously operating from an invariable distance, the structural therapist constantly changes positions, oscillating between the objectivity of the removed observer and the intensity of the direct participant. From any of these two vantage points, families are seen not as passive mechanisms that resist the therapist's input, but as active organisms that need to be joined, explored, and expanded.

PHILOSOPHY OF TRAINING

The first trainers of family therapy did not need to pay much attention to the specifics of alternative paradigms. They were vanguard explorers, marching in different directions, somewhat ahead of their disciples, but participating with everybody else in the overriding excitement of a revolutionary, somewhat underground movement. They were expanding the frontiers of therapy, deriving techniques from new concepts and concepts from new techniques. Then, as the field grew in scope and respectability, the explorers "staked the unmarked corners with their trade names" (Minuchin, 1982), and schools developed. Today, clinicians are trained not just in family therapy, but in the structural, strategic, systemic and/or other model of family therapy—each one separated from the next by differences in the conceptualization of both families and therapy.

Mission of Training

The diversification of family therapy has brought about a rapid increase in available technology—and with it a danger. The numerous and heterogeneous techniques developed by various schools are sometimes presented to the beginning therapist as an assortment of free-standing tools, each one endowed with its own efficiency, independent of the conceptual frame from which it emerged. Such an approach can generate a field

> full of clinicians who change chairs à la Minuchin, give directions à la Haley, go primary process à la Whitaker, offer paradoxes in Italian, tie people with ropes à la Satir, add a pinch of ethics à la Nagy, encourage cathartic crying à la Paul, review a tape of the session with the family à la Alger, and sometimes manage to combine all of these methods in one session. (Minuchin & Fishman, 1981, p. 9)

The problem is that techniques do not work by themselves. Knowing how to join, reframe, or unbalance is useless if one does not know when and why to do it. Therapeutic competence requires a synthesis of many different and even contradictory abilities; the structural therapist needs to engage clients intensely and also to keep an efficient distance from them; to accept and disrupt the ways of the family; to be a leader and a follower, firm and flexible, poised and humble. In order to choose, organize, and time specific interventions, the therapist needs to rely on the master blueprint, the therapeutic world view that is provided by the structural paradigm. The heuristic value of the paradigm as a propeller and organizer of the therapist's operations surpasses the efficacy of any collection of techniques, and therefore its acquisition constitutes the main mission of training. Technical skills need to be learned as a natural expression of a consistent paradigm (Colapinto, 1983).

Training Strategy

The early emphasis on techniques in the teaching of structural family therapy was a reaction to the limitations of traditional training, with its deductive sequence from theoretical constructs to specific interventions; the availability of live and videotape supervision exposed the huge discrepancies that may exist between the apparent understanding of concepts and the actual behavior of the therapist in the session. The idea then, as Minuchin recalls, was to teach the "steps of the dance," to focus on the specific skills of therapy "without burdening the student with a load of theory that would slow him down at moments of therapeutic immediacy." Theoretical integration, it was hoped, would emerge spontaneously: "Through an inductive process the student, in 'circles of decreasing uncertainty,' would arrive at the 'aha!' moment: the theory." (Minuchin & Fishman, 1981).

Experience with this approach eventually showed that spontaneous theoretical integration was the exception more than the rule. The tactic of concentrating on the practice of skills while leaving conceptual understanding for later may require from the student a strong and lengthy attachment to the teacher. In Zen and other Eastern models of learning (often cited as an inspiration by family therapy trainers) the student is sometimes even prevented from attempting to practice the master's teachings in the real world while in training (Herrigel, 1953). But in our world of licensing boards, third-party payers, and workshop show business, the relation of trainer to trainee offers little room for pure aesthetic contemplation and personal renunciation. Apprentices just will not wait for the master's anointment.

The student of structural family therapy should not be expected to infer the theory from the practice any more than the other way around. The conceptual understanding of the model and the practical operations in the therapy room need to be taught simultaneously and as an integral paradigm. A mere "balance" of theory and practice—such as the interspersion of theoretical seminars in a clinical program that otherwise focuses strictly on the practice of skills—is not enough, and may in fact defeat the purpose of integration by maintaining "theory" and "practice" as separate realms. A real integration of theory and practice can occur only in the arena of supervised clinical work, and the best opportunity for the supervisor to facilitate it is immediately before or during the therapeutic encounter with a family—when the therapist is at the highest point of motivation and alertness.

Pragmatics and Aesthetics of Training

The integrated approach to training presented in these pages offers one possible answer to the debate about the aesthetics and pragmatics of family therapy. Some authors (Allman, 1982; Keeney & Sprenkle, 1982), reacting to the pragmatic lure that "cookbooks" of techniques may exert on therapists, have argued for a more "aesthetic" attitude—one that would temper or counterbalance the pragmatic trend by enhancing a more contemplative understanding of underlying patterns of interconnectedness. The opposition, however, is a false one. The cookbook approach thrives not on excessive, but on defective pragmatism. Therapists who only learn techniques that "work" turn out to be as "practical" as actors who only impersonate others: the effectiveness of their performances diminishes as a function of their narrowed creativity. An awareness of "underlying patterns of interconnectedness"—like the ones depicted by the structural paradigm—is necessary, not to temper the therapist's pragmatic goals but to improve his or her chances of achieving them. Aesthetics, far from being the opposite of pragmatics, constitutes its highest form.

To help the therapist develop an aesthetic perspective, the trainer must begin by acknowledging and respecting the therapist's pragmatic concerns. If a trainee is anxious to learn how to do better therapy, attacking his or her motivation as being too pragmatic will not help in promoting a paradigm shift. But the trainer also can and should challenge the trainee's notion of *how* this pragmatic concern is to be satisfied. For instance, if the trainee attributes his or her performance deficits to ignorance of the right "recipe," the trainer can demonstrate that what is needed is better thinking; the pragmatic motive thus provides the incentive for a more integrated, "aesthetic" learning. This training strategy is evocative of the structural model of therapy, which accepts the focus on the presenting problem while repositioning it within a structural frame: the clients' immediate concerns with their symptoms are acknowledged and respected, but the clients are also told that in order to get rid of these symptoms their transactional patterns and views will need to change.

TRAINING CONTEXT

The training philosophy presented in the previous section has been implemented through several training programs. The example to be presented here is the Extern Program, a clinical practicum offered by the Family Therapy Training Center of the Philadelphia Child Guidance Clinic, and designed to teach generic concepts as well as specific techniques of structural family therapy.[2]

Extern students meet one day a week, from October through May. Organized in groups of eight, they work together with two supervisors for the entire training day. The program is structured around live supervision of family sessions that are also observed by the colleagues in the training group and subsequently reviewed on videotape. An additional one-day seminar, where all groups participate, is held every month.

Setting

The Family Therapy Training Center is part of the Clinic's Department of Training, which also offers other practica as well as internship programs for psychiatrists, psychologists, and social workers. In addition, a continuing education program offers workshops and conferences led by both Clinic staff and guest speakers. The Philadelphia Child Guidance Clinic is a large facility created in 1925 that provides outpatient and inpatient treatment to children and adolescents within a family perspective. The ecosystemic orientation of the services provides the Extern program with a "friendly" environment that facilitates consultations, transfers, and other communications within the broader context. The Clinic is the primary source of mental health services for a large catchment area and has access to the entire range of mental health problems, which permits direct supervision of treatment as a preferred training modality. A close liaison has been established with the Children's Hospital of Philadelphia in the areas of psychosomatic dysfunctions and chronic illnesses.

Each group of eight students and two supervisors has permanent access to two videorooms with observation and videotaping facilities. Group discussions and review of videotapes are conducted in a separate conference room. A student room functions as a relief office for paperwork, phone calls, and individual review of videotapes. The program also makes extensive use of the video and library department, which includes hundreds of edited and unedited videotapes of sessions conducted by Salvador Minuchin and other experienced therapists. Students have the same responsibilities as regular staff members concerning the medical records of the families in treatment.

Trainers and Trainees

The core faculty of the Extern Progam consists of supervisors who have been associated with the Clinic, in various clinical capacities, for periods ranging from 4 to 13 years. Their varied experience in the practice of structural family therapy within different contexts and populations is complemented by other members of the large and multidisciplinary Clinic staff, which covers nearly the entire range of specialities in the mental health field and is available for backup supervision and consultation.

Students are required to possess a master's degree or equivalent in a mental health area, and a minimum of one year's experience in the practice of family therapy. They need to be currently employed in an agency setting where they must carry a minimum of five families. Applicants submit a letter of interest, letters of recommendation, and curriculum vitae. A preliminary screening of the written applications leads to the exclusion of candidates with insufficient academic and/or experiential background; the rest of the candidates are interviewed by at least two faculty members, and final decisions are made by a selection committee. Typically, the therapist who joins the Extern program is acquainted with the concepts of structural family therapy through readings, workshops, and edited videotapes, but is not consistently operating under a structural paradigm. He or she may juxtapose straightforward structural moves with psychodynamic interpretations or paradoxical injunctions, and not recognize the differences and eventual incompatibilities between the structural and other models.

TRAINING FORMAT

The Extern program begins with a three-day seminar on structural family therapy, intended to set a basic common ground for the training process. The seminar also provides the faculty with an opportunity to observe the students' responses to the concepts and clinical material presented, and compare their understanding of families, the process of change, and the role of the therapist to the structural paradigm. The rest of the program revolves around direct supervision of the trainees' work with families. Clinical work is conceptualized as the arena where an integration of theory and practice can best occur. Each trainee conducts one or two sessions per day under live supervision, and receives on the average an additional half hour of videotape supervision for each hour of therapy. The unit of training is a cycle that includes a presession discussion, live supervision, postsession review, and videotape review.

Presession Discussion

The preliminary discussion of hypotheses about family dynamics and therapeutic strategies, based on intake information or the previous session, provides an opportunity to examine the trainee's thinking—how the trainee organizes the available material and perceives his or her own role. For instance, when the intake information on a case of school avoidance mentioned that mother had been beaten by her boyfriend, one trainee automatically focused his attention on mother's own "pathology." The supervisor then offered an alternative perspective, establishing a conceptual boundary between the woman's presumed incompetence in choosing partners, and her potentially competent role as a mother.

To facilitate the exploration of a trainee's paradigm, he or she is encouraged to participate actively during the presession discussion, presenting ideas and objections, as opposed to passively receiving instructions for the conduct of the session.

Initial interviews are minimally structured in advance; they are mostly devoted to entering the system, listening, and redefining the problem. As therapy progresses, presession discussions may focus more on specific treatment and/or training goals ("Today you should make an effort to mobilize the siblings subsystem"). Role playing may be utilized to enhance the trainee's understanding of complex therapeutic processes, such as unbalancing or entering into multiple alliances. The primary roles of the supervisor in this stage are to help the therapist develop a structural frame for the upcoming session ("What do you think the daughter is doing that keeps mom ineffective?") and to correct faulty frames ("You won't get very far if you keep regarding mom as a 100% slob").

Live Supervision

In the session, the previously discussed structural frame helps the therapist to keep one foot out of the system; for instance, it prevents him or her from being organized into thinking of mother as a slob. Overviewing the process of the session to make sure that the trainee protects that frame from homeostatic pulls or distractive contents is one of the functions of the supervisor at this stage. Other functions are to assist the therapist in dealing with unexpected developments ("My wife and I decided to divorce yesterday"), to correct the course if the unfolding of the session requires a change in focus, and to take maximum advantage of opportunities to enhance the process. For instance, when a depressed mother who has all but given up on her family lights up a cigarette, the supervisor suggests, "Challenge her to refrain from smoking; make it a test of will."

DECIDING TO INTERVENE

Sometimes supervisor and trainee can preplan the entire sequence of stages in a session, including a few "walkouts" by the therapist at specified times, for consultation purposes. The most frequent scenario in structural family therapy, though, is one that requires on-the-spot planning in response to feedback from the family, as the session progresses. Thus, live supervision usually demands quick decisions as to whether, when, in which way, and to what degree to interfere with the process in the room. The supervisor who expects the session to flawlessly follow his or her own conceptualization—and proceeds to "proofread" it from behind the mirror—will at best make a puppet out of the therapist, and at worst ruin the process of therapy. Allowance needs to be made for the idiosyncrasy of the student, whose course of action may not totally agree with the supervisor's, but may still aim at the same goal. On the other hand, if the supervisor is too passive and accepting, both treatment and learning may suffer. Like the structural therapist, the supervisor is both an observer and an active participant in the process of change.

In extreme cases, such as when the continuity of treatment or the well-being of the family are at risk, the need to intervene may be obvious. More frequently, however, the decision is not simple. A typical situation might be the "inconclusive maneuver," where the therapist begins to unbalance the structure but falters halfway, allowing the system to reestablish homeostasis. In such a case the supervisor needs to decide whether to "let it go" or insist that the job be finished. Numerous factors are weighed in the decision: the more or less serious implications that an aborted unbalancing could have for the family; the strength of the therapist; the status of his or her relation to the family and the supervisor; whether there will be a next time; whether the supervisor's intervention really has a chance of bringing about success.

Another example is the "golden opportunity," where the therapist is not in error but the supervisor sees a chance of moving the process of training and/or therapy one notch up. For instance, while the therapist may be doing a good job of helping a family with teenage children negotiate curfews or schoolwork, the supervisor may react to a tender remark by the 15-year-old daughter, and indicate a change of subject—to her relation with the apparently distant father.

FORMS OF INTERVENTION

The supervisor can choose among various modes of intervention: talking to the therapist on the phone; calling the therapist out of the room for a quick consultation; entering the therapy room. (The same alternatives are of course available for the therapist at his or her request.) If the same goal can be achieved through any of these methods of intervention, the least disruptive should be chosen. However, an ostensibly intrusive intervention like walking into the room is not always the most disruptive. If the supervisor needs to communicate a brief message ("I think that father has the answer to this one") in the middle of an intense discussion, calling the therapist out of the room or on the phone might cause an undesired distraction. It may be better for the supervisor to join the session briefly, without even taking a seat, offer his or her input, and leave. If, on the other hand, the therapeutic moment is so complex that the supervisor's message would either be too long ("Talk to father even if the girl cries. When she stops ask her about her mother, but if she does not stop, or if father gets distracted . . ."), or require minute-by-minute interruptions of the session, the best solution may be for the supervisor to demonstrate the idea directly.

In the context of the Extern Program, where both families and trainees get used to the presence of the supervisor and the group behind the mirror, these interventions can be assimilated into the therapeutic process as a form of ongoing consultation or cotherapy. Families are informed at the beginning of treatment that the therapist is part of a team, which provides a rationale for the interventions of the supervisor and minimizes the risk of a negative impact on the family's relation to the therapist. When the supervisor walks into the room, he or she frames the intervention as a cooperative effort ("I came here because I wanted to tell mother that . . ."), and/or addresses the therapist in a collegial way ("You know, Susan, I think that . . .").

CONTENT OF INTERVENTIONS

If the supervisory intervention consists of a dialogue with the trainee (a phone call or a consultation behind the mirror), the supervisor needs to pay special attention to the *content* of the message. Ideally, it should include a request for a specific action, with a rationale for that action, as a way of promoting the integration of paradigm and technique: "Husband needs to feel your support as he stands up to his wife [rationale]. Move your chair closer to him [action]." Occasionally, however, the supervisor will need to prescribe an action without offering any rationale. One therapist, for instance, had been struggling unsuccessfully to motivate a 16-year-old girl to fix a dinner for her family. The family was already leaving when the supervisor rang and told the therapist;

"Ask the girl if they have candlelight at home". Puzzled but appropriately curious, the therapist asked the question; the girl then nodded slowly, looked intensely at the therapist, and answered, "I see what you mean." ("What did I mean?" asked the therapist of the supervisor after the session.) But these are exceptions, justified when time is running out or events are unfolding too rapidly. Of course, as supervisor and trainee progress in their mutual understanding, the rationale may not need to be explicit: "Spend some time talking to the boy about his friends" may implicitly carry the comment, "You need to join the identified patient." Conversely, it may be the specific action that does not need to be detailed. When a trainee is told, "You are losing mother," or, "The kids have too much power in this family," that may be enough for him or her to implement the appropriate therapeutic interventions.

Postsession Review

Immediately after the session there is a short debriefing, limited by the time that remains until the next family arrives. Emphasis now shifts to the therapist's progress in training. Successes and failures are briefly discussed and linked to the paradigm: "You really joined mother today; that is what we mean when we insist that joining is not necessarily being nice," or, "I think the reason why you couldn't engage grandma was that you saw her only as a saboteur." This stage is also an opportunity to explain the reasons behind the supervisor's interventions, if they could not be provided during the session itself: "I asked you to mention the candlelight because they were really talking about wanting to be closer, not about chores." Finally, the trainee is instructed to locate specific segments in the tape for later review.

Videotape Review

The review of the session videotape, prior to the next appointment, facilitates a more thorough discussion of the trainee's perceptions and actions. Rather than reviewing the entire session, segments are chosen that highlight the family's dynamics and/or the therapist's performance; in-depth analysis of the implications of microsequences is preferred to an extensive overview. In this way the supervisor can concentrate on specific training needs of the therapist as reflected in the concrete clinical experience. The supervisor may ask various questions to assess and eventually correct the therapist's perception: "What do you see happening here? What can you tell, from that dialogue, about the relation between husband and wife? Did you notice any differences in the responses of father and mother to the girl's temper tantrum?" Other questions, such as, "Why did you decide to support father?" or, "Do you think it was necessary for you to teach mom how to control the kid?" address the trainee's understanding of his or her own role. The supervisor may also comment on the family ("I don't think this is an overinvolved dyad; look how mother responds to the child"), and on the therapist's performance ("You created an instant climate of comfort, but then became too careful not to risk it").

The trainee, in turn, asks for specific inputs: "What is going on in this family?" "How can I be less central?" He or she is primarily motivated to improve performance—in general and in the next session. The supervisor capitalizes on this legitimate interest and stimulates the therapist's integration of action and thinking, turning "what-should-I-do-next" questions into opportunities to develop the therapist's paradigm. The focus is on the clinical practice, but not in a theoretical vacuum: "Yes, you can go for the differences between mother and father, but are you clear as to why that is important at this point?" or, "I think you are not pushing father enough because you think too much of the function that the child's symptom may have for the couple."

The Group Format

The group format is essential to the process of supervision in the Extern Program. The group functions as a sounding board for the relation between the supervisor and each individual trainee, contributes useful suggestions and observations, and provides a safety net of mutual support. Through its comments, questions, and sheer presence, the group helps the supervisor to keep distance from the therapy itself and to maintain the perspective of a trainer—particularly during live supervision, when the immediacy of the therapeutic process might blur that perspective. Alternating between the roles of thera-pist and observer, the group members learn both through the intense experience of conducting a supervised session, and through the more relaxed participation in the dialogue between the supervisor and other trainees.

On the other hand, the group context places extra demands on the supervisor. When reviewing a videotaped session, for instance, the supervisor must double as a group leader, balancing the need for group participation with the need for a focus on the specific training needs of the individual trainee. In live supervision, the supervisor has to be careful not to become subtly induced by the group into taking too much control of the session ("Is Carl doing what you asked him to do?"). By maintaining an equidistant relation to all members, staying clear of coalitions, and sticking to the function of guiding the trainees' learning, the supervisor fosters group cohesiveness and discourages destruc-tive competition.

TRAINING CONTENT

The Extern trainee learns primarily in response to the requirements of clinical practice. Rather than following a prearranged curriculum, the program is shaped by the needs of the families in treatment and those of the trainees. The emphasis that the structural model places on cooperation with and accommodation to the family dictates, in princi-ple, a natural sequence. Issues related to joining, entering the family system, and forming therapeutic alliances tend to be dealt with before those related to challenge, unbalanc-ing, or confrontation. But some families or trainees may require an earlier focus on these latter issues, and it may also be that the more a therapist learns about changing families, the better he or she "reads" them in the beginning—and the better the reading, the better the joining.

The integration of theory and practice follows a pattern of alternation: the trainee works with a family, receives corrective feedback from the supervisor, returns to the family, and so on. Generic concepts, such as joining, unbalancing, or enacting, are intertwined with the discussion of specific clinical situations throughout all the stages of the training cycle, particularly during videotape reviews when there is more time to do so. This integrative approach is occasionally complemented with readings, assigned in accordance with the needs of each trainee; videotaped sessions of experienced clinicians, which the supervisor discusses to illustrate specific points; and the monthly one-day seminar where all students and supervisors meet to talk among themselves and with guest presenters.

The trainee may frequently feel, "Ah! This time I got it." Then he or she will experience failure, and the supervisor will introduce yet another correction. The experience can be frustrating, particularly for the student who expects to learn by continuous increments—that is, to expand his or her already acquired knowledge without having to put it into question. Instead, the process of learning a new paradigm typically adopts the form of a spiral, where elating experiences of insight are followed by the feeling of being "back to square one." It takes time for the student to realize that each new turn of the screw finds him or her, after all, at a higher level of competence.

This spiral pattern of learning is consistent with the notion that structural skills, as part of an integral model, are interdependent. They can not be taught and learned as free-standing techniques; on the contrary, the student must be consistently reminded of the relation that each technique has to the other, and of the places the techniques have within the structural paradigm. The paradigm needs to impregnate training as a constant presence, a point of reference that confers meaning to each instance of learning. If the goal of training is to form autonomous therapists, its content must be dominated not by "how-to-do" questions and the practice of discrete techniques, but by "what-for" questions and the understanding of how specific interventions are dictated by the larger structural goals. The following discussion of some of the typical problem areas in the teaching of structural family therapy illustrates these points.

Learning to See Structures

The ability to bring about structural change depends on the ability to "see" structures. A special scanning attitude is required so that data are gathered and organized in a way that will trigger structural interventions.

A trainee who was assigned the case of a violent 12-year-old boy learned during the first interview that the boy's father had died two years before. The therapist immediately focused on mother's feelings of loss, and did not have much trouble in finding confirmation for his hypothesis—that pathological mourning was causing the mother, via depression and hopelessness, to be ineffective as a parent. By gathering information according to a psychodynamic paradigm, the trainee was setting the stage for a therapeutic strategy based on helping the mother to work through her bereavement, so that she would become more available to raise her son.

The trainee was called out of the room and asked to find out how the family context (the structure) was contributing to the unresolved mourning *and* to mother's ineffectiveness. This time the trainee elicited structural information: mother's brother had been trying to help by volunteering anything from running errands (when mother did not feel like leaving the house), to half-fathering the boy. In the second interview, which was attended by the uncle, the trainee could also appreciate mother's complementary role in monitoring help:

by summoning her obliging brother whenever a minor difficulty arose, she was cooperating in the pattern that kept her depressed and unavailable for parenting. The stage was now set for a therapeutic strategy aimed at changing the dysfunctional system.

Instructing the therapist to elicit context information is one way of encouraging him or her to perceive structures. Other ways include the use of visual aids such as mapping (Minuchin, 1974) and the metaphoric depiction of complex patterns, like the "accordion" and other types of families (Minuchin & Fishman, 1981). Constructive approaches, however, are not enough. The trainer often needs to disrupt deep-seated assumptions about the explanation for dysfunctional behavior ("Is mourning the reason that mother can not handle her son, or is that just a copout?"), the direction of change ("Couldn't the boy's needs be utilized as leverage to extricate mother from her exclusive preoccupation with widowhood?"), and the therapist's own role ("Are you there to help them express their feelings, or to help them solve the violence problem?"). Underneath these questions and their alternative answers lies the more fundamental level of value judgments on what constitutes good—or better—family functioning. A family structure is always seen, assessed, and eventually modified by reference to an ideal model, connoted by such concepts as "clear boundaries," "flexibility to transform," or "developmentally appropriate patterns." Sooner or later in training, the supervisor needs to gain access to this deeper level.

In the case of our example, the therapist succeeded in moving his focus away from mother's mourning and toward context, once he came to see his function as one of helping mother and son restructure their relation in a way more appropriate to the present stage in their family life cycle. In the words of the trainee:

> The notion that impacted me the most was that this boy was at a crucial developmental spot, and could not wait for his mother to work through her individual stuff. When I went back to them (after consulting with the supervisor) I kept repeating to myself: "12 years old," and "7th grade." And asking myself: "What would be the right context for him now? What needs to happen between him and his mom, that is not happening?"

As the therapist looked at the family from this vantage point, it became apparent to him that they were not working as a good team. There was too much nurturance going from the boy to the mother, and too little guidance the other way around; they were not dealing with each other because they were both more connected to father's ghost. The health-oriented search for the missing pattern organized the therapist's quest for structural information.

Learning to Join

Because structural family therapy requires the cooperation of the family, it is essential for the therapist to participate actively in the formation of a therapeutic system (Minuchin, 1974; Minuchin & Fishman, 1981), where he or she temporarily joins the family in a position of leadership. The structural therapist needs to relate to family members in a way that validates their experience but does not preclude a challenge to the status quo. This is not an easy task. A frequent misconception among therapists in training is to view joining as just a preamble to "real" therapy—a social ritual that needs to be observed but can be quickly disposed of. Particularly vulnerable to this mistake are therapists previously trained to think strategically; they tend to plan their moves several steps ahead of the family's immediate feedback and may react impatiently to the supervisor's request that they slow down their thinking and "wait for the family."

Disregard for the complexities of joining often results in a superficial or an undifferentiated relation to the family: the therapist starts by smiling, being nice, and indulging in small talk, and ends up either in a peripheral position (without engaging the family) or inducted by the family process into a powerless predicament. The latter was the case for a trainee whom I shall call Mrs. Murphy.

Outside the session, Mrs. Murphy could articulate a rather sophisticated description of the family structure and its relation to the presenting problem. In the presence of the family, though, she appeared to lose that structural perspective. It was easy for her to engage individual members (she would, for instance, connect to children much better than their parents could), while the rest of the family watched appreciatively. Families liked her, but their compliance with her prescribed tasks and other recommendations was low, and no significant change would occur. As a therapist, Mrs. Murphy positioned herself at the center of a starlike configuration from where she made herself available to each individual member in succession, but she could not grasp the family system as such. Thus, the focus of her work changed constantly, following the pulls and pushes of the different family members.

In this case the therapist was hindered by her own ability to establish quick rapport with individuals. On entering the family system, she entirely trusted her spontaneity and failed to recognize the need for conscious, purposeful joining, which would have enhanced her leadership and ability to promote change.

The example is also illustrative of the close relation between the ability to join and the ability to see family patterns unfolding in the session.

But taking joining too casually is not the only mistake that a therapist in training can make. The nearly opposite misconception is to approach joining as a special technique or set of techniques that can be learned by practicing the appropriate sentences, voice intonations, gestures, and body postures. The therapist may then become overinvolved with his or her own maneuvering and lose touch with the family, thus defeating the very essence of joining and failing to develop the proximal relation to clients that structural family therapy requires.

A challenge for the supervisor, then, is how to call the trainee's attention to the dynamics of joining, while at the same time discouraging a "technical" approach. One possible avenue is to prescribe the trainee's behavior during the initial moments of therapy in a way that will facilitate joining, without disclosing this particular goal until later. For instance, a therapist who had a tendency to jump prematurely into "the problem that brings you here" was asked to slow down and make sure that he contacted everybody in the family before addressing the problem. The supervisor's instruction, originally framed as a way of eliciting necessary information, helped the therapist to join better and was discussed from this second point of view after the session.

In other cases the trainer needs to reach for the deeper level of the trainee's basic perceptions and attitudes. One therapist who generally liked children but distrusted parents would almost invariably ignore the presence of a mother in the room. The supervisor therefore instructed the therapist to start an initial session by addressing the mother, and to obtain any information about the daughter only through the mother. The therapist complied, but within less than one minute she had managed to convey her disapproval of the way in which the mother was talking about her daughter. Here, the supervisor had underestimated the pull of the therapist's attitudes, which organized her to operate as a child rescuer. A therapist thus organized usually has difficulties in joining because he or she is always ready to protect the child from any insinuation of scapegoating within the family, and thereby loses structural perspective. The supervisor should have detected and addressed the more basic paradigmatic issues: "Do you think that mother can give you that information?" "Is your role to protect the daughter from the mother, or to help them develop as a more viable unit?" In general, the skeptical therapist who routinely expects incompetence, resistance, uncooperativeness and/or malevolence will find them—and will not be able to join families as required by the structural model, even after trying the most sophisticated techniques.

Joining is not the outcome of a calculated technique, but the outgrowth of a positive attitude toward families. To encourage such an attitude, the supervisor needs to nurture the therapist's curiosity about the inner workings of the family ("What kind of animal is this?" "How is it that they cannot solve this problem?") and his or her confidence in the availability of latent resources within the family ("They are larger than what they are presenting to us"). In the case of Mrs. Murphy—the therapist who was too central—this proved to be the turning point. Initially, the supervisor had worked on increasing Mrs. Murphy's awareness of certain dynamics in families that would organize her to become central, and on how to avoid them. With the help of much self-discipline and a few reminders, she managed to keep her centrality in check. But then a new problem surfaced: she looked uninterested and disconnected from what was taking place in therapy, and one family began to miss sessions.

The supervisor found out that in spite of her familiarity with the literature and her preference for the structural model, Mrs. Murphy did not really believe that family members could have a beneficial influence on each other. She had been professionally trained to distrust the resourcefulness of clients, and to think of herself as the only "healer" in the room. Against the background of such a paradigm, the exercises designed to counter her centrality had resulted in skepticism and a lack of interest: once removed from the central position, Mrs. Murphy could not see herself as a therapist and, accordingly, would not expect any "real therapy" to occur.

This trainee's basic attitudes toward therapy could not be dealt with by just practicing techniques; a different context was needed. The length of her sessions was extended so that she would give families a chance to prove their strength, with the provision that she could always conduct "real therapy" in the last half hour if needed. The focus of the dialogue between Mrs. Murphy and her supervisor turned to their contrasting views on the level of strength available in each family, and what was needed from the therapist. During the sessions, Mrs. Murphy was directed to explore and push for the family's resources and for alternative configurations of the family structure. Her work began to show sustained progress. Her skepticism first acquired a different quality—she was intrigued with the possibility of altering her perception of her own role—and soon was replaced by a new intensity. Her curiosity became more invested in the process than in the individual pathologies, in the search for strengths rather than in the identification of weaknesses.

Learning to Challenge

The mobilization of family resources, an essential feature of the structural approach to change, requires the active involvement of the therapist as a protagonist more than as a mere commentator. In the process of motivating family members to try alternative patterns of transaction, the therapist often needs to challenge, more or less intensely, the family members' perceptions of their reality and/or their responses to it. Given that most therapists come to train in the structural model after having learned a more traditional definition of their role, the ability to challenge is usually regarded by both trainers and trainees as the most difficult to develop.

Like good joining, good challenging is the natural result of an attitude and cannot be taught or learned as a technique. Consider the therapist who by her own recognition was "too nice" and decided to practice a more challenging style. She wanted to help a passive adolescent to become angry at his mother for overcontrolling him. She tried variations of the same message: "You should react, you should get her off your back." The words were harsh, but the therapist maintained a casual posture that conveyed that she did not really expect the boy to deal successfully with his mother. Her "challenge," performed from a safe distance, sounded more like a put-down. In a situation like this, asking the therapist to lean forward or otherwise to reduce distance from the client would not be enough, because what is lacking is not a technical subtlety but the therapist's commitment to her actions. Had she been more tuned in to the family's predicament than to the practice of a technique, she might have glimpsed a streak of competence beyond the apparent stubbornness of the adolescent, adding decisive force to her intervention—and, by the way, she would have leaned forward without even planning it.

Challenging, to be effective, must be predicated on the client's strengths. Contrary to a common misconception, it is not the "opposite" of joining. Joining and challenging need to be seen as simultaneous qualities in any therapeutic intervention. Good joining includes a dimension of challenge: the intrusion into the clients' lives. Good challenging strengthens joining by cementing the alliance between the therapist and the "better side" of the challenged individuals. Both qualities express the same basic attitude, of curiosity, commitment to change, and confidence in the family's latent resources, that is a natural corollary of the therapist's adhesion to the structural paradigm.

Thus, the belief in the worthiness and attainability of structural goals sustains the therapist in his or her challenge to the established ways of the family. Without it, the therapist will most probably falter in the face of intensity, back off, and diffuse conflict. For instance, the father of a truant teenager would routinely escape from the pressures of parenthood by bringing up in sessions some ongoing feud with his wife. The therapist understood the supervisor's directive to block the distraction, but could not bring himself to challenge the father. It occurred to the supervisor that the therapist, having previously been trained to automatically refer any child problem to a marital conflict, might be in fact reacting sympathetically to the father's shift of focus. Following a discussion where the supervisor argued against the policy of leaving children's needs on the back burner, and in favor of an immediate correction of the organizational flaw that was responsible for the truancy, the therapist was able to develop a more challenging stance toward the father.

The basic ingredients of a challenging attitude can be developed in the trainee by encouraging critical observation. The therapist needs to discipline himself or herself to watch and listen to the family's transactions with a questioning disposition, not taking anything for granted. Patterns of transaction that may seem obvious to the family should be met with a silent or overt interrogation. How come Billy doesn't care about bringing pink slips from school? How come father doesn't know more about Joanna's friends? How come Vicky doesn't try to talk her way out of being grounded? The "how-come" mode of inquiry implies that patterns of transactions might, and maybe should, be different, and that it is within the power of the family to change them.

Because of the difficulties involved in conveying the meaning and role of the challenge, the supervisor is often in the position of teaching it by demonstration. When the supervisor enters the therapy room and challenges a family to move beyond its imaginary constraints, the purpose of the demonstration is not so much to show the trainee how to do it, but that it is possible to do it—that the family can be challenged without the entire therapeutic project falling apart. The subject of the lesson is the worthiness and viability of the challenge, more than its specific shape. As with any other demonstration, the subsequent explanation of the intervention and its relevance within the wider strategy is a crucial ingredient of the learning process.

Understanding the structural model of change is vital not only to sustain a challenge, but also to avoid the pitfalls of *compulsive* challenging—which has reached epidemic proportions among therapists trained by "practicing techniques." The structural therapist does not routinely block the intrusive member of a triad, but does so only when some therapeutic gain can be derived from that challenge; lenient parents of manipulative children are not invariably made angry, but are incited by the therapist only when their anger can be bound to the structural goal of increasing distance among subsystems.

Learning to Enact

Asking family members to do something in the therapy room may appear to be a simple, if sometimes awkward, endeavor. Yet because of its apparent simplicity, the procedure can easily become overtechnified, and the therapist can lose sight of the two functions that enactment plays within the structural model. One is to identify relational patterns that need to change; the other, more important, is to help the family experience that such change is both desirable and possible. The two functions need to become clearly understood and integrated by the trainee, to avoid some of the most common pitfalls in the practice of structural therapy.

A typical example is the unilateral emphasis on "bringing the problem into the room," whereby the therapist may try to get a 7-year-old to display his temper tantrum before anything else happens—and then not know what to do once the tantrum is in the room. Or the therapist may initiate a change-oriented enactment but fail to direct it to a successful conclusion. This is often the case when too much emphasis has been placed on the techniques of therapy and the trainee becomes overly anxious to "introduce" an enactment. For instance, a trainee has been told that he is too central and should practice "disengaging," so he eagerly moves to set up a conversation between two family members. They begin to talk, but the therapist does not know what to do about the process that is developing before his eyes. He may be thrilled by the release of emotional communication, the "husband finally being able to talk," and so on, or he may become fascinated with the content of the discussion, but he does not know where to go. The experience ends in failure. Emphasis on technique causes the therapist to lose sight of the fact that an enactment is only as good as the experience that it generates.

In helping the trainee to overcome these pitfalls, it may not be enough for the supervisor to restrain him or her from "premature enactment." A more comprehensive training strategy involves fostering an understanding of each enactment as a "sentence" in the script that the therapist is creating with and for the family. The therapist's punctuation of the experience generated by the enactment—the periods, commas, and footnotes that define the experience in one among many possible ways—is more relevant to the therapeutic process than the enactment itself. The structural therapist looks at an enactment as a building block to be used in the construction of a therapeutic reality. Consequently, the supervisor that directs a trainee to an enactment needs to supply a clearly stated goal. It is not enough to get father and son to talk to each other; the therapist needs to be aware of and focused on what is to be accomplished by the talking. Instructions for the enactment need to include ways of monitoring progress in relation to the goal ("Once they are talking, watch for what makes it difficult for them to maintain focus"). During the transaction itself, the trainee may need to be made aware of unfolding transactional patterns ("Did you notice that son lowers his head when Dad starts lecturing? Get one of them to do something different").

TRAINING EVALUATION

The Extern Program is monitored by the faculty during weekly meetings. Feedback from the trainees is gathered continuously—particularly at evaluation times: midterm and end of the program—from both informal verbal comments and written answers to questionnaires. As a result, various aspects of the program such as group composition, time allocation, and type of leadership have changed over the years.

The individual student's performance is evaluated by the supervisors according to his or her ability to keep families in treatment, diagnose problems, and help families to change. Ongoing evaluation proceeds as the supervisors follow the students' cases in live and tape supervision week after week. Also, "before" and "after" segments (from sessions conducted early in the program and toward the end) are used to evaluate progress. The trainee's colleagues in the supervisory group contribute their opinions to the evaluation. Specific remedial work with some students is planned by the two supervisors when needed; individualized goals are then set, which are periodically reevaluated by supervisors and trainees. Particularly difficult situations are brought to the attention of the faculty. The possibility of a student being requested to leave the program is built into the format but has very rarely been used.

The profile of the "ideal graduate" from the Extern Program includes the generic ingredients of a systemic paradigm: a disposition to make sense of problems by referring them to the dynamics of the family rather than the isolated reality of the symptom bearer; a belief that positive change is facilitated or made difficult by rules of interaction rather than intrapsychic forces or poor learning habits; and a preference for releasing the healing strengths of the family—by promoting functional processes and discouraging dysfunctional ones—rather than directly healing the individual. In addition to these generic qualities, the ideal profile also contains the specific marks of the structural paradigm: the ability to conceptualize problems in spatial terms (distance/proximity, inclusion/exclusion), to gather data that allow for a diagnosis of the "organizational flaw," to imagine possible structural rearrangements that might eliminate the problem, and in particular to adopt an active role in engaging, motivating, and leading the family toward change.

TRAINING RELATIONSHIP

While the supervisor works toward producing such ideal graduates, the trainee may have a different view of his or her own needs. Some implications of the resulting conflict are briefly examined here.

The relation between Extern supervisor and trainee is colored by a creative tension, an oscillation between harmonic and conflictive encounters. A basic assumption of complementary cooperation sets the general tone: the trainee, no matter how experienced, is here to learn and the supervisor to teach. This hierarchical arrangement is prevalent through the entire training process; the level of dependence of the trainee on the supervisor may vary over the course of the year, but real autonomy for the trainee comes with the final disengagement as marked by the "end of the course" ritual.

There are naturally areas of conflict where the basic complementarity is challenged. The trainee's expectations may ask for a gradual, reassuring accumulation of skills (to be built upon his or her existing competence), while the supervisor's own assessment may call for a drastic, and possibly unsettling, paradigmatic shift. From the trainee's point of view the supervisor's comments and directives may at times look senseless, arbitrary, irrelevant, or disruptive. To the supervisor, the trainee's objection may reveal paradigmatic "errors," non-structural thinking that needs correction. In such cases a sort of power struggle is likely to occur, where the trainee will tend to repudiate the structural approach and fall back into one where he or she feels more comfortable, while the supervisor may insist, "But you are here to learn our way." The rules of the game are biased in favor of the supervisor's position, because they allow maximum intrusiveness in the trainee's handling of the cases.

In teaching the structural paradigm, the supervisor will alternately support and push, encourage and restrain the therapist. This does not mean evenly balancing kicks and strokes but, rather, identifying and responding differently to strengths and weaknesses. The goal of learning is given priority over good feelings; a certain level of stress is accepted as a natural component of the process, which includes the possibility that the student may temporarily lose his or her sense of competence. Performance fears, misunderstandings, resentment, and opposition are to be expected, but not allowed to prevent learning. The supervisor must be careful not to promote unnecessary anxiety that might block learning, but also not to abdicate the interests of learning just because the trainee might become anxious. For example, a trainee breaks down after 20 minutes of waiting for her family: if they do not arrive, it will be the third family in a row that has dropped from treatment. Tearful, the trainee claims that families "leave" her as soon as she challenges them—implying that the structural approach "is not for her." The supervisor insists on the need to discuss the upcoming session since the family may still show up. The therapist continues crying while examining with the supervisor alternative ways of challenging the mother in the family without making her feel attacked.

The family eventually arrives and the session opens with one of the daughters announcing that she will not attend any more sessions. Through the one-way mirror, the therapist looks shaken. The supervisor phones in and instructs her to establish the daughter's attendance as a condition for the continuity of treatment. After the session, the therapist reports that the intervention removed her from her usual begging stance and helped her to both challenge and keep the family.

This particular incident involved only the trainee and the supervisor. In a more typical scenario, the group of trainees would be in charge of meeting individual emotional needs at times of crisis; by spontaneously providing the necessary support, it frees the supervisor to focus on the demands of the task at hand in his or her own relationship to the trainee.

As the training relation progresses, the cumulative experience of the trainee, and the growing understanding between trainee and supervisor, contribute to reduce the incidence of anxiety and interpersonal tension. Differences between supervisor and trainee, however, persist until the very end. And when the training relation comes to a close, the supervisor finds out that the student did not learn exactly what he or she had intended to teach, but something less, or more, or at any rate different. The supervisor is then reminded of the words of William Morris: ". . . men fight and lose the battle, and the thing they fought for comes about in spite of their defeat, and when it comes it turns out not to be what they meant, and other men have to fight for what they meant under another name . . ." (Morris, 1948).

Notes

1. The author was affiliated with the Philadelphia Child Guidance Clinic from 1976 to 1986.
2. The Extern program is periodically revised and updated, and the description offered here reflects the program as it was in the mid-1980s.

References

Allman, L. R. (1982). The aesthetic preference: Overcoming the pragmatic error. *Family Process, 21*, 43–56.
Aponte, H. A., & VanDeusen, J. M. (1981). Structural family therapy. In A. S. Gurman & D. P. Kniskern (Eds.), *Handbook of family therapy*. New York: Brunner/Mazel.
Bateson, G. (1972). *Steps to an ecology of mind*. New York: Ballantine Books.
Colapinto, J. (1982). Structural family therapy. In A. M. Horne & M. M. Ohlsen (Eds.), *Family counseling and therapy*. Itasca, IL: Peacock.
Colapinto, J. (1983). Beyond technique: Teaching how to think structurally. *Journal of Strategic and Systemic Therapies, 2*, 12–21.
Herrigel, E. (1953). *Zen in the art of archery*. New York: Pantheon Books.
Keeney, B. P., & Sprenkle, D. H. (1982). Ecosystemic epistemology: Critical implications for the aesthetics and pragmatics of family therapy. *Family Process, 21*, 1–19.
Minuchin, S. (1974). *Families and family therapy*. Cambridge, MA: Harvard University Press.

Minuchin, S. (1982). Reflections on boundaries. *American Journal of Orthopsychiatry, 52*, 655–663.

Minuchin, S., & Fishman, H. C. (1981). *Family therapy techniques*. Cambridge, MA: Harvard University Press.

Morris, W. (1948). A dream of John Bell. In D. H. Cole (Ed.), *William Morris: Selected writings*. New York: Random House.

Nichols, M. (1984). *Family therapy: Concepts and methods*. New York: Gardner Press.

Scheflen, A. E. (1978). Susan smiled: An explanation in family therapy. *Family Process, 17*, 59–68.

Umbarger, C. (1983). *Structural family therapy*. New York: Grune & Stratton.

3

The Milan Training Program

SERGIO PIRROTTA
Mental Health and Retardation Services, Inc., Lawrence, Massachusetts

GIANFRANCO CECCHIN
Centro Milanese di Terapia della Famiglia, Milan, Italy

The Milan team, made up of Mara Selvini-Palazzoli, Luigi Boscolo, Gianfranco Cecchin, and Giuiana Prata, initially developed their systemic therapy approach as a treatment of families and couples. Their book, *Paradox and Counterparadox* (Palazzoli, Boscolo, Cecchin, & Prata, 1978), was first published in Italy in 1975, and presented the conceptual framework and methodology of their family therapy. In 1977, Luigi Boscolo and Gianfranco Cecchin began a training program designed to teach that systemic framework and family therapy method for the treatment of psychiatric disorders. A detailed history of the Milan team's early years and the family therapy methodology they taught is beyond the scope of this chapter, but has been described at length elsewhere (Boscolo & Cecchin, 1982; Tomm, 1984a, 1984b). What is of interest is that after several years of this training experience, the trainers began to notice some unexpected negative consequences. The trainees began to return to the Center with reports of treatment failures and disappointment. In some cases, the student's experiences were disastrous, as attempts to introduce this kind of therapy within their own working contexts resulted in stirring up the wrath of co-workers, their administrators, and their clients. Many had faced the ridicule of colleagues and disciplinary action from their superiors not only for treatment failures, but also for what was often seen to be unorthodox and perhaps dangerous conduct in the therapeutic contact with patients and their families.

The training team was forced to reexamine its program on the basis of this feedback. It became clear to them that they had made a major epistemological error. In their attempt to impart to their students that very family therapy technique which had been so successful for the Milan team's clinical work for so many years, they had overlooked the fact that their technique had been developed within a context quite different from that within which the students worked.

The Milan Center is a private clinic, staffed by recognized experts in the field of family therapy, and cases are referred there only after a history of treatment failures with traditional treatments. Further, being privately funded, with no administrative or political ties to any other institution, the Center is accountable only to its clients and to itself. In contrast, the students typically worked as line therapists or doctors in the public sector; they were most often in positions low in the organizational hierarchies of their institutions, and were often accountable to many (and sometimes conflicting) institutional, political, or administrative forces. The definition of the client's request for service, the definition of the clinician's role, the definition of appropriate outcome and expectations, and the definition of who is allowed to decide what should be done and how it should be done, were all questions that in the trainees' work settings had a variety of different, confused, and often contradictory answers. These were certainly quite different work settings from the Milan Center. A particular kind of therapy as innovative and different as systemic family therapy, with its radical perspectives and interventions, took on very different meaning when transposed to each of these different contexts.

At this same time, the Milan team was undergoing some radical changes in its own thinking about systems. Stimulated by continued study of Bateson's writings (Bateson, 1972, 1979), the Milan trainers were beginning to alter the focus of their analysis of systems. Until this point, the Milan clinicians had seen the therapeutic process as the therapy team observing the family system in order to understand it and act on it. The ideas of working as a team, of the mirror, of circular interviewing, and of utilizing systemic analysis to describe the family's interactional map, were all inventions to try to ensure that the therapist could remain separate from the family being observed. The intervention was also seen as an insertion of a change-inducing informational unit by the therapeutic team into the pathological system. This sort of analysis and approach was later labeled by them as "first-order cybernetics."

Through a rereading of Bateson's work, the Milan clinicians began to shift their focus to not only the system being observed, but also the context of that observation itself, and hence the observing system as well. Whereas in first-order cybernetics there is a distinction arbitrarily drawn between the family and the therapist, as though they were two distinct systems, the Milan clinicians began instead to see the family in the context of the therapist's interaction with them. In short, they saw this as the co-creation of a new reality. This new reality involved a second level of observation concurrent with the first— the observation of the system created by the therapist–family interaction within the context of the therapeutic encounter. This second level of observation has been termed "second-order cybernetics" (Tomm, 1984a).

This shift in their theoretical understanding of systems, coupled with the feedback they were receiving from their trainees' experiences in the field, led the Milan trainers to begin to focus on the contextual effects in making meaning from phenomena, and on observing the observer (in their case, the therapist) in the process of interacting with the family in the therapeutic context. They began to redefine their training mission as that of teaching their trainees to think systemically regardless of their contexts. The analysis of one's own work context became a prime concern in the training. Instead of simply studying the interactional patterns of family members, they began to teach their trainees to consider the feedback loops developed between the interviewer and the interviewees, or between the worker and the client.

This chapter will describe the training methods currently being utilized by Luigi Boscolo and Gianfranco Cecchin in their Center.[1] Because of this change in focus away from family therapy methodology in favor of teaching their trainees a new way of perceiving human problems and intervening in human service situations, much attention will be given to the basic epistemological tenets of the Milan school, and how the program guides the students to make this epistemological shift.

THE TRAINING CONTEXT

The Centro Milanese di Terapia della Famiglia is located in the city of Milan, a major industrial and financial center in northern Italy, and it attracts trainees mostly from the northern half of the country. Trainees are from the disciplines of psychiatry, psychology, and social work, and must have a minimum of three years of postdegree work experience in order to be eligible for participation. There is an expectation that students will be working in the field concurrently with their participation in the training. In fact, most are working in the public sector, either as school psychologists, or in community inpatient units in local hospitals, or in community clinics mandated to provide a wide variety of social assistance as well as clinical services to the public free of charge as part of the country's socialized medical system. Student selection is made by the senior trainers each year. Students pay a tuition, usually out of pocket, although some may be reimbursed in part or fully by their work agencies for the training.

The families seen at the Center come from all over the country, although, predictably, the largest number tend to be from the greater Milan area. They span the full range of the socioeconomic spectrum, but tend toward the upper income range, as the therapy is paid for out of pocket without the benefit of insurance reimbursements. Families are usually referred by other professionals and by current or former students of the Center, or by other informal channels. There is no public advertising of the Center's therapeutic activities.

The training sequence is composed of three years of biweekly sessions, exclusive of the summer months. One day of training every two weeks allows trainees to participate in the training with the minimum disruption of their work. The total number of training sessions is usually about 52 to 54. In the first year, the training sessions are of one-half day's duration. The last two years are full-day sessions. Training groups tend to remain together throughout that time, and are often urged to take a six-month to one-year interruption of the training sequence between the second and third years in order to integrate their learning into their own work setting.

The training resources of the Center include a therapy room with a contiguous observation room connected by a one-way mirror, a videotaping setup with a wide-angle camera in the therapy room and a manually operated zoom lens camera controlled from within the observation room, and a control panel that switches cameras operated by the video technician. There is no telephone hookup between the therapy room and the observation room. Interruptions during a session are made by calling out the therapist with a knock on the door.

The full-time staff of the Center consists of the two senior trainers, who are the founders of the Center, an administrative assistant who is also the video technician, and a secretary. In addition to the senior trainers, there are other part-time instructors, all of whom are graduates of the Milan training program. There are 4 junior instructors who are responsible for all but the clinical portion of training for the groups they run, and 10 other assistant instructors who help the senior trainers with running the advanced groups. The senior trainers directly surpervise any family session that is conducted in the Center. The increase in the size of the staff is a recent phenomenon, for until 1982 all the training was done exclusively by Boscolo and Cecchin.

BASIC THEORETICAL CONCEPTS UNDERLYING THE TRAINING

The training structure and methods of the Milan Center embody, to a large extent, an attempt to teach the Batesonian view of a systemic, circular epistemology through the very process of how that epistemology is transmitted to the students. In order to understand how that is done, it is first necessary to examine the Milan team's view about the essential elements of that epistemology. Although for the purposes of clarity it is useful to discuss these concepts as separate and discrete, they are in fact interrelated in a theoretical world view. Readers who are familiar with a systemic epistemology will correctly note that the separation of these concepts, and the author's choice in selecting these as core concepts to be considered in training or therapy, represent an arbitrary and idiosyncratic punctuation.

The Emphasis on Epistemology

The Milan team's method of therapy and training emphasizes the notion of epistemology rather than that of a clinical, empirical science. Following from Bateson's use of the term, the Milan team chooses not to focus on what the world is but, rather, on how we think about it, how we understand it and know it. In viewing families and human interactions, the team is concerned with how clients in therapy understand their existence, their relation with one another, their actions and attitudes toward each other, the problem behavior, and the rest of the world, including the helping professionals. Similarly, the therapists are concerned less about what we know about families, and more about what we believe, think, and observe about human interactions.

The epistemological approach, then, focuses more on ideas and beliefs than on the qualities of the individuals or the systems and subsystems of skin-bounded entities. What the therapist does with a family, the conclusions drawn from his or her observations of interactions, the interventions utilized, all spring from the way the therapist makes sense of the phenomena observed.

An extension of this emphasis on epistemology is the shift of focus from traits of the individual or the system to relationships and differences. For Bateson, a relationship is defined best through differences, and human beings understand things best through the perception of differences. The human mind thinks, or develops ideas, through the perception of differences that make a difference. These perceived differences are information, and information creates ideas (Bateson, 1972, 1979).

In the study of human behavior, there are many relationships that are important to consider: relations between one person and another, between one aggregate of persons and others, between a belief and/or idea and another, between perceptions of event at one point in time and another, and so on. For the therapist in the process of developing an understanding of the system being observed, it is essential to create maps of these differences. The maps can be created through a process of continual observation and interaction cycles. The cycles are seen to be necessary because the therapist, as an observer, can only approximate an understanding of the reality being observed. In the process of making the observations, the therapist is necessarily changing or co-creating the reality being observed. This last idea is a relatively new one, involving an understanding of the cybernetics of observing systems. It will be described elsewhere in this chapter. Through the observation/intervention cycles, the therapist/observer is able to create a map and then test it in a series of continuing feedback loops between himself or herself and the family.

Circularity

An important property of the Batesonian epistemology is the concept of circularity. In moving from a mechanistic, trait-oriented, empirical organization of the world of percepts to a systemic epistemology based on information, one moves from a linear, causal view of phenomena to a circular, reflexive notion of reality as a creation. Systemic therapists are well aware of the significant difference between a linear and circular model of viewing the world, and hence it is not necessary to outline it here.

The Batesonian view of circular epistemology does make a point that is emphasized by the Milan group, however, and therefore bears closer scrutiny. In his writings, Bateson does not appear to be saying that there are two different ways of viewing the world, the circular and the linear. Rather, the implication is that a linear viewpoint is a partial view of events, and represents not so much a straight line of causality as, rather, an arc, or partially circular view.

The concept of circularity, as used by the Milan team, is an attempt to add together these partial views into a more holistic, more total map of reality. Still, even a circular view is only a map, a creation, an approximation of reality, albeit a more complete one. The Batesonian and Milan view of reality will be discussed next.

The Relativity of Truth

Another extension of Batesonian thinking is a radically different notion of the nature of truth and reality. Unlike the classical Aristotelian notion that truth exists and must be discovered, Bateson and other systemic epistemologists see truth as relative and arbitrary, dependent on the point of view of the observer and the context in which the observation is made. It can be seen that this view is consistent with the previously mentioned premises of a circular epistemology. Bateson goes one step further in his ideas about truth and reality. He sees that the way in which we know is determined through a perception of differences that becomes articulated through the interaction of a person with his or her social, physical, and metaphysical environment.

In therapy, or in the analysis of social behavior, the view of reality is likewise constructed through this process. Again, what is constructed is a map of reality, an approximation of the truth, and not truth itself. Bateson warns that the most typical error in our Western way of thinking is to mistake that map for the territory itself.

Linguistic Conditioning

Epistemological mannerisms are influenced by the language and structure of language with which Western cultures communicate. Bateson has pointed out that Western linguistic usage reflects a concept of mind as existing inside a human being, and that linear causality is almost always implied when describing events in common parlance. In addition, Bateson states that language is almost exclusively geared to the transmission of digital communication, and therefore is not easily adaptable to describing and understanding relational messages.

In their book *Paradox and Counterparadox*, the Milan clinicians devote a brief but significant chapter to what they call "The Tyrany of Linguistic Conditioning," (Palazzoli *et al.*, 1978). Expanding on Bateson's assertions, and quoting Shands, the Milan authors describe the epistemological errors that tend to occur under the influence of this linguistic conditioning. Because of the linear and digital nature of language, a person is said to own characteristics, or moods—as, for example, when therapists say, "The father was a distancer," or "He was depressed." Language then implies a linear, causal, and moralistic view of transactions. People are said to act on other people, as in the statement, "She made her mother angry." This statement implies a subject from whom the action begins, an object who is the recipient of the action, and a result.

The Milan trainers are cautious with the use of language, both in their therapy and in their training. They are careful to emphasize the use of words and phrases such as "seems," "acts as if," "appears," "has the effect of," and others to describe the behavior of family members and of therapists being observed. In this way they avoid making linear, causal implications in describing the phenomena they are observing.

Information versus Traits

An important difference that is readily apparent between clinicians who have been taught individualistic, intrapsychic, or illness-oriented therapy models, as opposed to those who approach therapy from a systemic relational view, is the degree to which the former describe a case on the basis of the individual traits of the family members. In psychiatry, as in common parlance, people are identified by their traits. For example, a person is said to be an abuser, a borderline, or a schizophrenic. In psychiatry, such a trait is then expanded to include correlate traits, often with a complete etiology. Some people, such as classical psychoanalytic theorists, believe that all of a person's personality structure is determined within the first five years of life, so that these traits are essentially crystallized in childhood.

This view is in sharp contrast with the systemic epistemology of Bateson, who believes that people act and react on the basis of the perception of information, and that "mind" does not reside within the individual, but in the interactive circuit between the brain, the body, and the social and physical environment (Bateson, 1972). According to Bateson, what activates the mind is the perception of differences, and, for him, the news of a difference is information. Information can activate the mind to generate behavior, thus starting a recurrent loop of action–feedback–reaction in relation to an object or person in the environment. Bateson's classic example of this concept is that of a man felling a tree with an axe, where the total system of tree-eyes-brain-muscles-axe-stroke-tree is seen as the locus of the "mind" circuit. This is sharply contrasted to our common notion that there is a self that acts purposely to cut down a delimited object, (i.e., the tree).

The clinical implications of this epistemological distinction are profound. This shift justifies the change of focus from the intrapsychic makeup of the self to an analysis of relationships between and among the interacting components of a system. Further, since the locus of the problem is no longer seen to be within the psychic makeup of an individual, individuals cannot be seen as the cause of the problem. The problem lies within the network of relationships and the patterns of behaviors that become established in this network over time. Clinicians are forced to shift their attention from the traits of each individual to relationships among individuals, to perceive the flow of information across these networks of relationships, always with a mind to Bateson's tenet that information lies in differences and the perception of differences.

It is not only social relationships that produce information within a system. Information can come from perceived differences between objects, ideas, beliefs, and events, as well as between persons. In Bateson's example of the man and the axe, it was the perceived difference in an object's (the tree's) condition between axe strokes that represented the critical information to guide subsequent strokes. In Milan systemic therapy, attention is given to all forms of differences—between individuals, relationships, beliefs, events—over time. The effect that an event may have on a person's ideas or beliefs is as important as changes in relationships. The interaction of ideas and beliefs becomes as important as the interaction of people.

Evolving Systems

Among theoreticians who have embraced a systemic view of behavior, there has been a controversy between the followers of a General Systems view of a system and those who view systems as open and constantly changing and evolving (Hoffman, 1981). In recent years the controversy over this aspect of systems theory has progressed to the point of claims about the epistemological purity of each theorist (Coyne, Denner, & Ransom, 1982; Dell, 1982; DeShazer, 1982b; Keeney, 1982; Keeney & Sprenkle, 1982). In the last four years the Milan team has undergone a quiet change in their theoretical orientation on this issue. In the days of the collaboration with Palazzoli and Prata, the Milan team held a view of the family as having both the qualities of homeostasis and those of morphogenesis. In that period, it was thought that the pathological family system was rigidly stuck around the symptom and that the symptom acted as a homeostatic mechanism to prevent change. The object of therapy was to discover the so-called nodal point that held the system crystallized, and explode it with powerful, counter-paradoxical techniques, thus allowing the family a chance to discover new patterns of interaction. The therapist was seen as separate from the family system, a separation that was reinforced by the connection to the colleagues behind the mirror. Through this separation the therapist could remain detached, inject an intervention, and retreat into an observational role.

As described in an earlier part of this chapter, Boscolo and Cecchin began to view systems as being open, constantly in flux and influenced by other systems with which they come into contact. Embracing this view of second-order cybernetics, they now are concerned with understanding how the observer helps to co-create the reality of the family in the process of interacting with it. A family comes to seek therapy because their system has formed insoluble contradictions which create a state of distress. These contradictions may be with the outside world, the extended family, or within the familial system itself between various subgroups, coalitions, or beliefs. The job of the therapist is to understand the nature of these contradictions, and also how the therapist fits into the existing belief system of the family.

When the family comes to therapy, a new system is formed; family-plus-therapist. The dynamics and behavioral patterns around this new system are necessarily different, and can have an effect on the family's previous structures, beliefs, and behaviors. Because of this, the therapist has a unique opportunity in the early stages of therapy to introduce to the family the possibility of new ways of thinking about and relating to their problems. At this stage of therapy the therapist and the family co-create a new system that can incorporate the old system and change it, or can be incorporated by the old system and become a new loop in the repetitive spiral of the family's behavioral patterns, perhaps to introduce a new level of complexity in that redundancy. This latter scenario occurs most often when the family's contradictions involve professionals who help maintain the pathology. Instead of helping to resolve the family's contradictions, the therapist can inadvertently continue or exacerbate them.

The early stage of therapy, if approached with care, can afford the therapist the opportunity to co-evolve a process of understanding the family's situation in a manner that leaves open avenues to change. In order to exploit this opportunity, the Milan clinicians insist that the most appropriate therapeutic stance should be one of neutrality. This stance will be discussed next.

Neutrality

"Neutrality," as used by the Milan team, has two separate but related connotations. The first is the therapist's maintenance of nonalliance with any particular part of the system. The Milan team believes that in order to be therapeutically effective, the therapist must make an equal alliance with every part of the significant system. This is manifested in the therapeutic interview by the approximate equality of time afforded to each member of the family to respond to the therapist's questions, and the equal import given to the answers.

The second aspect of neutrality is that the therapist maintains a neutral stance with regard to ideas proposed by the family. This has two components in practice. The first is that the therapist does not accept either the role of a teacher or that of a moralist. (Exceptions to this, of course, occur when the therapist is called on to be a social control agent, at which point the therapeutic position is momentarily lost.) The second component is the therapist's simultaneous acceptance and nonacceptance of the ideas, opinions, and explanations given by each family member. This stance of listening but suspending judgment, accepting statements as information but not accepting the conclusions implied by them, is a very important part of neutrality. This stance has been described by the Milan clinicians as a scientific attitude. The therapist knows that he or she does not *know* what is happening in the family, but seeks to discover this through the process of therapy. It is active state of curiosity, wherein the therapist tries to understand how the system became what it is, without formulating what it *should* be.

Both these aspects of the neutral stance of the therapist have a theoretical root in the notion that in order to be helpful toward change, the therapist must know and understand the family's map of their relational and ideological reality but not accept it. To accept that map is to mistake it for the territory, that is, to accept that how the family perceives things is the truth. In so accepting, the therapist loses the opportunity to help the family create a new relational and ideologic reality, to co-evolve a new and different system that does not rely on the symptomatic behavior around the identified patient.

The Milan clinicians see the stance of neutrality as therapeutic in itself. It leads the clinician to a position of blamelessness and clears the way for the introduction of circular thinking into the family's own map of reality.

Levels of Communication and Levels of Reality

The studies of the Mental Research Institute (M.R.I.) in the 1960s led to an articulation of the notion of multiple levels of logic within which people communicate (Watzlawick, Beavin, & Jackson, 1967). Based on the pioneering work on double-binding communication and schizophrenia published a decade earlier by Bateson, Jackson, Haley & Weakland (1978, 1956), the M.R.I. group's notion was primarily concerned with what they identified as the two most commonly ascertainable levels in communication, the content level and the command level (Watzlawick *et al.*, 1967). In schizophrenic transactions, they postulated, there are always two logically contradictory messages being transmitted or perceived, one at the content level and the second at the so-called command or relational level.

The Milan clinicians make a similar distinction between levels of communication. Although they most often utilize the content-level versus relational-level distinction in analyzing behavior, they are also aware that a given behavior can have a variety of different meanings in different contexts, and to different persons within a single context. In fact, it is often a situation of logical contradiction at several levels within a family's system and ecosystem that brings the family to a crisis of pathology. The clearest articulation of this concept is what occurs when the family enters into interaction with a helping system whose own communicational levels are fraught with contradictions. The Milan clinicians emphasize that a systemic analysis must be flexible enough to include a variety of different levels of context, as often it is at these other levels that the family remains stuck in their pathology. This concept has been most clearly articulated recently by the work of Cronen and Pearce (1985) in their analysis of the Milan team's therapy, and by Tomm (1985) in his work on circular questions in systemic therapy.

TRAINING METHODS

In this section, a variety of features of the Milan training program will be described in order to illustrate how the basic theoretical concepts of the model that have been listed in the previous section are transmitted to a student in the process of training. An analysis of each of these features will demonstrate how they function to get across particular concepts. Once again it must be emphasized that the listing of these methods and the analysis of their efficacy is an arbitrary segmentation of the actual reality of training for the purposes of explication. In fact, the Milan clinicians do not perceive themselves as utilizing discrete methods to teach particular skills. It is the whole gestalt of the program that, in the end, allows the student to learn to think systemically.

Structure of the Training Day

The structure of the training day reflects the training priorities of the Milan program. The day is divided into three parts: the first is devoted to theory, the second to the application of that theory to a variety of contexts, and the third to clinical work in live family therapy sessions. This division of the day emphasizes the various aspects that are seen to be essential in helping to change the student's epistemology.

The first such aspect is the focus on theory. Students are assigned readings that include the writings of Bateson, Watzlawick, Haley, Hoffman, Ashby, Dell, Keeney, the Milan group's own writings, the writings of a variety of contemporary Italian and other European therapists and theoreticians, and many selections from former students of the Milan program. Two students are usually assigned to report to the rest of the group on the reading for that day, and the ensuing discussion will begin from comments or critiques that the presenters themselves make regarding the material.

The next part of the day is devoted to the application of systemic theory to analyze and change human systems in a variety of contexts. It is during this part of the day that methodology is most often addressed, yet always with an eye to how methodology is at the service of a systemic analysis of human interactions rather than solely as a clinical tool for family therapy.

Two types of training activities are utilized, and are usually alternated from meeting to meeting. The first is presentations of cases currently being seen by students in their own work settings or situations. These presentations and the ensuing discussions are meant to be illustrative departure points for the exploration of issues and questions about the application of systemic methodology. They are not seen as, nor do they serve the function of, clinical supervision, and there is no systematic follow-up in the ensuing meetings of cases presented by students.

On alternating weeks, this part of the day is devoted to clinical exercises involving either role playing or videotapes of therapy cases. These occasions constitute the only time when specific attention is given to the teaching of clinical methodology per se, and even here the focus is more on observation, analysis, and hypothesizing than on the learning of clinical skills by the student-as-therapist. The use of role playing will be discussed in more depth later in this chapter.

The third portion of the day is the participation in the treatment of live family therapy cases from behind the one-way mirror. Each group usually follows the progress of treatment of several families throughout the training year. For first-year groups, the students are primarily in an observational role, and participate only nominally as a treatment team. In the first year of training, the family is seen by one of the senior clinicians, and the junior instructor plays a dual role as a "supervisor" for the therapist as well as group leader and teacher for the training group. In the second and third years, families are assigned to trainees, and the group members become in effect the treatment team for their fellow students. The use of a team as a training tool will also be discussed in greater depth later in this chapter.

Case Presentations

On alternating weeks, a portion of the training day features case presentations of problematic situations encountered by students in their own place of work. These cases do not always involve families seen in therapy: for example, the case presented might be from an inpatient unit of a hospital, where the problematic system is seen as the patient, therapist, ward staff, and hospital administration; or from a social worker in the public clinic whose job it is to manage all the needs of a client, from social assistance to therapy.

In the case presentation, the student is asked to begin by defining the context of the case. What is the student's role and position at the clinic? What does the clinic expect of him or her? What does the client expect? What do others in that same role do with such cases? What does the agency do, and what do others think it does or should do? Is the client seeking help for a self-perceived problem, or has he or she been defined by someone else as deviant, sick, or needy? Is the client coming in to seek a given service or the answer to a simple question, such as, "Which program can I send my handicapped child to?"? Is it the systemically oriented therapist who is interpreting the client's request as more complex, perhaps reading into it a request for change of the whole family system? Who is sending the client, or is the client coming of his or her own accord? Why here and why now?

It is this definition of the context that the Milan group considers such a crucial foundation for the understanding of the ensuing interaction that occurs between a helper and the client, and which defines the nature of the relationships in the client–helpers system. Many situations of impasse, therapeutic failures, or therapists' own malaise or pathology can be traced to an inadequate understanding of the context of the helping interaction or the larger system that surrounds that interaction. In some cases, what may appear to be a discrete system (the family) seeking help from an individual helper (the therapist) may actually be a far more complex situation. The helper may consider himself or herself a therapist, but the client does not. Or the client may have a different notion of the kind of help being sought, or the helper may have been described by the referring source in a manner that sets up given expectations on the part of the client. All these considerations will be crucial to an eventual definition of the helping relationship.

It is not the function of the case presentation and the subsequent discussion to resolve the case, to give advice or supervision, or even to dissolve the impasse. Rather, the case is a departure point for an analysis of how systems in general operate, and how a problem can be seen from several different levels of a single system. Such an analysis usually has the effect of not only teaching a more flexible notion of systems to the trainees but also enlightening the student to the unseen influences contributing to that student's frustration in the work setting. From the experience of several years of training, the Milan group has discovered that the students typically find themselves in a triangulated position between the client or the family and other professionals. These professionals often have dual roles—as helpers addressing the client's perceived distress and as social control agents whose task is to reduce deviancy. The therapist or helper is often placed in the middle. He or she can easily become drawn into a position of advocacy for the client, totally accepting the pathology and defending the deviancy in the face of the larger society that seeks to oppress the client. On the other hand, the therapist can find himself or herself positioned on the side of the larger system, tending to view the client as a deviant and to reduce him or her in some manner, often by force or coercion, into normality. A systemic analysis and intervention often can offer the student a way out of this bind, at least for the moment, while the helping system itself goes through changes. It is a side effect of the training that the students often become more content and competent in their jobs without feeling that they must first change their work systems or their hierarchical position in the system before they can begin to be clinically effective.

Role Plays

Often, after the discussion of a case, the training day will continue with a role play of a given case. This role play may enact some aspect of the case just presented, or of another student's case. Again, the purpose of the role play is to explore some aspects of a system in interaction; it is not meant to reproduce the actual situation or to offer clinical solutions to the case. Role plays can involve families in a therapy situation or some other service-oriented meeting with a helper, or clinical team interactions around a given case or issue, or larger system interactions around some case-related issue. If the role play is of a therapy session or a case management meeting, a student is selected to conduct the interview, with the rest of the group functioning as a treatment team and an observation team. The role play always begins with the interviewer's introducing himself or herself and describing the setting in which the interview occurs. The role play is stopped by the instructor at various points, either around a moment of impasse, or at a moment when a new line of questioning should be pursued, or when the interviewer feels stuck or in need of consultation. Both the effects of the interviewer's questions and interactions, and the observed messages from the interviewees, are commented on by the group. Initial hypotheses are offered to guide further inquiry. Suggestions are made for new directions in the interview, and usually another student picks up the interview from that juncture. At some point in the interview, the instructor will stop and ask for a discussion to process the team's observations and to construct a more complete hypothesis.

If the role play has been of a family interview, the hypotheses developed are of the family system, often with a component that takes into consideration the family–interviewer system. Potential interventions are discussed and analyzed for the particular effects at which they are aimed. In these cases, care is taken to examine the effects of each intervention in the particular context being simulated. If the role play was of a meeting with a school psychologist and a family, for example, what effect would a given intervention have on the classroom teachers, or on the principal?

In role plays of clinical meetings or larger consultations, the analysis often offers valuable information about the nature of each participant's position in his or her own system, and in the relational system created around the case or issue under discussion. Such role plays can uncover conflicting hierarchies; hidden agendas dictated by professional, disciplinary, or administrative demands; or situations where political pressures can contradict the exigencies of the treatment situation in covert and double-binding ways. This helps the students to understand how their own therapeutic teams function, how they are affected by problematic cases, how their team's relationship with the rest of their agency affects and is affected by the way in which they deliver their treatment to their clients, and how they are affected as a team by the clients themselves. This represents a higher logical level of analysis of systems, one that includes an understanding of more of the ecosystem around the treatment process.

Blind Simulations: The Co-creation of Realities

Another important type of role play used in training is the so-called blind simulation. Normally in a role play the players are given a description of their roles and some of the rules by which their system functions, often based on an actual family or case presented by a student. In contrast, the role players in the blind simulation are not given any predetermined roles or interactional rules. They are given only the instruction to invent a system and to interact spontaneously.

To start the exercise, the student who plays the part of the interviewer is asked to identify himself or herself and the work context within which the simulated meeting takes place. As the role play unfolds, the system slowly begins to take shape as the players respond to the interviewer and to each other. The observers and team operate as they do in other role plays, but with more careful attention to the information that is fed back into the system in the form of questions, and to the therapeutic stance of the interviewer. At the end of the role play, the team hypothesizes how the newly evolved system operates, and about the part the interviewer has played in this evolution. The players are then interviewed out of role to determine how their particular roles developed during the role play, and what they felt determined the development of relational rules and redundancies that created their system. The affective reactions of each player at key moments of the role play are also elicited in order to explore all the effects of other members' relational moves, as well as those of the interviewer.

This sort of role play illustrates the part the therapist or interviewer plays in the co-creation of the reality that subsequently guides the therapeutic meetings in family therapy. The effects of assumptions, judgments, opinions, and values with which the interviewer conducts the interview, and the effects of the interviewer's questions on the other players, are studied to highlight how the interviewer not only becomes a part of the system under study, but very much affects it. A microanalysis of these effects serves not only to drive home the role of the interviewer, but also as convincing proof of the usefulness of a stance of neutrality and the generative power of circular questions.

Collaborative Teamwork

One of the important aspects of the training program is the emphasis on teamwork in the development of systemic observations and hypotheses during the live family sessions. The team is seen as a collaborative entity without any formal hierarchy. During the sessions, the therapy team collaborates directly with the therapist or cotherapists, providing the systemic factory for the production of observations and ideas that, when worked and reworked in the group's discussion process, develop into systemic hypotheses that will guide the conduct of future sessions. This process is quite telling in itself, because it embodies the Milan team's basic view of Batesonian realities.

At the beginning of the team's discussion, each member is encouraged to make his or her own observations of the interactions observed in the therapy room. No attempt is made to correct people's observations or to force students to be circular or systemic in their initial opinions. In fact, this stage of the discussion is often referred to as "an orgy of linear hypothesizing." The belief is that linear observations are necessary parts of the reality observed, and that exercising one's linearity in a group demystifies the process of developing systemic hypotheses. The Milan trainers believe that circular hypotheses cannot be hatched fully developed from the heads of Western therapists, because they are conditioned to think in linear, causal terms. They see that circular hypotheses are built from piecing together linear arcs from various members of the team. Comments are made about relations, usually dyadic, within the family. As more observations are expressed, other dyads become illuminated, and triadic relationships become more apparent. Each member of the team can introduce different punctuations of the events just witnessed in the session, and as the discussion continues more and more members of the family, more behaviors, and more ideas get interconnected in a variety of ways.

From these discussions, two or three different relational hypotheses or epistemological maps of the family emerge. These hypotheses provide a connection between many or all of the members of the family, and all or many of the facts and pieces of analogic and digital communication witnessed during the session.[2] The process is one of a subtle evolution, from simple, linear, causal ideas to more complex, circular, and systemic hypotheses. No attempt is made to determine which is the "right" solution, or the most "correct" solution, or even the best or most systemic hypothesis. It is considered a rich and productive session if the team emerges with several plausible hypotheses. From these hypotheses, one is chosen to be tested through an intervention designed for this purpose. The choice of hypothesis is often made on the basis of several factors. The hypothesis chosen can be the one that appears to best fit the facts that have emerged from the observations, or it can be the one that is most practically feasible from what the family has indicated they will allow the therapist to do, or it can be the one that best combines two opposing qualities—that is, an idea that is the most different from the family's own perception of the problem while at the same time the most plausible for the family to accept without disqualifications.

Much has been written by others about the collaborative team as a therapeutic tool and as a training tool (Breunlin & Cade, 1981; Coppersmith, 1980; DeShazer, 1982a; Roberts, 1981; Tomm & Wright, 1982), but several aspects of its use as a training vehicle in the Milan training program bear some closer scrutiny. As indicated in an earlier section, the Milan program places a strong emphasis on the distinction between *information* and *traits*. The use of a team in therapy is exploited in order to help emphasize this distinction. The team is not structured hierarchically; instead, everyone is seen as an equal member in an attempt to emphasize the notion of ideas prevailing over individual personal traits. Each member of the team works toward the creation of an idea, a systemic hypothesis, that incorporates all the relevant bits of information observed at various levels of observation.

It is the strong belief of the Milan group that through the team process, hypotheses are generated that are at a higher logical level than those generated by a single individual, no matter how skilled that individual may be in the systemic model. By not seeing linear and circular thinking as opposites, the group avoids the tendency to create a belief that linear thoughts are wrong and circular thoughts are right. As the team's collective generative process works to weave a circular hypothesis, attempts are made to incorporate all or many of the partial observed linear arcs by seeking a superior logical level that will encompass them. The process of struggling to find the logical level that incorporates all the lineal arcs is a purely systemic one. If a single circular hypothesis cannot be generated to incorporate all informational elements, alternative hypotheses are generated, which then become the guiding structures for further inquiry with the family in subsequent sessions. Further, because it is not the intent of the team to generate a model of what is the actual reality of the family's system at any given moment, but, rather, to create a map that is useful in the exploration of the relational territory being observed with the goal of therapeutic change, it is not inconsistent to generate multiple hypotheses.

A side effect of this attitude of emphasizing ideas over individuals is that no judgment is made on the rightness or wrongness of a trainee's observation or idea. Those ideas useful in the creation of an overall hypothesis are utilized, and those which are not are set aside by the group, at times to be resurrected in a later discussion when the current operating hypothesis has proved to be inconsistent with emerging information. The students themselves, then, are not subject to feeling blamed or stupid for "incorrect" observations or ideas. In this way, the Milan group's concept of neutrality is serendipitously transmitted in the process of learning.

Students are encouraged to incorporate idiosyncratic points of view, biases, and experiences into their observations and discussion, insofar as these are related to the family in question. This incorporation is the introduction of new information, triggered by the perception of information during the observing process in the session. The team acts as a filter to accept, modify, or reject various ideas as it compares the new information coming from the individual to the information already lying on the table in the discussion. Information is kept from straying too far afield from the family's reality by keeping in mind that the team's ideas will be fed back to the family in the process of asking circular questions, offering opinions, delivering rituals, or performing other interventions. If the family responds to this feedback with blank stares or confusion, the team will modify its intervention accordingly. In this way, a fine line is held between ideas that are too foreign to the family to be registered and those that are too similar to the family's own map of reality to bring about any change.

Therapy Team and Observation Team

One important characteristic of the Milan training program is the separation of the group into a Therapy Team (T-Team) and Observation Team (O-Team) during their clinical work with families. It is not until toward the end of the first year of training that the group is judged to be sufficiently experienced to divide into two teams behind the mirror. At that time, a group of four or five students are randomly selected to function as a treatment team, while the rest of the group and the instructor become the observation team. It is the function of the T-Team to assist the therapist (who, in the first year, is always one of the two senior clinicians) in the conduct of the session by making observations, developing lines of inquiry or potential hypotheses, and planning possible interventions. The role of the O-Team is to observe all interactions, both inside the therapy room and in the observation room, without interacting with the T-Team.

In the early stage of training, any interruptions of the session on the part of the T-Team are done through the instructor. If the team has a particular line of inquiry or critical observation to make to the therapist that may affect the course of the session, they will discuss it with the instructor, who will determine whether or not to call out the therapist for a brief conference. When they become more experienced, usually by the second year of training, the students themselves will make the decision to interrupt the session. During such brief in-session conferences, the O-Team once again observes without interacting with either the therapist or the T-Team.

Toward the end of the session, the therapist will come behind the mirror to confer once again with the T-Team in a longer intra-session discussion to develop a working hypothesis and a strategy for creating an intervention to be delivered to the waiting family. The O-Team meets in a separate room with the instructor in order to discuss its own observations of the family, the therapist, and the T-Team. It strives to develop alternative hypotheses and potential treatment plans and interventions that take into consideration these observations. Not bound by the same pragmatic constraints as the T-Team, which has to deliver a timely intervention to the family, the O-Team often discusses its observations and hypotheses more fully, and may arrive at more than one intervention.

The intra-session discussion can range from 5 to 45 minutes, and concludes when the T-Team has come up with a therapeutic plan for the therapist to bring back into the session, usually in the form of a systemic opinion or a ritual prescription. The two teams then return to their posts behind the mirror while the therapist concludes the session.

The whole group then meets with the therapist. The O-Team begins the discussion with its observations and alternative hypotheses and interventions. The T-Team will discuss the thinking behind its chosen intervention, and the therapist will comment on the affective feedback felt in the treatment room. A discussion ensues that serves to integrate the ideas from the three positions, as well as to attempt to understand the immediate reaction of the family to the intervention. This discussion is invariably cut short only by the end of the training day.

The separation of the group into T-Team and O-Team was designed to create and emphasize the notion of different levels of analysis of interacting systems. The family itself represents one level of analysis; the therapist in the room with the family represents a second level. The T-Team, behind the mirror, has the vantage point to observe and hypothesize about the interactions within the family system, as well as the family–therapist system. The O-Team, sitting behind the T-Team, has an even higher vantage point, and can observe and hypothesize at all three levels: the family system, the family–therapist system, and the family–therapist–team system.

A second advantage of this feature is that it allows for the recognition of the two simultaneous contexts within which the family session occurs. The first is the context of clinical treatment, and the second is the context of training. The T-Team, by necessity, is confined by time pressures and practical considerations to the clinical treatment context. It must be able to help the therapist help the family in order to remain consistent with that context. During their observations, and their intra-session discussions, the members of the T-Team are goal-oriented and under pressure to come up with an immediate functional hypothesis and intervention that will further the treatment of the family. The O-Team is less affected by these requirements, and can therefore explore more possibilities at different levels of analysis. The only drawback the O-Team is hampered by is their lack of freedom to intervene directly on the system to test ideas during the session, and so must confine themselves to speculations based on their observations.

The T-Team is bound by the nature of their relationship with the therapist to be helpful and to be attuned to the needs and emotional constraints of the therapist in his or her relationship with the family. Their interventions, whether in the form of questions, lines of inquiry, rituals, prescriptions, or opinions, are limited to what is practically possible for the therapist within the definition of the relationship with the family. For example, if a family has responded with an emotionally charged reaction to a line of inquiry about a particular relationship—say, the relationship between a father and his in-laws—this might make the therapist loath to focus directly on that relationship. The T-Team is likely to accept that as a given and to explore other directions that might be more likely to protect the therapist from undergoing the discomfort of the family's reactions around this topic. The O-Team, which is not as directly bound by the same relational considerations, will be able to observe and comment on this process, and perhaps even suggest alternative strategies for future use. This "meta-level" commentary also allows the trainees to begin to develop an ecosystemic appreciation, as often patterns of relational behavior observed at the level of the therapist–family relationship, or the therapist–team relationship, can be seen to be isomorphic to the relational patterns within the family itself. It is not unusual for, say, a protective relationship between the T-Team and the therapist to reflect a similar protective relationship between the identified patient in the family and some key family member, usually around some particularly charged issue that is intricately enveloped in the maintenance of the symptomatology.

The O-Team's position serves a vital function in the teaching of this epistemology, for it embodies the constant reminder that the system observed during the conduct of the session is not just the family's, but the therapist's system as well. In essence, there are two systems, the family and the therapy team, that intersect in the therapy session to create a therapeutic system that is itself a new reality. The O-Team's observations, when done effectively, keep a focus on the overall contextual message being given to the family, and can be an avenue for the development of a meta-level view at a logical level that is superior to that developed by the T-Team. The final postsession discussion feeds back the O-Team's information from their observational context into the overall therapy system. In future sessions with the same family, the therapy will benefit from that information, for not only is the information available to the entire team, but trainees who were previously on the O-Team may find themselves on the T-Team in a subsequent session. By its very existence, the O-Team allows the student not only to learn about, but also to experience the idea of multiple levels of logic under which the therapy session operates in this systemic model.

Clinical Interviewing and Cotherapy Experiences

A part of the training experience for the students involves actual clinical interviewing experience with families. Starting in the second year of training, students begin to volunteer, as they feel ready, to take on a clinical case at the Center. This is normally done in cotherapy teams at a time that a new case is referred to the Center. Those who volunteer are assigned the family on intake, and will continue to be the family's primary therapists throughout the treatment, while the rest of the group remains behind the mirror along with the supervisors, making up the therapeutic and observation teams. This practical clinical experience allows each student the opportunity to apply the interviewing skills learned in the process of training (through role plays, as well as live and videotape observations of other therapies).

Normally, in the course of the three-year training period, each student has the opportunity to pick up only a single case as the primary therapist, since the training groups are large (15 to 18 trainees) and the available hours of direct clinical time are limited. Working in cotherapy with a colleague, however, will allow each student the opportunity to see at least one family case.

There are other benefits of cotherapy assignments. The first is that they provide the students with a moral collegial support in what, for many, is a rather stressful situation. For many students, entering the room with the family for an initial interview represents a series of firsts. It is often the first time they have sat down for a family therapy session. Often, too, it is the first time that they have not been alone in a clinical situation. For almost all of them, it is the first time they have been in front of a one-way mirror, observed not only by fellow students, but by supervisors as well. It is usually the first time they have been videotaped in a clinical session. Finally, for most of them, it is the first time that they are applying their newly learned systemic skills in a live clinical session. To be able to share such a potentially stressful situation with a partner alleviates much of the anxiety.

Cotherapy is also useful for students because it allows each therapist more time to observe and process feedback from the family during the session, working in a sort of tag-team fashion; as one therapist is actively engaged with the family, asking questions and interacting with them, the other can have time to review the evolving information, formulate additional questions, or determine new areas of inquiry. Cotherapy can serve to create a smoother running session, as it is not necessary to halt the session in order to consult with the team. One therapist can leave to consult with the team, while the partner continues the interview. There is an understanding that the therapist returning from a consultation will be bringing in new information, or a new line of inquiry, or possibly a new hypothesis to be tested out, and hence will be given the floor by his or her partner.

A final advantage of cotherapy in this model of therapy is that it continues to deemphasize the individual in favor of the collaborative approach. The therapist feels and functions as part of a therapeutic team, and is better able to accept therapeutic errors as treatment-system errors rather than to personalize them. Likewise, he or she is able to work more collaboratively rather than competitively.

Through the clinical experience, trainees are able to practice the process of asking circular questions, of maintaining neutrality in the face of the influence of the family's epistemology, of making connections, of observing patterns of interaction, and of creating and revising relational hypotheses in the midst of interaction with the family system. Students are also able to develop their own style of interaction with the family, and to utilize their own idiosyncratic skills and characteristics in the process of therapy.

In order to aid this process, and to reduce the anxiety of the therapists in the room, the supervisors utilize what is known as the 30-minute ritual. This is a rule that allows the cotherapists to conduct the first 30 minutes of the session without any interruptions from the therapy team. In this manner, the therapists in the room can work out their initial jitters on their own, as well as establish a rapport, a style, and a rhythm in the session before introducing suggestions from behind the mirror. An additional benefit of this ritual is that it maintains the therapist's influence in the eyes of the family, who might otherwise wonder why the therapists need to be so closely guided by the supervisors behind the mirror.

The message transmitted to the trainee by such devices as the 30-minute ritual is as important as any other practical effect. It is meant to reinforce the notion that there is no "correct" way of doing therapy, nor are there particular character traits or behavioral skills prerequisite to a systemic therapy. The only emphasis placed on skill learning is the teaching of the difference between conducting a useful therapy session and a mere conversation with the family. A useful therapy interview is one that allows the team to understand the family's epistemology without buying into it; one that allows the team to draw distinctions between family members, between the past and the present, between the family's behaviors around certain issues or events, usually having to do with the symptomatology; one that allows the team to create a relational map of the family; and one that allows the team, through the therapist's questions, to introduce microchanges in the family's belief system. The basic principles of the conduct of an interview that the Milan team described in their 1980 article remain the guidelines that they teach their trainees for the conduct of the interview (Palazzoli et al., 1980). Within those guidelines, however, there is ample room for the development of individual styles, methods, and skills.

Instructors' Attitudes toward Trainees, Training, and the Process of Learning a Systemic Epistemology

An important training component of the Milan group is not a method but, rather, an overall attitude that the instructors, particularly the two senior instructors, have toward their students and the process of learning. Much of this attitude has already been alluded to in the description of various training techniques and procedures, but it is useful to emphasize it here, as it is a major factor in transmitting to the trainees the ideas inherent in a systemic epistemology.

In the process of selecting students for the training program, the clinicians of the Milan Center make their first and most important distinction. The criteria for selection, which require prospective trainees already to be at a professional level with at least three years of postdegree work, and to be interested and motivated enough to make the effort to negotiate the time off from that work, ensures a certain level of professional competence and motivation toward learning. From the point of selection, the instructors assume the trainees to be competent and able to learn systemic theory. This allows the instructors to think of their training groups as they would think of a family system. They see each student as having the same status as any other member of the team. Each person's idea or observation is considered important and is incorporated into the discussion of the team. By avoiding judgment of the students or of a particular idea, they have found that contributions that at first might appear trivial or stupid can, when reconsidered by the team's discussion process, become important and significant for the future direction of the therapy.

This attitude toward the students and their ideas and contributions has significant effects on two levels: at the level of increasing the efficiency and motivation of the participating trainees, and at the level of epistemology. The trainers' nonjudgmental attitude toward their trainees, and their deemphasis of the individual in favor of the team process, allows the students more quickly to transcend the relational level of their participation in the training, and to focus on learning instead. There is no processing of the training group's interpersonal dynamics, as the group is seen as an epistemological tool rather than an end in itself. It is not considered important to examine how the individual fits into this particular group, or how the group process affects individuals. The group remains focused on its sole purpose—that of collecting individual observations and linear bits of information to make circular connections in order to build a circular, relational hypothesis about the phenomenon being observed. The team itself is never the object of study, except inasmuch as it reflects isomorphic features from the system observed, whether that be a family or a group simulation.

On those occasions when the group is functioning well, the experience for the students is exhilarating, as they become part of a larger organism that pushes each to make connections between ideas and persons in the observed system, in what can best be described as a rarefied systemic atmosphere. The hypotheses created from such a process do not belong to anyone, as they have evolved in a process in which the individual mind does not seem to exist as an identifiable entity. It is at this point that the student has the opportunity to experience the Batesonian concept that mind is social, thereby making the phenomenological connection between what they have learned about systemic epistemology, what they are observing within the family system, and what they are experiencing in the team's discussion process itself.

Another effect communicated by the Milan trainers by way of their attitude toward their students is that they do not expect students to discard their own manner of thinking or to disqualify their work in their own work contexts. The students' experiences in their own settings, and the experiences that they go through in the process of training, become important feedback to the systemic model that the trainers are trying to elaborate and to the training program they are in the constant process of revising. The student is seen as, and is made to feel part of, a continual process of evaluation of ideas and methods, which again is isomorphic to the concept of continual cybernetic change that both Bateson and the Milan team espouse. Just as their process of therapy is a continually circular one— observation of feedback, creation of hypotheses, testing of hypotheses through questions or interventions, and once again observation of feedback—their process of training involves a continual monitoring of feedback, and adjustments.

The trainers' respect for the work and ideas of their trainees is also witnessed in the yearly papers that are required of the training participants. These papers are often collaborative efforts on the part of several students, and compel the students to articulate how they have assimilated what they have learned into their own work, or to think creatively about theoretical or methodological topics. The Milan Center also sponsors a yearly conference where current and former students are invited to present their work to each other in an atmosphere of wide-open systemic exploration and study. The trainers view these presentations as potentially important contributions at the cutting edge of systemic research, both to theory and to the application of theory to a wide range of contextual laboratories. Conference papers are published yearly by the Milan Center, and some become reading assignments for discussion in the following year.

EFFECTS OF THE TRAINING

In this section, some of the effects of the Milan training program will be discussed, on the basis of observations made during visits to various work sites of current and former students of the program, as well as through discussions with current trainees, graduates, and junior instructors. No formal follow-up study or survey has been conducted by the Milan group to quantify the effects of the training.

The dropout rate of students is a rather steady 8 to 10% each year, with indications that most drop out for practical rather than ideological reasons. For those who stay, there appears to be a common progression of reaction to the training. Initially, students appear dazzled by the therapy and theory, and become disciples of it. By the second year, however, the initial awe and mystification about systemic therapy has become tempered by the student's frustrating experiences in attempting to convert others in their work sites to this model of therapy. During this period, students often voice their frustrations in the training groups and appear to lose much of their initial enthusiasm for the model of therapy. Although the message of the trainers to the students is always one of caution about transposing interventions and techniques from the Milan Center context to their own work context, many students go through a period of difficulty while they struggle to integrate what they are learning to settings that may be quite hostile to their new ideas. Often by the middle of the second year of training, however, this integration appears to be well underway as students find their own unique solutions to how to apply systemic thinking to their own work settings.

This struggle to transfer the systemic theory and interventions to the varied settings in which the students work is a central issue often discussed by the students and instructors. There is great concern among the trainees that the assumptions made by the Milan approach to systemic thinking cannot be transferred easily within other contexts where the function of the therapist is too ill defined, or in those where the roles are too rigidly defined by long-standing expectations or predetermined legislated functions. This was felt in particular by trainees who, within their work settings, found themselves near the bottom of the organizational hierarchy. These trainees felt quite restricted in what they could do in their agencies, since their behavior was prescribed by "the powers that be." For these individuals, their work setting created a sort of double bind with the training program. Motivated by a wish to climb out of the lowest positions in the hierarchy, they seek training in Milan to learn new techniques that might allow them to excel and advance in their work setting. When, in the course of training, they begin to perceive the consistent message of the trainers that a systemic intervention begins by first accepting the context as it is, they find themselves in an apparent contradiction with their initial intent in seeking the training. For some, this contradiction appears to be very difficult, perhaps even intolerable. Future investigations of trainees who drop out of the training may shed more light on this issue. Presumably, for others the resolution of this contradiction is one that allows them to function more effectively in their settings even without immediately affecting their hierarchical status in their organizations.

Another issue that appeared to be of concern for students was that the Milan program focuses very little on the development of the therapeutic skills of the individual. In their emphasis on "ideas over individuals," much time is spent on examining the *process* of interviewing, and hypothesis making, circularity, and neutrality as principles in that process, but there is very little opportunity for the individual student to focus on developing interviewing skills or style. In the course of the three years of training, each trainee will usually have had the opportunity to be the therapist for only one or perhaps two families. Over that span of time, each trainee may also be involved in the role of therapist in four or five short role plays. However, in the live family interviews, as well as in the role plays, only a minor part of the focus is on the interviewing process itself, and the ability of the trainee to perform or not perform adequately is seldom, and never directly, addressed. Videotapes of a trainee's interviews are theoretically available to him or her for review; but, for practical reasons, seldom do trainees have the time or opportunity to study their own interviewing technique. Thus a rich source of self-corrective feedback is not utilized to its fullest potential.

One additional problem with the Milan training program that was observed but not directly commented on by the trainees interviewed was that the emphasis on the collaborative group process left individuals to fend for themselves in their own learning process. For some trainees this problem may have been attenuated because they attended the training with one or more colleagues with whom what was learned in the training could be further articulated, experimented with, and debated. These students could have study groups, collaborative teams, and research groups in their work setting, where the systemic approach learned at the Center could be better developed within the particular exigencies of that work context. For those students who were alone while attending the training, however, this opportunity was not available, and thus they were more likely to flounder.

In order to address some of these problems, the Milan trainers have discussed the possibility of developing advanced or postgraduate training groups to focus on particular topics that are not adequately covered in the course of the three-year training. In this way, graduates who see families would form a training group to focus on the development of family therapy skills. For others, whose work requires the analysis of larger systems, the training group would focus on the development of those techniques. Another group might focus on the special problems of working with the deinstitutionalized population. The addition of special topic training groups would allow the Center to become more like an institute, where the work of graduates of the program can be fed back into the research and thinking of the Milan group, as well as the teaching of the next generation of systemic therapists.

CONCLUSION

The process of systemic therapy is a process of creating feedback loops between the therapist and the family. During this mutually influenced process, the therapist is constantly forced to adapt the working hypothesis to perceived feedback, and the subsequent questions and interventions become stimuli for further reactions from the family system. The process of training systemic therapists can be seen as a similar phenomenon. As an open, living system, a training program can and should be influenced by the feedback it receives from its students. The Milan program has been profoundly influenced by the experiences of its early trainees, and the result has been a further articulation of the theory on which it is based, and of the methodology of producing change. This chapter represents only one segment of that continuing process.

Notes

1. This article was first written in 1985, and describes the training program at that time.
2. Pertinent relational information about a system comes not only from the content of what is said in the session, but also from communications about communication, which usually come from nonverbal and contextual communication. For an excellent discussion of digital and analogic communication, the reader is referred to Watzlawick, Beavin & Jackson, *Pragmatics of Human Communication* (1967).

References

Bateson, G. (1972). *Steps to an ecology of mind.* New York: Ballantine Books.

Bateson, G. (1979). *Mind and nature: A necessary unit.* New York: Bantam Books.

Bateson, G., Jackson, D. D., Haley, J., & Weakland, J. (1978). Toward a theory of schizophrenia. In M. M. Berger (Ed.), *Beyond the double bind.* New York: Brunner/Mazel. (Originally published 1956.)

Boscolo, L., & Cecchin, G. (1982). Training in systemic therapy at the Milan Centre. In R. Whiffin & J. Byng-Hall (Eds.), *Family therapy supervision: Recent developments in practice.* London: Academic Press.

Breunlin, D., & Cade, B. W. (1981). Intervening in family systems with observer messages. *Journal of Marital and Family Therapy, 7,* 453–460.

Coppersmith, E. I. (1980). Expanding uses of the telephone in family therapy. *Family Process, 19,* 411–417.

Coyne, J. C., Denner, B., & Ransom, D. C. (1982). Undressing the fashionable mind. *Family Process, 21*(4), 391–396.

Cronen, V. E., & Pearce, W. B. (1985). Toward an explanation of how the Milan method works. In D. Campbell & R. Draper (Eds.), *Applications of systemic family therapy: The Milan approach.* London: Academic Press.

Dell, P. (1982). Beyond homeostasis: Toward a concept of coherence. *Family Process, 21*(1), 21–41.

DeShazer, S. (1982a). *Patterns of brief family therapy.* New York: Guilford Press.

DeShazer, S. (1982b). Some conceptual distinctions are more useful than others. *Family Process, 21*(1), 71–84.

Hoffman, L. (1981). *Foundations of family therapy: A conceptual framework for systems change.* New York: Basic Books.

Keeney, B. (1982). What is an epistemology of family therapy? *Family Process, 21*(2), 153–168.

Kenney, B., & Sprenkle, D. H. (1982). Ecosystemic epistemology: Critical implications for the aesthetics and pragmatics of family therapy. *Family Process, 21*(1), 1–20.

Palazzoli, M. S., Boscolo, L., Cecchin, G., & Prata, G. (1978). *Paradox and counterparadox.* New York: Jason Aronson.

Palazzoli, M. S., Boscolo, L., Cecchin, G., & Prata, G. (1980). Hypothesizing-circularity-neutrality: Three guidelines for the conductor of the session. *Family Process, 19,* 3–12.

Roberts, J. (1981). The development of a team approach in live supervision. *Journal of Strategic and Systemic Therapies*, 1, 24–35.

Tomm, K. M. (1984a). One perspective on the Milan systemic approach. Part I. Overview of development, theory, and practice. *Journal of Marital and Family Therapy*, 10, 113–125.

Tomm, K. M. (1984b). One perspective on the Milan systemic approach. Part II. Description of session format, inteviewing style, and interventions. *Journal of Marital and Family Therapy*, 10, 253–271.

Tomm, K. M. (1985). Circular interviewing: A multifaceted clinical tool. In D. Campbell, & R. Draper (Eds.), *Applications of systemic family therapy: The Milan method*. London: Academic Press.

Tomm, K. M., & Wright, L. (1982). Multilevel training and supervision in an outpatient service programme. In R. Whiffen & J. Byng-Hall (Eds.), *Family therapy supervision: Recent developments in practice*. London: Academic Press.

Watzlawick, P., Beavin, J. H., & Jackson, D. D. (1967). *Pragmatics of human communication*. New York: W. W. Norton.

4

Training in Bowen Theory

DANIEL V. PAPERO
Georgetown University Family Center

The human quest for knowledge is subtly and intricately connected to the urge to communicate that knowledge, particularly that part seen as new, to someone else. An honest effort to pass what is known on to some other person tends ultimately to highlight what remains unknown. The gaps in knowledge and the questions they produce then come into clear focus. The unknown is extremely important. It promotes curiosity, investigation, and occasionally humility.

One generally assumes that training involves the transfer of information or skill from someone who knows to someone who does not. The function of the known in highlighting the unknown can be easily overlooked, so that the instructor presents knowledge as if all questions were thereby answered. When this happens, learning becomes rote, and the motivating power of curiosity is dampened. The teacher is overvalued (or overblamed), and the learner is not sufficiently challenged to define his or her responsibility for learning.

Yet the separate roles of teacher and learner are not mutually exclusive. Astute teachers continually learn from their students. If the training process could be seen as a mutual quest for knowledge on the part of teacher and learner, the responsibility for learning could rest more clearly with each, and the interaction between them might further drive the pursuit of knowledge.

To achieve such an interplay in a real sense is extremely difficult. How does teacher or learner maintain respect for what is known while remaining aware of and alert to what is not? How does one use human capacities to the fullest without supplying imaginary answers to complex and difficult questions? How does each brain go as far as possible toward knowing without denying ignorance?

Such questions must at some time or another bedevil anyone who contemplates any facet of learning. They continue to be important questions for teachers and learners of Bowen theory, who attempt to communicate a different way of looking at the world and understanding what one sees. That viewpoint, which has been called systems thinking, requires that both teacher and learner revise and review long-held and firmly implanted views of the world and the nature of man.

Bowen theory guides the training process in the same manner that it guides therapy. One cannot attempt to convey the essence of the training regimen without first addressing the basic ideas themselves. Consequently, a succinct introduction to the Bowen Family Systems theory will precede the specific discussion of training in Bowen theory.

BOWEN THEORY

Bowen theory is the product of an effort to see the human being from a broad perspective. Bowen's initial interest in the attachment between mother and child led him to see the family as a unit. As his perspective broadened, the multigenerational family came into view. He began to see functioning of any nuclear family as a product of, and influenced continually by, the generations preceding it. He realized it was not possible to see the nuclear family without also viewing its connections to the past.

Differentiation

At the core of Bowen Family Systems theory, and by extension at the core of any effort at training in that theory, is the concept of differentiation of self. Despite its importance, this concept is often poorly understood and is one of the very difficult ideas to communicate. It shapes, however, the entire effort of training.

There are many levels of the concept of differentiation. It addresses the way organisms differ in terms of sensitivity to an environment and the automatic or instinctive behavior that accompanies such sensitivity. For the human, differentiation also concerns the degree to which the individual has some choice about or control over the kinds of feeling states and behavior that result from interaction within an environment.

On another level, differentiation concerns the distinction between intellectual and emotional functioning or, more precisely, the balance between the two in a person, in a group, or even in society. The use of the term "emotion" in this context has a specific connotation. It is intended to be synonomous with "instinct," and to refer to an automatic guidance system within the organism, a feature that *Homo sapiens* has in common with other forms of life. Intellectual functioning refers to cognitive processes more colloquially addressed as reflection or thought.

The distinction between emotion and thought is elusive. Some sorts of cerebration are clearly related to intense automatic processes. Easily recognized examples include the thoughts commonly labeled paranoia, those associated with revenge, and even more simply those connected with panic or intense anxiety. Characteristics of such emotionally based mental processes include a narrowing perspective frequently marked by polarized perception (an either–or dichotomy), ambivalence, confusion, and a reliance on what "feels right" or on whatever relieves discomfort. Often such processes revolve around another person, or, more accurately, around the real or imagined impact of the other on the self. One can only see where the other is wrong, stubborn, insensitive, or in some other manner generally unreliable. Frequently such fantasies have a degree of accuracy within that narrow perspective. They often form the basis of an overt or covert effort to force change upon the other. While acutely aware of the impact of other on self, the person is rarely attuned to the impact of self on other.

In contrast to emotionally based mental activity, a kind of clear thought is also available to the human on a limited basis. It is marked by a broad perspective from which several variables can be followed. Such a perspective allows complexity to be appreciated and minimizes simplistic efforts to assign blame or causality for an event. Moreover, from such a perspective the viewer can get some idea of his or her own role in the situation. One is more aware of the impact of self on the other or others. With reflection, the person is often more clearly aware of what is important to him or her. One can be clear about plans to maintain that stand. Life direction can also be more carefully considered; principles or beliefs, anchored in careful thought, can be worked out as a means of calibrating one's course in life.

One could also attempt to present the distinction between the intellectual system and the emotional system in terms of objectivity and subjectivity. Since all perception must pass through the brain, the human can never become totally objective. Nonetheless, it is possible to distinguish between a narrowly subjective focus and a broader focus called objective. The former would define self as the center of the universe and the measure of all that occurs. The latter would have a broader view of self as a responding part, with quite limited importance, of a larger world.

The level of differentiation for any individual has to do with the degree to which he or she has the ability to choose between intellectual and emotional functioning. The balance between the two in a given person, or the range of choice between emotion and intellect, is determined by a number of factors. Of primary importance is one's family. On a theoretical level, one cannot be much different from one's parents in terms of level of differentiation. One can have slightly greater or slightly lesser degrees of choice.

At any given point in time, environmental factors play a role both in the present and into the future. This is a simple point, yet it is often difficult to picture. The emotional system, as an internal guidance system, has evolved across time in response to the demands on each organism to survive and to reproduce. Yet each guidance system fits, in a sense, with every other in a particular environment.

This interdependence can be recognized most clearly in the attachment between predator and prey, or in mating behavior within a species. Hunter and hunted evolve together. The guidance system of the prey is geared in part to avoiding the predator, and the hunter's guidance system is geared toward catching its meal. A recent article by Horner (1984) describes an ancient example of this basic point. In the late Cretaceous, in what is now Montana, a particular species of herbivorous dinosaur established a nesting ground on the shore of a shallow lake. The dinosaurs created nests in which the eggs were deposited. Various pieces of evidence suggest that these nests were guarded by adult animals who then associated with the nestlings after hatching. In essence this would be an early demonstration of the biological roots of the family. Horner presumes the grouping occurred to protect the young. But what were they to be protected from? Within the nesting ground, among the circular nests of the herbivores, fossilized eggs of a different sort, laid on the ground in a straight line, provide evidence that a species of carnivorous dinosaur also used the nesting ground. The young carnivores, upon hatching, could prey upon their vegetarian cousins. The nesting behavior of each species had evolved based upon that of the other.

The emotional system and the environment evolve together. A sustained change in organism or environment has the potential to alter both. Thus the functioning of the emotional guidance system of any individual, and the emotionally based behavior of any group at any point in time, is the product of the evolutionary history of organism and environment, as well as of the particular interplay of the two in the present. The automatic or instinctive behavior of any person is in part related to the interaction of his or her grandparents with their world. The balance between thought and emotion in a person is related to the history of that person's family and the environmental factors of the present.

Among mammals a clearly visible movement toward group functioning can be noted, particularly in the presence of perceived threat, whether real or imagined. It is also evident in mating behaviors of a wide range of species. Examples of this phenomenon are easily noted in the behavior of ungulate herds in the presence of predators, or of primate bands in the presence of unknown humans. Bowen called this tendency in the human a "togetherness force."

There is with people an automatic tendency for the togetherness force to heighten emotional functioning to the detriment of intellectual functioning. Stated differently, the togetherness force intensifies emotional functioning in the human and can override intellectual functioning.

It would miss the point, however, to assign negative value to emotional functioning and positive value to intellectual functioning. The emotional system in the human is as old as evolution itself, and represented a major step forward for early mammals. It is not only useful but necessary for an organism to have an internal guidance system operating generally beyond conscious awareness. Mating and bonding are as much emotional system functions as are hostility and aggression. Togetherness, or the functioning of individuals as a unit, may be necessary to the sustenance of life itself for the human. The blending of emotional functioning in a group, or the joining of one emotional system to another, may lie at the core of the concept of support throughout much of animal life.

Yet it is equally clear that too much togetherness can create problems both for the individual and for the group. Individuals can become too sensitive to one another. Behavior can become so much determined by the group as a whole that the capacity for an independent life course becomes impaired. Organisms can arrive at a point where they cannot function without one another, a fairly simple definition of *symbiosis*. In response to togetherness pressures, individuals can be swept into directions and activities they would not have chosen themselves, and that may even be detrimental to them.

But each individual also moves naturally toward greater individuality and autonomy when the togetherness pressures fade. That same movement toward separation and autonomy, when colored by anxiety, can surface as rebellion. Between the extremes of complete togetherness and individuation, the person bounces along. Each surge toward togetherness is met by a countersurge toward individuation. If the person moves too much toward individuation, automatic pressures toward togetherness come to bear; too much movement toward togetherness sets up corresponding pressures toward individuation.

Anxiety, or the perception of real or imagined threat, is a critical variable affecting the balance of togetherness and individuation. Anxiety may accompany the togetherness force, and the advantages of togetherness may not always relieve the anxiety. If the anxiety is sufficiently intense, people may attempt to distance themselves from the togetherness pressures. They may appear independent, yet their independence is based on their aversion to togetherness.

Differentiation has to do with the ability of the individual to maintain a degree of autonomy in spite of the pressures for togetherness. The differentiated person understands the advantages of both togetherness and individuation. Differentiation is manifested in a person's ability to be close to another and yet at the same time be separate. Differentiation does not deny the connectedness of people.

The family from which one came is an ideal field for the work on differentiation of self. Contact with important family members can illuminate one's sensitivity to others and trigger the feeling states and mechanisms that operate automatically to reduce discomfort. It is a ready laboratory to which one can turn repeatedly to learn about one's own connectedness to others and about the struggle to be relatively autonomous within such attachment. The goal is not to change the family but to learn about the part one plays in family processes and, if one chooses, to alter that role.

Although clinical practices have been derived from theoretical thought, Bowen has worked to communicate his thinking rather than to focus on the techniques of clinical practice. A training program nonetheless grew up around this thought. In addition to medical residents in active training, staff of Georgetown Medical Center began to attend Bowen's seminars, and later began a weekly program for mental health professionals. Since 1976, training activities in Bowen theory have been conducted at the Family Center, a division of Georgetown Medical School's Department of Psychiatry.

The basic focus of the training programs on theory has never changed. A certain thrust is evident in the training presentations; humans are seen as more similar to other life forms than different. This implies that other species have a great deal to teach about human behavior, and the training programs have reflected this interest in a broad range of life. All nature in some manner presents information about natural systems, and Bowen theory is based on the observation of the natural system of the human. To begin to see this system, one must look at what people *do* rather than what they *say* about themselves or others; it may be a fact that a parent speaks about a child as being a problem, but what that parent actually says may not be a fact. This distinction is sometimes described as the difference between content and process.

If the concept of differentiation of self is the "sun" of Bowen theory, seven other concepts are its "planets." Six of them describe how levels of differentiation affect specific areas of family functioning. The seventh extends the thinking to similar processes that operate in society. Each of these seven concepts will be briefly presented in relationship to the concept of differentiation. Readers interested in a more thorough discussion of them may consult Bowen (1978) or Toman (1976/1961).

Triangles

The level of differentiation of any person indicates his or her sensitivity to others, the intensity of the feeling states and responses that accompany such sensitivity, and the degree to which automatic or instinctive processes override or decrease that person's ability to guide behavior with careful reflection or thought. The less differentiated a person is, the more his or her life decisions are rooted in sensitivity and response to important people. The more such sensitivity governs the behavior of each party to a relationship, the more the pair acts as a unit rather than as separate individuals. When adequate anxiety is present, such a unit behaves in a predictable manner. The triangle describes this process.

A two-person relationship is essentially unstable. When sufficiently anxious, one of the two will automatically involve a third. This movement is predictable and can be known in great detail. When such involvement of a significant outsider is insufficient to reduce anxiety, additional outsiders will be drawn in through a series of interlocking triangles. The knowledge of triangles is an important factor in working toward increased differentiation of self.

Nuclear Family Emotional Process

The more two people function as a unit, the greater the loss of autonomy for each. There are pressures both for greater closeness and greater distance, particularly when one or both people are anxious. Certain processes automatically come into play to regulate closeness and distance and to minimize the disruption of balance in the unit. The greater the undifferentiation in the individuals, the greater the vulnerability of each to loss of autonomy in the flow of togetherness and distance.

The core of the nuclear family, the marital unit, employs four mechanisms to manage the anxiety it generates and/or absorbs. The mechanisms may be unobservable during periods of low anxiety, but automatically appear as anxiety mounts. Families may use a mixture of such mechanisms, or one may become primary. The four mechanisms are emotional distance, marital conflict, dysfunction in a spouse, and the involvement of a child.

When the nuclear family emotional processes are not able to maintain the balance of closeness and distance, the triangle, described above, comes into play.

Family Projection Process

In any family some adult anxiety may "spill over" to involve a child. A major factor in this process is the parents' level of differentiation of self: the greater each parent's level of undifferentiation, the more difficult it is for each to see the child's reality. Feeling states pass between the parents, and between parent and child, and the child comes to be an integral part of the family group, with corresponding loss of autonomy.

The projection process operates through the parents' anxiety about the child, often present even before birth. The parent, often the mother, relates to the child on the basis of that anxiety rather than from a realistic awareness of the child's needs. The process quickly becomes reciprocal, with the child behaving in a manner that triggers parental anxiety. Again, how the father relates to the mother, and she to him, is an important variable in the process. The child who has been the object of the family projection process tends to emerge with a lower level of differentiation than other, less involved siblings.

Multigenerational Transmission Process

The family projection process, operating across the generations, results in branches of families that move toward greater and lesser levels of differentiation. People tend to pick as a mate a person of about the same level of differentiation of self. If a person, as a consequence of the family projection process, grows up with a lower level of differentiation than the parents and marries someone with a similar level, that next generation will emerge with a lower level of differentiation than that of the original parents. In this manner, across time, sections of families move toward greater and lesser levels of differentiation.

Sibling Position

In 1961, Walter Toman published *Family Constellation* (Toman, 1976/1961). Toman presented behavior profiles of the characteristics of individuals occupying specific sibling positions in families. This work consolidated and clarified an entire area of Bowen's thinking. The information about sibling position, along with a knowledge of triangles, made it possible to see the mechanisms of the nuclear family more clearly than previously. It also provided one link between the behavioral patterns in a nuclear family and similar patterns in previous generations.

Toman's work focused on normal families, and it does not take into account the processes by which a child becomes involved in the parents' lack of differentiation. It does, however, suggest some of the postures people assume in their efforts to manage undifferentiation in a relationship.

Emotional Cutoff

A basic element in the concept of differentiation of self is the notion of unresolved emotional sensitivity to one's parents. To manage the loss of autonomy in the relationship to the parents (and other important figures in the family), the person maintains a certain distance. The distance can be intrapsychic or measured in actual miles. The distance may insulate one from the effects of undifferentiation, but it does not change one's level of differentiation. Although the individual appears to handle the relationship to the parents, he or she remains vulnerable to loss of autonomy in other important relationships.

Emotional Processes in Society

This concept extends Bowen theory to social behavior. Bowen became interested in the way anxious, poorly differentiated parents deal with teenage behavior problems, and the way society, through its representatives, deals with the same phenomenon. Essentially similar processes operate in society and in the family, and reflect the pressures of the forces for togetherness and individuation. The status of emotional processes in society at any point influences the functioning of the family.

Several of the eight concepts seem easily understood, particularly the nuclear family emotional system and sibling position. The concept of differentiation of self and of triangles appear much more difficult for people to grasp. Yet to communicate to learners the importance of these theoretical ideas is a central task of the training process.

In clinical training at the Family Center there is little focus on "interventions" or on precisely what technique one applies in the clinical session. Although many skilled clinicians think about, formulate, and firmly believe in the value of interventions, this viewpoint represents a different thrust from Bowen theory in clinical practice. There are, to be sure, techniques, but these are considered less important than the manner in which the clinician understands the family.

The single most important idea to be communicated in the clinical arena is that when the clinician can relate to an anxious family without becoming a part of the emotional process within it, the family will automatically grow less anxious and more thoughtful. Over the years this idea has been conveyed with the word "detachment," yet this disregards the other important notion of contact with the family. People confuse distance with differentiation.

A second important idea has been that of the clinician as researcher. When the clinician can remain interested in the family and focused on understanding rather than changing it, the family members begin to emerge as individuals who are prepared to think differently about their problems and find their own ways to handle them.

BOWEN THEORY IN THERAPY

The methodology of Bowen theory in therapy is relatively uncomplicated. It does not require the presence of all family members. Often the husband and wife are seen, although further theoretical developments have led to a method of seeing only one member of a family in the clinical session. There are four main functions for the clinician when working with the marital unit: (1) defining and clarifying the relationship between the spouses; (2) keeping self detriangled from the family emotional system; (3) teaching the functioning of emotional systems; and (4) demonstrating differentiation by taking "I-positions" during the course of therapy. Each of these functions represents a theoretical perspective.

In the late 1960s Bowen presented an account of his efforts in his own family to a conference of well known family clinicians, and the ideas from the presentation filtered into his teaching. Shortly thereafter Bowen discovered that students were applying these ideas in their own families. Furthermore, they were making faster progress in their own nuclear families and in their clinical work than others, even those in weekly family therapy. His conclusion was "that families in which the focus is on the differentiation of self in the families of origin automatically make as much or more progress in working out the relationship with spouses and children as families seen in formal family therapy in which there is a principal focus on the interdependence in the marriage" (Bowen, 1974, pp. 82–83).

Coaching

From such observations a method of working in the family emotional system evolved. In this method, referred to as "coaching," the clinician functions more as a consultant and teacher than as a therapist. Coaching often occurs with only one member of a family. Progress comes from the efforts that member makes toward differentiation of self in the family. Sessions are often infrequent, sometimes at intervals of a month or more. The focus is primarily on the family of origin, and the responsibility for the effort remains with the person, not the coach.

The work is directed in four general areas: (1) an effort to become a more accurate observer of self and the family; (2) the development of person-to-person relationships with each member of the family; (3) an effort to increase one's ability to control emotional reactivity to the family; and (4) a sustained effort to remain neutral or detriangled while relating to the emotional issues of the family.

TRAINING CONTEXT

The Family Center is affiliated with the Department of Psychiatry of the Georgetown University Medical School. The Family Center is located a short distance from the Medical Center in its own office space. Medical students and residents in various phases of their training receive instruction at the Family Center. For medical students the time at the Family Center is one of several possible elective courses. The Center also offers a fellowship to psychiatrists in their fourth year of residency, which lasts a year or more, with the Fellow involved full-time at the Family Center.

In addition to the instruction of medical personnel, two training courses are open to mental health professionals who have completed their academic training. Those living in the Washington area may attend a weekly course lasting an academic year. It meets one evening a week for three hours. Professionals outside the Washington area may participate in a program meeting four times yearly, three days at a time, at the Family Center. In the interval between visits to Georgetown, participants maintain contact with their Georgetown-assigned supervisor. With the completion of several years training, participants may serve as interns at the Family Center.

Trainees come from all established academic disciplines generally associated with the area of mental health. Most have completed their graduate degrees in a particular discipline prior to their acceptance into the training program, and almost all are working in some capacity as a mental health professional. All applicants must fill out an extensive application form, and those in the Washington area are requested to come for an interview.

Selection of candidates for admission to the training programs is carried out fairly rigorously. Applicants who appear to be unfamiliar with family theory in general and Bowen theory in particular are advised to spend a year reading extensively in the field and attending meetings to get a better idea for themselves of training directions and programs available. People deeply involved in personal therapy of any variety are asked to reapply when their therapy has been completed. Generally the interviewer or reviewer looks for a person who seems genuinely interested in the pursuit of knowledge about the family and has some notion of the importance of his or her own family to the process. Specific experience in family therapy is not necessary for admission.

Three hundred sixty-eight people have completed at least one year of the training program. This group can be described by discipline according to the following percentages: nursing (22%), social work (35%), psychology (14%), medicine (5%), clergy (9%), other (15%). (The category "other" includes a number of probation counselors without a degree in a traditional mental health discipline, as well as a few other individuals with degrees that do not fit easily into established tracks.)

Interns and Fellows receive referrals from the Family Center Clinic. Families seen represent all socioeconomic levels and almost any presenting problem imaginable.

Participants in the professional training programs provide their own clinical families, whether through the agencies in which they work or through their private practices. A requirement for admission to the professional program is the availability to the participant of families for clinical practice.

The processes described by Bowen theory seem to be universal in families. They are not significantly affected by race, religion, or ethnic background. While the economic status of a family may influence its level of anxiety, the basic processes remain the same. The concept of differentiation is applicable to all families. The intensity of the anxiety and the level of differentiation may vary from family to family.

The basic thinking that guides clinical practice, derived from Bowen theory, does not change in response to socioeconomic factors. The primary task is to be in contact with the family while remaining separate from it. The higher the level of anxiety and the lower the level of differentiation in a family, however, the greater the challenge to the clinician to maintain his or her own level of differentiation while in contact with the family.

There are currently 15 faculty members at the Family Center; Six psychiatrists, five nurses, and four social workers. All are volunteer, receiving no salary for services in the training programs. Faculty are generally available for consultation weekly if required, although not all are involved in supervision of learners at the same time. Several of the faculty are at the Center daily, maintaining at least a portion of their private practices there. All faculty have had a long-term involvement as learners in one of the training programs prior to appointment to the faculty.

TRAINING PROGRAM

Training is seen essentially as a person-to-person effort, with the instructor having as much to learn as the learner. In a sense the training process becomes a dialogue between engaged minds, at least when it is occurring most efficiently. The instructor must be able to be close enough to the learner that his or her presence alone has an effect. At the same time he or she must be separate enough to respect the struggles of the learner, and humble enough not to interrupt that effort. In short, the instructor, along with the learner, continually works on differentiation of self.

The single most important goal of training is to assist the learner in understanding the concept of differentiation of self and to assist each person to go as far as he or she is able toward increased personal differentiation. These are interrelated tasks of equal importance. In clinical practice, differentiation is manifested in the clinician's ability to be in contact with a family, as close as desired, while remaining a separate, autonomous individual. Such an effort is seen as a long-term project. Clinical skill is believed to derive directly from the effort with one's own family.

A second primary goal is to communicate to the trainee the ideas of natural systems and to aid the trainee in thinking differently about old and new phenomena. This general area is referred to as "systems thinking" and is difficult for most people to keep in view.

Each of the training programs at the Family Center is comprised of a didactic and a supervisory component. The primary format for the presentation of didactic material is the lecture followed by discussion. Instructional videotapes may accompany a lecture to illustrate a point or convey an idea. The content of a lecture may focus on an aspect of Bowen theory, on a specific clinical example, or more broadly on the natural sciences and the importance of natural systems.

The Family Center has an extensive library of instructional videotapes available to faculty and learners. These tapes present interviews with Dr. Bowen about theoretical points, and edited composites of clinical sessions that illustrate a particular point. In addition, an already large collection of clinical tapes grows monthly as new tapes are made. Still, precisely how to use this resource is unclear; people seem to equate seeing a videotape of a clinical session with learning, which ignores the basic thrust of training toward a person's work within his or her own family. Viewers seem to focus more on what the therapist says or does and to miss the function of the tapes in contributing to theoretical understanding. As a result, the clinical tapes are rarely shown in the training programs.

Little use is made of role play or live supervision to present theoretical and didactic material. The Family Center has no observation rooms or one-way mirrors. Where observation occurs, the visitors are present in the room so that the family is aware of their presence and sees their faces. Role play and live supervision fall into the category of techniques that are employed to help people learn what to do. The thrust of Bowen theory has always moved toward helping people to think and to go as far with their cognitive abilities as possible toward differentiation of self in their own families. The major effort occurs outside the walls of the Center.

If one believes that very little is understood about the functioning of the human family, then the effort to focus on thinking, theory, and the expansion of knowledge that lies at the core of training in Bowen theory comes into clearer perspective. To see phenomena clearly is a continual challenge; the human brain repeatedly defines the world in terms of itself, and it is extremely difficult to see beyond one's preconceived notions. The emphasis on theory represents an effort to work with one's own limited perception to see beyond the limits of one's background and training.

Systems thinking always focuses on the part the self plays in any situation, rather than on the other person. Such a focus does not deny the other's role. The human emotional system tends continually to see, sometimes with accuracy, the locus of a problem outside itself. The effort to change another person is characteristic of anxious families. Training in Bowen theory works always to clarify one's own role in a situation and to step beyond the inclination to change another person. When one can be clear about one's own role and how one intends to manage oneself in a situation, the other has the freedom and the responsibility to find his or her own way.

The level of differentiation of the clinician has a great influence on a family's response. When a clinician is caught up in the emotional reactivity of a family, anything he or she says or does, no matter how therapeutically based, tends to drive the family toward greater reactivity and turmoil. By the same token, when a person is able to maintain contact but remain relatively differentiated, virtually anything he or she contributes tends to be beneficial to the family. The focus of the clinician, at least in Bowen theory, is always on the level of differentiation of self and not on a particular technique to aid the family.

A fundamental respect for the human family, and for its ability to handle almost any difficulty, underlies all efforts at the Family Center. Bowen observed early in his research that families appeared to make greater progress when dealing with the researchers who merely tried to understand the family and to ask objective questions about it than they did when working with the psychotherapists who were actively attempting to help the families. One could call the effort to be as objective as possible and to learn more about a particular family a technique. It is directed toward the clinician's management of self, however, rather than toward changing the family

Four or five trainees meet weekly with a faculty member for supervision. Each has an opportunity to present material either from clinical practice or from efforts with his or her own family. The faculty supervisor and others may ask questions, make comments, or offer a suggestion or thought. The effort is to tap the most objective thinking of each person rather than to activate feelings and automatic emotional processes. Although a major emphasis is on differentiation of self in one's own family, trainees are encouraged to make videotapes of their clinical work for review by their supervisors. In a general way supervisor and trainee attempt to see in the tapes how the clinician becomes caught up in the emotional processes of the family, and how such involvement reflects the clinician's own level of differentiation. From time to time the trainee may meet alone with the supervisor for consultation and evaluation.

Didactic and supervisory activities are intended to assist the trainee in the effort toward differentiation of self in his or her own family and in clinical practice. Clear understanding of theory, particularly of differentiation of self, seems to be of greater assistance in the long run than do specific techniques. Theory points out the need for self differentiation, while simultaneously highlighting what one does not know about a particular family. Families vary, and what is effective in maintaining neutrality in one family may not work in the next.

It is extremely difficult to assess differentiation of self on a short-term basis. Experience in a Family Center training program only represents a beginning. People could not be expected to have acquired a new level of differentiation of self as a result of their efforts in the training progam. It is reasonable to expect, however, that they have a working understanding of the concept and a way of recognizing their own lack of differentiation in the family from which they came, in which they live, and in the families seen in their clinical practice.

The four areas of effort described earlier in the discussion of coaching form a general framework for evaluating the work of a learner: (1) the effort to become a more accurate observer of self and the family; (2) the development of person-to-person relationships with each member of the family; (3) the effort to increase one's ability to control emotional reactivity to the family; and (4) the sustained effort to remain neutral or detriangled while relating to the emotional issues of the family.

During the course of supervisory sessions a learner's understanding of theoretical material and the efforts made toward differentiation of self in one's own family can be assessed. Much more is involved than simply the frequency of visits made to the family and what is said during the visit. How well does the trainee understand his or her own role in the family processes? What sort of efforts has the trainee undertaken to increase understanding? Does the trainee show respect for the power of emotional processes in the family? Is his or her focus on self in the family or on "fixing" the family's problem, that is, changing someone else in an effort to improve family functioning?

The distinction between management of self in an intense emotional field and the effort to change others in that field is fundamental and should again be emphasized. Systems thinking is always focused on the role and contribution of self to a system. Families have ways to deal with those who set out to change them. Differentiation is learning for one's self within the laboratory of the family.

Another area of evaluation concerns the quality of thinking the learner displays. This is a difficult and elusive area. To "think systems" is not an easy task. How well can the learner see a big picture and not become enmeshed in details? Does the trainee have an appreciation of complexity, or is he or she caught up in simple answers to difficult problems? Does the individual have a way of monitoring his or her own subjectivity? To what extent can the person entertain ideas for their own merit without automatically trying to integrate them into an existing mode of thinking? Does the trainee appreciate the long-term nature of the effort toward differentiation of self?

Evaluations are generally conducted on a person-to-person basis between the supervisor and the trainee. While each instructor varies somewhat in terms of criteria, he or she tries to give the learner specific suggestions for further work and future directions.

The nature of the relationship between a given faculty member and a particular trainee eludes easy description. Each person is different, and the nature of the training relationship varies greatly. The teacher has to have a way of challenging the thinking of the learner while simultaneously listening for what he or she has to contribute to a broader understanding of a phenomenon.

Each person in the position of instructor struggles with his or her particular version of dogmatism, subjectivity, and lack of respect for the learning dilemmas of the other. At the same time, the effort to maintain a clear definition of self in the face of the learner's tendency to integrate quite different ideas and thoughts in an eclectic manner can be extremely challenging.

The notion of resistance on the part of a trainee is not often heard at the Family Center. It belongs to a different way of thinking about training and about human functioning, and suggests that the barrier to learning lies with the trainee rather than with the faculty member. People at the Family Center are no more immune to this view than anyone else. Nonetheless, to focus on the problem in another is the antithesis of systems thinking.

Learners often react strongly to a teacher's dogmatism or lack of perspective. Even more subtle is the instructor's effort to make the student different, to push through a change in his or her thinking that the learner is unwilling or unable to accept. If such an interaction between instructor and trainee is called resistance, one must address the forces or pressures in the instructor that help propel the process; to place the locus of the problem in the learner is to recreate the projection process so characteristic of family interaction.

The general guideline for Family Center faculty is to manage self in such situations rather than to focus on the other. Such a posture does not deny or minimize the part another plays. It is in accordance with the basic systems idea, outlined above, that the management of self takes precedence over the effort to change another. This is difficult to do and requires a great deal of effort. It requires working against the tendency of the emotional system to project the problem onto another. When one can control the part of self that contributes to greater levels of anxiety in a family, every other person has a new degree of freedom and responsibility for his or her own self. When a Family Center training program is working well, all faculty members attempt to minimize their own tendency to project. This is an ongoing challenge.

It is difficult to recognize the role a teacher plays in a learner's lack of understanding. Anyone who teaches has the potential to inhibit another's learning. The Family Center is not immune to this dilemma. An element of the problem lies in the nature of the relationship formed between teacher and learner. Like many other people, teachers struggle with their own level of differentiation, in relation to a trainees and to each other. When an instructor loses sight of differentiation of self and the continual effort required, the atmosphere of a clique clouds the teaching process. One can hardly blame trainees for reacting to the faculty's togetherness. The continual focus on theoretical material also plays a role. Many trainees find it difficult and irrelevant to their interests. They want to know what to do with families, and find the point of theory difficult to grasp.

From time to time problems appear in the training programs and/or between a teacher and a learner. There is no easy formula for resolving these disagreements. Often a complaint rests on very valid criticisms. Where possible such criticisms are acknowledged. Honest people can disagree, however. As far as possible, the Family Center faculty recognize the right of another to hold his or her own opinion, and ask only that the same recognition be acknowledged in return.

The concept of differentiation of self is not easily understood, and many trainees initially understand only a piece of it. Even so, they often acquire ideas that are useful to them in their clinical practice and which they integrate into their existing way of thinking about human problems. With repeated exposure and effort, their understanding becomes more sophisticated and new levels of ideas become apparent.

A small number of trainees maintain contact with the Family Center for long periods of time. Some work with a particular supervisor or attend the general meetings and symposia the Family Center sponsors each year. Many of these people make important contributions to further theoretical understanding of complex clinical issues and human behavior in general.

There really is no such thing as a "standard" or "prototypical" trainee. Ages, backgrounds, and experiences of trainees are quite varied, as are their reactions to the training process itself. Few standard problems recur from year to year and from trainee to trainee. In part this may be due to the fact that each trainee's family is somewhat different, and the dilemma or bind that one trainee faces is different from that of another.

The length of time a trainee spends in the program is also quite varied. The work on differentiation of self is considered a lifelong task, and a set period of time in a training program cannot measure progress. Many trainees continue in "coaching" with a faculty member long after they have ended their participation in formal training program. Others will end their contact with the Family Center within a year or so. There seem to be no standard reasons for leaving at a particular point in training. Some people find that the focus on theory and on one's own family is not what they are looking for. Still others find that the commitments of time, energy, and resources required for participation are greater than they had expected or are able to meet.

Perhaps a discussion of the prototypical trainee can best be summed up with reference to the concept of differentiation of self. Each trainee and each faculty member vary in terms of the level of differentiation of self. The nature of training, the difficulties encountered, and the time spent are directly related to those varying levels of differentiation.

TOWARD THE FUTURE

Bowen's development of a theory of the natural system of the human family rested on the assumption that *Homo sapiens* was more like other life forms than different. That perspective still guides thinking and study at the Family Center. It makes the work of all natural scientists of great interest, not only work exclusively or even primarily directed toward the human family. This broad range of interest and study is reflected in the list of invited guest speakers to the annual Georgetown Symposium on Family Theory and Family Psychotherapy. Their topics have ranged from genetics to cellular behavior to the culture and behavior of whales.

The broad phenomenon generally referred to as "emotional reactivity" is of great interest, and is being approached from several directions. An important tool in such research is biofeedback, and the Family Center includes a biofeedback staff involved in a number of research tasks. Recent projects have attempted to investigate the role of reactivity in physical processes like diabetes and in measurable intelligence.

Social processes are another area of attention, with people attempting to understand how society functions and how such functioning relates to the broad scope of life on earth. Nature appears always to have had a way to deal with those species and life forms that fouled their nests, and there is no reason to expect the human to be above Nature. Seen from the perspective of the age of the universe, evolution moves very rapidly indeed. Whether humankind will develop the ability to step beyond the instinctual processes that drive predation and the exploitation of the planet remains an open question.

Further development of a theory of natural systems is of major importance, and all work at the Family Center is in one way or another directed toward that goal. Specific applications of theory, while always important, are somewhat secondary. Yet the involvement with theoretical thinking seems to bring a continual freshness and interest to clinical work.

CONCLUSION

Family therapy is presently more popular than ever before. Training programs, workshops, and clinical programs spring up around the country and multiply like the kudzu that threatens to overrun the South. But proliferation marks only fecundity. It conveys little about longevity or capacity to contribute significant improvement. The lasting importance of the field will be determined, I believe, by its ability or inability to curb the tendency to overstate what it knows at the expense of what it does not. Family theory raises far more questions than answers.

No matter what the future of family therapy, however, the reproduction of species, the circling of the earth around the sun, the position of the solar system in the galaxy, and the apparently expanding universe will be little affected. The human family and human family therapists are as much creatures of Nature as any other life form on the planet. The potential of systems is to provide a way to better understand the interconnectedness of all life with the earth and the forces that shape and govern the interrelationship.

References

Bowen, M. (1974). Toward the differentiation of self in one's family of origin. In P. Lorio & F. Andres (Eds.), *Georgetown Family Symposia* (Vol. I, pp. 70–86). Washington, DC: Department of Psychiatry, Georgetown University Medical Center.

Bowen, M. (1978). *Family theory in clinical practice.* New York: Jason Aronson.

Horner, J. R. (1984). The nesting behavior of dinosaurs. *Scientific American, 250*(4), 130–137.

Toman, W. (1976). *Family constellation: Its effects on personality and social behavior* (3rd ed.). New York: Springer Publishing. (Originally published 1961.)

5

Training in the Brief Therapy Model

RICHARD FISCH

Brief Therapy Center, The Mental Research Institute, Palo Alto, California

The model of Brief Therapy is one that evolved from collaborative clinical research over a 20-year period at the Brief Therapy Center of the Mental Research Institute (M.R.I.) in Palo Alto, California. A basic tenet of the approach is a relativistic, or constructionist, view of reality: that the "true" nature of things cannot be known and that what are usually regarded as "facts," "discoveries," and "truths" are conceptual constructs to explain why or how something "works" or "doesn't work"; these constructs might be called "mythologies," "maps," or "models." Such maps or models are necessary or, rather, unavoidable, as frameworks for operating in one's milieu. In this formulation of "reality," then, the validity of a model is measured not by its "truth" but by the achievement or nonachievement of desired results. In the work at the Brief Therapy Center, we have discovered nothing, but, instead, have constructed a model, just as, in our view, other innovators have constructed models, be they psychoanalytic, behavioral, biochemical, and so on.

MAJOR FEATURES OF THE MODEL

The model itself is simple, attaching importance to only a few elements to explain how problems arise and how they are maintained (Fisch, Weakland, & Segal, 1982; Watzlawick, Weakland, & Fisch, 1974; Weakland, Fisch, Watzlawick, Bodin, 1974). It is its very simplicity that allows for brevity of treatment but creates difficulties for therapists in training who have been utilizing more complex models. Many of the agendas they are accustomed to dealing with in treatment sessions are regarded as irrelevant and they are, initially, inclined to feel that important "dynamics" in a case are being neglected, for example the "function" of a symptom in a family. The simplicity and its difference from other models derives from two major features, a nonpathologic and non-normative view.

Nonpathologic Aspect

By nonpathologic we mean that the formation and persistence of problems does not imply that individuals or families have anything inherently wrong with them. We do not see clients as being more vulnerable to problems than others in the general population, nor do we place importance on the origination of their problems, seeing the occurrence of difficulties as inherent and unremarkable events in the course of people's lives in their transactions as family members, workers, and members of a community. However, we do attach importance to the *persistence* of problems, viewing such persistence as the logical outcome of the very attempts the identified patient, and/or others involved in the problem, are making to resolve that problem—what we refer to as the "attempted solution." We do not view those attempts as reflecting any pathology or deficiency but, rather, as expressions of generally held notions of how to deal with problems, what might be called "common sense." One part of common sense is the idea that if one does not succeed at first, one should redouble one's efforts—more of the same—rather than question the attempts at solution. Common sense also dictates that if, after repeated attempts and repeated failures, the problem persists or gets worse, then the problem is to be regarded as one lying outside the capabilities of the average person and, therefore, as requiring the expertise of a therapist—in other words, that the problem is some form of "mental illness."

Non-normative Aspect

By non-normative we mean that we use no criteria to judge the health or normality of an individual or family. As therapists, we do not regard any particular way of functioning, relating, or living as a problem if the client is not expressing discontent with it. Therefore, our only criterion is whether someone is *complaining* about some situation or state of affairs. Similarly, our only criterion for evaluating the resolution of a problem is whether there is an elimination or sufficient reduction of the complaint. (With many problems, the identified patient may not be the complainant, as is commonly the case in child- or adolescent-centered problems; in a small number of cases, neither the identified patient nor any other member of the family may be the complainant, but someone from the community might be, as in cases where an offender is ordered into treatment by a probation officer or the court. There are even some rare cases where *no one* is a complainant, for example, where a person has halfheartedly consulted a therapist, but decided after one interview that the effort and the cost are simply not worth it, that the problem is not that difficult to live with.) Thus, in our model, if no one is complaining, there is no problem.

By these two paradigms, nonpathologic and non-normative, the relevant agenda in therapy is enormously reduced, since only the complaint needs to be modified, and that modification, in turn, requires only that the client and involved others depart from their problem-maintaining efforts.

Problem-Solving Approach

Because the model dictates a problem-solving approach, one requiring that the therapist use *planned* influence to get the client to *do* something different, it presents different technical problems in the course of treatment than would be encountered in therapies using different models. These technical difficulties can pose problems for trainees accustomed to different roles with their clients. For example, a problem-solving approach necessitates that the therapist obtain a very clear and concrete picture of the complaint, as well as the "attempted solution." With many clients, it is quite difficult to obtain sufficiently clear data; the clients are vague, use generalities when specifics are asked for, shift quickly from one topic to another, qualify statements in a confusing way, and so forth. Trainees accustomed to an insight-oriented model will not feel it necessary to pin down data and will feel rattled during direct supervision when the supervisor keeps calling in to ask them to get the client to be more specific.

Since the emphasis is on getting clients to take some action very different than what they have been doing, another problem arises when attempting to gain their compliance in following a suggestion or task. As mentioned above, people tend to persist in an unsuccessful "solution" because it seems to be the only "sane," logical, or safe course within their frame of reference. Often it is no simple task to get them to abandon it, and very careful planning and explanation are required. That planning and explanation utilize the client's frame of reference. We believe it more efficient and effective to "talk the client's language" than to try to get clients to make a shift in their values or world view. While trainees can acknowledge the validity of that approach, it is the most avowedly manipulative aspect of treatment and they will feel very uncomfortable saying something to a client that they do not truly believe. Obviously, this is most difficult for trainees accustomed to an approach emphasizing "authenticity," "rapport," and "awareness."

ASSUMPTIONS REGARDING TRAINING

Just as our model is simple, our assumptions regarding training are few and not particularly complicated. First, our fundamental view is that the approach is teachable to any reasonably intelligent and interested therapist. We do not see skepticism on the trainee's part as an obstacle, as long as the trainee is not there just to disprove the rationale. So far we have not encountered that. Second, we anticipate that the biggest hurdle for the trainee is recognizing that a shift in frame of reference is required, and then making that shift. With little exception, trainees are grounded in models that have a pathologic base. For example, if it is a psychodynamic model, the symptom (the complaint) is seen as an expression of intrapsychic defense. In a family therapy model, the problem in the identified patient is considered necessary to maintain the stability of the dysfunctional homeostasis of the family. Thus, attempting simply to modify the complaint is strongly considered futile, if not dangerous, since the "underlying" support for the symptom has not been changed. Trainees may feel delinquent in their responsibility to the client if they do not pursue the understanding and resolution of these "underlying" factors, and may find it jarring to be told that there is no need for the symptom, nor is there any payoff for maintaining it. If parents argue about the correct way to deal with junior, the more traditionally oriented family therapist will view that as evidence of the marital conflict underlying their son's problem. It takes some time for our trainees to accept and operate on the notion that it is a *parenting* conflict, that is, that parents often have different points of view as to what is correct or effective in raising a child, and that this is an inherent, albeit troublesome, spinoff effect when parents have been doing what they regard as reasonable and there has been no change in the child's problem. For the same reason, trainees tend to delve into past history, since they are more accustomed to models that view problems as having a chronological course. Before they make a shift to the new model, they feel they are trivializing treatment, being too superficial, when the supervisor asks them not to bother with that "ancient history."

While many suggested interventions are seen as intriguing, they are at the same time, experienced by some trainees as puzzling or mysterious or insufficient.

Similar problems arise for trainees because of the non-normative fact of the model. On the theoretical level, they may confuse *non-normative* with *nonvalue*. They ask, quite correctly, how any approach can be without any value, since even "no value" is a value statement. We have to make clear that one *value* of our approach is not to use standards of "normality" in judging a problem and its resolution, on the presumption that once standards of normal functioning are created, for the individual or the family, then treatment is unnecessarily prolonged, since deviations from those standards must then be regarded as significant factors contributing to the problem. While trainees can accept that rationale, they nevertheless find it difficult to ignore clients' comments about their families or themselves when those comments indicate a deviance from "established" criteria of "mental health," "functional norms in families," and the like. It takes some getting used to to operate on the notion that if the client is not complaining about it, it is no problem, at least for the client. This aspect of the model, its non-normative feature, is a little less troublesome for the trainee than its nonpathologic base. For example, the trainee can more readily grasp the idea that in a marital problem the mutual agreement between the spouses to divorce is not necessarily a failure of treatment; in our society, divorce is a legitimate option for the resolution of conflict.

The difficulty in making a conceptual shift is compounded when the trainee is unaware that he or she has been operating from a model. Instead, trainees will view what they have been doing with clients as based on simple "fact" about the nature of problems, families, and individuals. Other schools of treatment are seen mainly as different ways of going about dealing with those "facts" or emphasizing different aspects of an individual or family problem. Thus they are inclined to talk about the "indications" for using family therapy, or the "contraindications" for using behavioral methods, or to describe their orientation as "eclectic." It would seem that in their original training, it had never been made explicit that the approach and technique they were learning was based on a conceptual framework, one of many frameworks promoted by different schools. For such trainees, "mental illness" is a given fact, not a conceptual construct, and they are confused when, in our training, we seem to ignore the "realities" of "mental illness."

We also assume that learning a new approach to treatment, both conceptually and technically, best comes about by *doing* that treatment, under guidance, with ongoing cases. While there is some initial didactic explanation of rationale and technique, the greatest bulk of the training involves direct supervision of treatment. We believe that direct guidance is superior to indirect guidance, although some time is given to indirect supervision of cases with which trainees are working in their own practices or agencies.

Finally, we place the greater emphasis on an understanding of the rationale and technique rather than on therapist "style," charisma, "giftedness," and the like. We believe that the artistry of the therapist can lend some advantage and character to his or her therapy, but that the principal effectiveness comes from careful and thoughtful implementation of the approach we offer. This is consistent with the approach itself, since, with little exception, interventions in cases are planned in between sessions and with a careful review of the relevant factors at any particular point in treatment. Flashes of brilliance and imagination during sessions are rare, and we do not believe these should be relied on for solid and efficient therapy. Likewise, we do not place great importance on the sex, ethnicity, or other personal traits of the therapist and do not assign cases on the basis of any of these factors. Certainly, we do not look at any of these factors as limiting the therapist; if anything, we prefer to see how any of these features might be *used* in working with clients. For example, a number of trainees who come from foreign countries have had difficulty with English and are tempted to try to obscure that difficulty from clients. Instead, we suggest that they make it very clear that they will be having some trouble understanding the client; this puts more pressure on the client to be clear in describing the problem and how he or she has been trying to deal with it.

The desired goal of the training is to provide trainees with a sufficient grasp of the underlying rationale and its derivative technique so that they can generalize applications from it to their own cases, both current and future. In particular, we want trainees to be able to demonstrate their understanding of what are relevant data and what are irrelevant, how to clarify those data with clients, how to identify the complainant in a case, how to use reframing as part of intervening, how to formulate the problem as well as the clients' efforts which maintain that problem, how to formulate appropriate tasks or interventions, and, finally, how to assess progress in a case without using normative values.

THE TRAINING PROGRAM

The training is offered at the Mental Research Institute in Palo Alto. Since its inception, the training program has been conducted by the author and John Weakland. The author is a psychiatrist and director of the Brief Therapy Center; John Weakland is a psychotherapist and clinical anthropologist and is associate director of the Center. They have worked closely together in their association with the Center since its beginning 20 years ago, contributing, along with others, to the development and refinement of the treatment approach.

The physical setting is a replication of that used by the Brief Therapy Center. Therapy is done in an informal consultation room with comfortable chairs placed around a low coffee table. In the center of the table is a microphone connected to a speaker and tape deck in the observation room, which is separated by a one-way mirror. Also on the table is an intercom phone allowing for communication between the therapist and observers. Clients are always informed of these special arrangements and that the therapist is in training. The client's written consent is obtained. Customarily, the trainee therapist is alone with clients during a session, although the trainer has the option to enter and leave the room. By the same token, the trainee can leave or be asked to leave the treatment room to consult with the trainer at any time during a session, although such conferences tend to occur toward the end of the session. Consultation between trainee and trainer, however, is usually via the intercom phone, such consultations most often being initiated by the trainer.

In general, phone calls entail only a few categories. In the early phase of treatment, the trainer will call in to ask the trainee to clarify some data, or obtain data that are missing. In this way, trainees learn what information is relevant, how specific and clear it needs to be, and some guidelines for obtaining clear data. Early in training, trainees will settle for imprecise or vague data, and more calling from "the back room" is needed. A second major category of calls involve directives to the trainee regarding making interventions, and in framing a rationale of the tasks to clients so they will more likely carry out those tasks or suggestions. Depending on the nature or complexity of the suggestion, the trainer may, at the same time, give some brief explanation to the trainee to fit in with the overall strategy for that session, or at least the interactions at that time. Otherwise, the trainer will wait until after the session is over to explain the directives. Beause it is a strategy-oriented approach and verbal communication is the principal means of influencing clients, precise and careful use of wording is regarded as a necessary tool; trainers will often ask that a directive be delivered to the clients in exactly the same wording given to the trainee. (Since trainees can never anticipate whether a call might ask them to obtain or clarify information, or be a general suggestion allowing them to "ad lib," or be meant as a precise directive, a useful code word can diminish that uncertainty. Thus, trainees might be informed that a call preceded by the word "quote" is meant to be a directive to be delivered to the client verbatim, or that "this is for information" means that some datum should be obtained or clarified.)

Trainees rotate in taking cases. Depending on the number of trainees, we usually run two or four cases in any one training session. Trainees not having a case or not having a session at the time will be in the observation room with the trainer. As much as possible, the trainer will make explanatory comments to them during the session, which are intended to highlight or illustrate particular points about the clients and the treatment. These comments tend to be few, since the trainer's concentration is first and foremost on guiding responsible treatment, secondarily on the needs of the trainee therapist, and lastly, on the observing trainees. Also, many such comments can be saved for the postsession discussion allowing the trainee–therapist to hear them also. (This tripartite concentration is always a factor and makes this kind of supervision quite fatiguing.) An hour is allowed for each treatment session, although the session can be shorter depending on pacing. For example, if the therapist has given the clients a task to perform at home and they have agreed to do it, the trainer may tell the therapist to terminate the session at that point even though there might be some time left before the hour is up. (Since ours is an action-oriented approach, we do not want to dilute the agreement to do an assignment by having some subsequent discussion.) Most often, however, the full time is used up. Following each session, a half-hour follow-up discussion is done with the observers and therapist–trainee. Most of this discussion is led by the trainer, who will start off with comments about the course of the session, critiquing the therapist's performance, and planning the next session. Other discussion stems from questions or comments made by trainees, both observers and therapist.

The Cases

In the training, each case is allotted eight weekly sessions. Patients have the option after that time to continued treatment with the therapist–trainee if that is feasible, or with a therapist in the M.R.I. clinic, or with any other therapist of their choosing. While such provisions are made, and while the cases are seen for a relatively short period, we have not encountered with trainees a mentality of "this is only a training case" or "this is not really treatment." Partly, we believe, this is because trainees are reminded that the average number of sessions in the Brief Therapy Center is only 6 or 7, and because trainers have been rather firm in having trainees do treatment "right." Cases for training are obtained from several sources: trainees' own caseloads, from their agencies, from the M.R.I. clinic and from the Brief Therapy Center.

The Training Session

The training is given in a 5-hour session once a week and for a total of 35 weeks, roughly a 9-month period. The first two sessions are devoted to a description of the model, general guidelines for data gathering and intervening, exemplification of the approach through playing audio- and videotape recordings of treatment undertaken at the Brief Therapy Center, and on occasion simulated treatment sessions with trainees. Additionally, trainees will have read or be asked to read some of the literature authored by members of the Brief Therapy Center, works that expand on the rationale and technique of the approach. Didactic input is limited to these two sessions and the reading, since we believe that truer understanding of the approach will mainly come about by doing it and watching other trainee–therapists do it, and by being guided during sessions by the trainers. The last training session is not a supervisory one, but a "windup" where students may voice any final questions or comments, as well as a "winding down" in the form of a simple party. In addition to that windup session, trainees are encouraged to make suggestions and criticisms of the training thoughout its course, since we would prefer to take corrective action when needed than after the fact.

The 5-hour training session is divided into two phases. The first three hours are devoted to direct supervision of two cases and a postsession discussion of those cases. (Since there are two observation and treatment rooms at M.R.I., a larger group of trainees can be split into two smaller groups allowing for work with four cases in an afternoon.) The latter 2 hours are devoted to indirect supervision. Even with a larger group of trainees, the entire group and both trainees meet at this time and trainees bring in tape recordings, which we prefer, or notes of sessions with their own clients outside of the training center. (So far, we have not felt it enough of an advantage to ask trainees to bring in videotapes even if they have them; the preponderant emphasis in treatment is on verbal and tonal exchange, and little or no importance is attached to nonverbal events in sessions.) In addition to indirect supervision, the latter part of the afternoon is taken up with questions trainees raise about general, theoretical, or technical aspects of the approach when these points are not clear.

Cotraining

A training group of 8 to 10 people is divided into two smaller groups, each of the trainers supervising a small group during the direct supervision part of the day. During the indirect supervision, the whole group and both trainers meet together. After each 8-week treatment cycle, the groups change supervisors. Halfway through the training course, the trainee groups are reshuffled so that all trainees will have an opportunity to work with each trainer and all other members of the trainee group. With fewer than 8 people in the trainee group, budget does not allow for this cotraining arrangement. In such a case, trainees will work with each other sequentially, with the supervisors alternating every eight weeks. In any case, all trainees have an opportunity to work with at least two cases under direct supervision in the course of the 9 months. Extra cases depend on whether, and how many, cases are terminated before the full eight sessions are up.

The cotraining arrangement is much more preferable to the sequential one. First, it allows more individual attention to trainees. During the course of the training, it also allows for inter-session discussion about and evaluation of the trainees. In our approach to treatment, inter-session planning is regarded as an important feature. Similarly, in the training of therapists, planning can be very valuable in aiding trainees who are having difficulties. For example, some trainees have trouble handling the stress of doing treatment under direct observation by a supervisor and colleagues. Their anxiety can interfere with their treatment of a case and with using suggestions or directives from the supervisor. Trainers can discuss this problem and formulate some intervention for the trainee so that he or she might be a little more relaxed during sessions; e.g., suggest they use their more familiar way of working "just for this next session so we can see what useful features of it should be retained"; or, decide to spend extra time in the treatment room with the trainee during sessions. (Thus far, we have not encountered a great variety of trainee "weaknesses." Aside from the expected initial difficulties in "getting the hang" of the approach, some trainees are inclined to take a "one-up" stance with their clients, that is, attempting to display self-confidence, tending to get into arguments with clients, and being too quick in expressing patronizing empathy. Other trainees overuse "supportive" comments and unwittingly alienate a client, or trivialize some point a client feels very strongly about. However, these kinds of difficulties have been handled by simple and direct discussion with the trainee.) Since each trainer will work with each trainee, trainers can compare their assessments and arrive at some agreement as to how best to help a particular trainee, should it be needed.

The coteaching arrangement has another useful feature. Often, trainees assume that it takes a certain kind of character or "artistry" to perform any innovative therapy well. This notion can be quickly dispelled, since neither the author nor Weakland have what might be called charismatic personalities and, in addition, both have very different styles in conducting a session. Further, when trainers have a dialogue with each other during the assessment of a case or an intervention, it affords an opportunity for trainees to hear how the process of therapy is arrived at, clarifying what could otherwise be seen as mysterious or requiring unique "giftedness." At times, cotrainers may suggest different interventions to implement a strategy, and this too gives trainees a chance to see that there can be more than one way to intervene in a case, that there isn't just one "correct" thing to say or suggest to clients.

The Trainees

Our trainees come from diverse backgrounds and experience, and from many parts of the United States as well as different countries. They have included psychologists, clinical social workers, psychiatrists, pastoral counselors and one person with a sociology background. All trainees are required to have a minimum of three years of clinical experience beyond their training, one year involving work with families or couples. (These requirements were waived for the sociologist partly because her inclusion was considered a training experiment and because she had considerable experience in organizational consultation, experience we felt was analogous to the problem-solving aspect of clinical work.) They are also required to be in current active practice, although absence from their home territory, as in the case of trainees coming from a foreign country or another State, necessitates a temporary "sabbatical."

We do not lay significant emphasis on selection interviewing of trainees. In many cases, such as when the applicant is living far away, it is not feasible. In such a case, we will conduct an interview over the phone. Our criteria for selection are not complicated and we are principally interested in the above-cited factors: the trainees' facility with English, their expectations regarding the training, and how they plan to use it. As in our approach to treatment, we put more emphasis on *how* to work with someone, rather than whether that individual is workable or not. As of now, we would prefer to look to improving our training methods rather than tightening up entrance requirements for trainees. Especially when we are oversubscribed, we will give weight to applicants working in an agency rather than those strictly in private practice. This is based on the assumption that doing therapy briefly can pose some economic consequences for therapists in private practice and thus tend to discourage them from using the training they will have received. For practical reasons, we will also give weight to applicants working locally, since they will be able to provide clients for the training. (Getting clients is a chronic problem, especially since our schedule and requirements are rather tight: clients must be available on a rigid 8-week schedule, willing to be seen early in an afternoon, willing to be observed and tape-recorded, and willing to be treated by therapists who are in a training program.) Finally, we will give priority to applicants working in an outpatient setting over those working in an inpatient setting. Again, this is because brief psychotherapy has its principal use as an outpatient approach and, as part of that approach, is designed to *prevent* hospitalization. For the most part, hospitalization is viewed as putting on hold most any form of problem solving therapy, since problems arise in the day-to-day milieu of people and need to be resolved in that milieu.

GOALS OF BRIEF THERAPY TRAINING

As mentioned earlier, the goal of the training is to instill in trainees a working grasp of the approach so they can utilize it on their own with their own cases. The process for achieving this requires two main efforts: unlearning their previous model and its derived techniques and, concomitantly, learning the new model we are presenting. It appears that the former is the more difficult yet more strategic part of the process. Again, this coincides with our overall view of problems in general: that the significant factor is identifying what is to be avoided, rather than searching for the precise solution. We believe that more is to be learned from the trainees' errors in the running of a case than in correct moves they make. Most often, these errors provide the best starting point from which to clarify the model the trainee has been using, and then to contrast it with the new model. The trainee can then see that, using that newer model, the intervention would have to be different. In the process of unlearning and learning, the major modality, whether in direct or indirect supervision, is constantly to relate technique with model. Whenever possible, a directive to a trainee is always explained on the basis of the model, at least after the session is over. Similarly, if we are making some correction of a trainee's intervention or performance, we will demonstrate how that intervention is an expression of the trainee's accustomed model; how that model is inconsistent with or discontinuous with our model; and, finally, how, from the newer model, a different intervention might have been made at that same point in the session. For example, a client giving information to the trainee about his problem may make some vague or qualified statement. The trainee will respond with "I see; uh huh," and then allow the client to proceed on an unclear narrative. The trainer might phone in and ask the trainee to interrupt the narrative and ask for some clarification of the earlier vague information. Later, in the postsession discussion, the trainer will ask what the trainee had in mind in conveying understanding of data that were obviously obscure. The trainee might explain that in that early phase of treatment, he or she felt it important to establish rapport with the client, and to have pressed for clarification would have seemed "cold" and unempathic. The trainer would say, "Establishing rapport is based on a model of therapy in which clients are viewed as partially helpless in dealing with an overwhelming problem. In that model, then, it is consistent to give priority to assuring the client that he has an understanding ally and thus to say "I see," even though the given data are unclear. However, that is not a view of the model you are trying to learn. There, we view the client as an active agent in his problem, *doing* something that maintains his problem. Therefore, priority is given to getting clear information as to what is the problem and, further, what exactly has he been doing that maintains it. So, at that point our response to unclear data would be 'I don't understand; would you explain that, please.'"

Often, the trainer might simply phone in an intervention and later explain to the trainee—and observing trainees—the rationale of that intervention in terms of the ongoing events of treatment, while emphasizing that intervention relates to the basic model. For example, "When I asked you to tell the client that one of us in the back room didn't believe he could really do what you asked of him in the coming week, I was keeping in mind his comment in the first session that he feels people underestimate him and he resents that. Now that is what we would regard as a "position" statement; that is, he feels strongly about some value. In our model, we do not attach importance to the client understanding his problem, but rather to getting the client to *do* something different than what he has been doing. Principally, ours is an influence model, not an insight model. Therefore, we are always looking for leverages to enhance the client's compliance with a task or suggestion and, in this case, it seemed that it would help if we utilized his motivation to prove that he should not be underestimated. At the same time, this frees you to be flexible, since the suggstion was not coming from you but from 'the back room.'"

In addition to relating technique to theory, we believe that emulation aids in learning. When we first offered the advanced training, the trainers were reluctant to enter the treatment room, believing that it would impede the learning process since the trainer would be "taking over" and doing the treatment for the trainee. However, on those occasions when we did go in, trainees often remarked that they felt this helped them understand things much better. This seemed to be borne out in subsequent sessions. Thus, over time, trainers have become more active and direct participants in the treatment. While it doesn't make up a significant portion of the treatment session, it is not unusual for a trainer to be in the treatment room at least once during a session; it helps the trainee to relax knowing that he or she isn't "in the tank" alone and that, if need be, the supervisor will "bail me out." (After having done treatment under observation for 20 years, it is easy to forget that it is a new and anxiety-laden experience for most trainees.) Most often, supervisors will enter the room when the trainee is running into trouble. Rather than handle such a situation over the phone, the supervisor will go in and "take over." For example, the trainee might have ignored some strongly held notion of the client's, and, in attempting to get the client to agree to a course of action, may have gotten into a subtle but troublesome argument. At that point of impasse, the trainer can enter the room and intervene. Addressing the client, the supervisor explains that he is unclear about some comment the client made earlier in the session (the comment having to do with the point the trainee has ignored). As the client reiterates his or her position, the trainer can express newfound understanding, can explain that understanding to the trainee and, before leaving the room, ask the trainee to explore that point "a bit further." Later in the session, the supervisor can phone in an intervention based on a nonargumentative explanation, and in the postsession discussion explain what was happening in the session and the rationale of what he did.

Evaluation

In evaluating the progress of trainees we will look to see whether or not they are incorporating previously discussed elements of treatment in a subsequent session with their clients. If they do, we will make explicit note of that; if not, we might ask if they were unclear about a previous explanation, or if they failed to see its application in that subsequent session. As direct and indirect supervision progresses, we may volunteer fewer explanations, and instead ask the trainees to try to explain why we suggested what we did. This is an additional way of checking progress. At times, we may pose hypothetical case vignettes and ask trainees, as a group, to discuss their thinking out loud: How do they see the problem? What is the solution attempted by the client? What position or positions is the client taking? What would they most avoid as a basic thrust of treatment? How would they intervene to interdict the client's problem-maintaining efforts? On occasion, we might even pose some nonclinical problem, such as how to deal with a guest who is always late or how to respond to being pulled over for a driving infraction. This not only helps convey the nonpathologic aspect of the model—that is, "problems are problems," and the distinction between "clinical" and "nonclinical" is an artificial one—but can serve as a way of checking how well trainees are picking up the elements of the approach by being able to apply them to very different contexts. Moreover, it aids in assessing how much they have departed from their accustomed ways of viewing and handling problems.

Trainer–Trainee Relationship

The relationship between trainer and trainee is close to the traditional academic or teaching context. This does not mean lectures, examinations, or grading, but rather the idea that the trainer has become accomplished in his craft (i.e., doing therapy briefly) and has sufficient ability to impart that knowledge to interested professionals. As with the traditional role of a teacher, we feel this view should include an openness to comments and suggestions by trainees, regarding both ongoing treatment of clients and the training itself. However, in decisions regarding both we assume the ultimate responsibility is the trainer's. Thus, our view of training is isomorphic with our view and practice of therapy: the therapist is primarily responsible for directing the course and outcome of treatment; the trainer is primarily responsible for directing the course and outcome of training. In direct supervision, this responsibility also includes the treatment of the client, since the trainer is the "metatherapist." For example, a therapist–trainee accustomed to using an insight-oriented approach might disagree with the trainer who is insisting that he or she get the client to be more specific about some data, the trainee believing that the client needs time to "ventilate." This disparity of view will be discussed with the trainee and, most often, the trainer will give reasons for pinning the client down to specifics and then insist the trainee go ahead with that plan. If necessary, the trainer will offer some suggestions as to how to expedite that effort.

Trainee Problems

What might be called "resistance issues" have not arisen because in training, as well as in therapy, we do not think in terms of resistance. This does not mean that trainees will not have difficulty in grasping or implementing the approach, but we attribute those difficulties to the trainees' frame of reference and, early in training, to an unawareness that they have been operating from a frame of reference. In addition, we assume that some of the trainees' passivity and awkwardness at interviewing stems from their self-consciousness in being observed. Most of the trainees are unaccustomed to such observation, especially when it includes peers as well as a supervisor. Thus, if a trainee is "flubbing" a message phoned in by the trainer, we do not assume he or she is being resistant, but that the trainee is anxious in the situation. We will discuss this after the session is over. In that regard, there is not a great deal we believe we can do to help the trainee to become significantly more relaxed, since it is a context inherently fraught with anxiety. Most often it seems enough to acknowledge that the trainees are in an extremely difficult spot, that anxiety and self-consciousness are to be expected, and for that matter that the trainers themselves are still not comfortable being observed after all their years of working under observation. Finally, the postsession and presession discussions of the cases the trainees are working on partly involve formulating a "game plan" for the upcoming session; these guidelines can also reduce anxiety on the trainee's part.

Problems arising from the trainees' frame of reference have been discussed earlier, but a summary of them at this point might be useful. They encompass a few general areas. First, some trainees enter the training with the misconception that the approach consists of just some body of clever, usually "paradoxical" interventions. Such trainees will attempt to use interventions inappropriately with their clients. To offset this expectation, we have been emphasizing, early in training, that the brevity of treatment depends primarily on the simplicity of the model—"knowing what not to bother with"—rather than on interventions per se. In earlier intensive training, we had not made that distinction clear. Another broad area of difficulty occurs with trainees accustomed to an insight-oriented approach. Such an approach is consistent with a more passive role by the therapist. However, in our strategic and problem-oriented approach, just the opposite role is necessary; the therapist needs to be in deliberate control of the overall treatment and its pacing. Problems in supervision occur when trainees allow clients to dominate the conversation and are hesitant to interrupt, partly because they are concerned about interfering with the client's "need to ventilate" and partly because they believe it necessary to convey "acceptance" to the client. Again, in insight-oriented models, the therapist is inclined to listen for the "meaning behind the meaning" rather than take time to ask the client for clarification of vague or contradictory comments. Helping trainees to become more active and intrusive is one of the major hurdles in teaching the Brief Therapy approach. The very format of direct supervision can aid the trainee in the desired direction, since it inherently involves interruptions by the supervisor. A significant percentage of the calls into the treatment room direct the trainee to ask the client for clarification of a statement. Moreover, in the postsession discussion the supervisor will explain the calls relating the pacing of that session and the activity required of the therapist to the basic rationale of the treatment approach.

A related difficulty is that trainees will ask for elaboration of data which are, in our model, irrelevant to the problem. Thus, trainers will ask the trainee to drop a line of questioning about tangential data and get back to the data revolving around the client's complaint. Again, we rely on the postsession discussion to aid the trainee in grasping the differences between the model they have been accustomed to using and the model they are attempting to shift to; that some kinds of data are relevant for some models but not for others. A trainee used to a normative model will attempt to get the client to elaborate on information mentioned regarding any variations from "the norm," even though it is quite clear that the client is not expressing dissatisfaction with those features of his or her life. The trainee, then, may be jarred when the trainer calls and says that such data are not important and to drop that line of investigation. During the postsession discussion we will explain at more length the non-normative feature of our model and the internal logic of not attaching importance to and pursuing such information.

Finally, a number of trainees will "resist" utilizing reframing as a deliberate maneuver to influence the client. This is because they have been accustomed to think of the therapist's role as an "honest" one, meant to point out to the client what the therapist believes to be "true," especially when the client is not "facing reality." Thus, the more avowedly manipulative aspect of our approach is uncomfortably alien to them. Even if they see the relevance of it, they will still hold back, believing that they couldn't pull it off believably. "I'm not that good an actor." The latter problem is easier to deal with, since trainees usually find that "poor actors" though they might be, the client, more often than not, will readily accept their reframing. The former problem is usually dealt with by reiterating the concept that, as ours is a problem-solving approach, we are interested in getting the client to *do* something different regarding the problem rather than to understand the problem. In that light, we need to use wording that will enhance the acceptance of and the carrying out of action suggestions. After some repetition of that paradigm, trainees have less trouble using the client's frame of reference, rather than seeking to alter that frame.

CONCLUSION

Since our program is relatively young (in operation only about 8 years), we are open to suggestions about and criticisms of the training by the trainees. We are not inclined to see those suggestions and criticisms as "resistance." For example, when trainees urged us to come into the treatment room more often rather than restrict communications to the intercom phone, we did not view this as an attempt to "get off the hook" from the responsibility of treating the client. We were not sure how useful or counterproductive it would be, but we were willing to give it a try, and it seems to have worked out well. Another group had asked us to limit the time spent in indirect supervision and, instead, add another case for direct supervision. We did so for the remainder of that group's training but found that it left too little time to discuss and digest what was happening in any one case; we were all too swamped simply keeping up with the clinical elements of the cases. Subsequently, we felt more assured in discouraging it when a later group asked for the same arrangement, giving them our experience and our reasoning for not continuing with it.

Because of the relative newness, for us, of this kind of training, we have not given much thought to future trends, nor of making controlled assessments of success or failure of training, desirable as those things might be. We have been content to persist in the main format and structure of the training, but have made an informal attempt to increase trainee input in the training as well as in treating their cases. Two other factors, in addition to the newness, have convinced us that there is no significant need to readjust the training. First, while we have discussed difficulties trainees have, for the most part they have shown evidence of profiting from the training in taperecorded sessions with clients they are working with in their own jobs and practices. At some point, we will probably want to get a more accurate assessment of changes in trainees' ways of conducting therapy. The second reason we are not in a hurry to formalize assessments and alterations in the training is that we have found ourselves learning from the very difficulties trainees have had. For example, we originally had assumed and taught that obtaining data about the complaint was simply *one* of the items of information needed along with some other items. However, listening to trainees' complaints about having difficulty with "where to go with this client," we became aware that the single most strategic element in their confusion was a lack of clarity about the complaint the client was registering. As a result, we have come to place prime importance on clarifying the problem, seeing that as the major and most strategic task of the therapy; all other aspects of treatment flow from that one datum. In less fundamental but still important ways, we have learned to tighten up our own understanding of the relationship between model and practice; this too has come from difficulties and challenging questions of the trainees. We hope this kind of learning continues to happen.

References

Fisch, R., Weakland, J., & Segal, L. (1982). *The tactics of change: Doing therapy briefly.* San Francisco: Jossey-Bass.

Watzlawick, P., Weakland, J., & Fisch, R. (1974). *Change: Principles of problem formation and problem resolution.* New York: W. W. Norton.

Weakland, J., Fisch, R., Watzlawick, P., & Bodin, A. (1974). *Brief psychotherapy: Focused problem resolution. Family Process, 13*(2), 141–168.

6

Training Strategic Therapists:
The Use of Indirect Techniques

JUDITH MAZZA
Center for Problem Solving, Bethesda, Maryland

Training a strategic therapist involves the design of a specific and individualized plan by the supervisor. The plan followed may be shared with the therapist or may be indirect and not shared. This chapter will discuss the conceptual process used during strategic supervision, and the techniques for achieving change.

ADMINISTRATIVE CONTEXT

Strategic therapists are generally trained "live." A small group of therapists meets to observe each other and discuss their work. The therapists who are observing may make comments or ask questions of the supervisor, but may not instruct or advise the therapist in any way. A clear hierarchy is established in which the supervisor is responsible for simultaneously training therapists and solving clients' problems. It is assumed that a therapist who brings certain life experiences to the therapy (such as raising a family, struggling with clinical issues, or developing a range of interests) will be more successful than an inexperienced therapist. Families are protected from the inexperienced therapist by the live supervision, and sometimes report that they look forward to knowing that more than one therapist is working on solving their problems. Each therapist is assigned a supervisor who discusses the intake and plans the initial phone call with the therapist. The therapist calls, sets the appointment, and arranges for the relevant family members to attend the first session.

Therapists have the opportunity to treat a wide range of clients, including those with acute and chronic problems, clear symptoms and vague dilemmas, from the needy and the upper class, and of all ages. The therapists must be trained to deal with each type of situation. After the first year of supervision, a therapist may not devise a brilliant strategy, but should be able to conduct a clear first interview with any client.

The Family Therapy Institute of Washington, D.C., follows the strategic model of Haley (1976) and Madanes (1981, 1984) in which the therapy is expected to be brief, problem-focused, with planned sessions and an active therapist. The supervisorial emphasis is on helping a therapist to have maximum success. While therapists in the group behind the one-way mirror are encouraged to make constructive comments, ask questions, and suggest interventions, they are prevented by the supervisor from making analytic or disparaging remarks about their colleagues. Nontrainee observers are not permitted behind the mirror on a regular basis; the privilege of observing another's therapy is earned by exposing one's own work. The goal of the training is to prepare therapists to work in a variety of settings, not be dependent on a team behind a one-way mirror.

INCREASING THE THERAPEUTIC RANGE

Each therapist must learn ways to change the families being treated, and be able to generate new strategies for future families. Training therapists in a directive therapy requires a directive training, in which therapists learn by doing. As the behavior of the therapist changes, his or her thinking about how to approach problems and solve human dilemmas will change. The strategic supervisor designs interventions to effect these changes. Being able to describe and teach therapy is a different skill than successfully solving a client's problem.

As a therapist works in front of the one-way mirror, providing a demonstration interview for colleagues, the supervisor is lecturing the group of therapists behind the mirror. In this way, the supervisor is constantly teaching therapists at meta-levels. Comments that are made in relation to the therapist working in front of the mirror are made also in relation to the therapists behind the mirror. Although therapists are taught specific technical skills, the training emphasizes the development of a conceptual framework. This framework provides a method of thinking rather than a method of therapy.

One goal of the strategic supervisor is to develop a framework for each therapist. This framework, or method of thinking, is individually crafted to make best use of that therapist's skills. A therapist who has a clear method of thinking will be more likely to generate clear interventions and strategies.

Every therapist has a range of interventions to use, and a range of therapeutic postures to assume, to implement a variety of interventions. A therapist should develop the capacity to be serious, humorous, light, heavy, democratic, authoritarian, flirtatious, humble, expert, and so forth. If a therapist has an increased range of postures that can be assumed, he or she will have increased the range of interventions possible, and will probably succeed with a broader range of clients. Part of developing this range includes teaching the therapist how to be humble, how to apologize, and how to take a helpless position.

A therapist should be comfortable being the central figure—so that all communication among family members goes through him or her—and comfortable being peripheral—so that the family interacts on its own. The therapist should be familiar with when to use each position. Another part of the development of the therapist's range is to be able to tell someone clearly and directly what to do. Therapists should be able to give a broad range of strategic directives in such a way that they will be clearly understood. The therapist, like the conductor of an orchestra, should be able to build motivation over the course of a therapy session, carefully laying the groundwork for the directives and interventions that follow. Alternatively, a therapist may seed ideas during one session and build to a major intervention over several sessions.

THE UNIT OF CHANGE

The unit considered for intervention by a strategic supervisor is broad. It includes the administrative context, the group of students behind the mirror, the therapist and family in front of the mirror, and his or her own involvement. A supervisor who thinks in terms of individuals may consider problems the therapist shows as being due to some personality problem of the therapist (he or she is too rigid, is too shy, has an unresolved conflict, etc.). In that way of thinking, the resolution of the therapist's problem would be found in some intrapsychic manner. A supervisor who thinks dyadically may consider the therapist's problem as the result of some difficulty with that specific client (he or she needs to get the father to talk more in the session). After making the conceptual leap to an interactional approach, the supervisor thinks contextually or organizationally, that is, looks at a sequence of events that may "require" the problem behavior. A naive observer of the supervision might think the supervisor is focused only on changing the therapist's behavior, and consequently consider the unit of change to be the therapist and the family. More careful observation indicates the supervisor must take into account a complex system involving the context of the client, the context of the therapist, and the context of the supervisor.

HIERARCHICAL CONSIDERATIONS

A basic premise of the strategic model is that pathology develops when there are confusions in existing hierarchies (Haley, 1976) that may be displayed in the form of simultaneously occurring incongruous hierarchies (Madanes, 1981). The existing hierarchical relationship between therapist and supervisor cannot be ignored, and is carried into the therapy room. The way in which the supervisor expects the therapist to behave toward the family being treated is directly related to the way in which the supervisor behaves toward the therapist being trained. If a supervisor were to develop a coalition in which he or she rescued the family and disenfranchised the therapist, it is assumed that additional problems would develop; the family might drop out of treatment, attempt to disqualify the therapist, or attempt to deal more directly with the supervisor. It is possible for the supervisor to enter the therapy room without disenfranchising the therapist. It is easier, however, for the family to respect the existing hierarchy when the supervisor avoids direct contact with the client and goes through the therapist.

The hierarchical relationship with the therapist must be considered carefully when the supervisor intervenes on behalf of the client. A therapist observing a mother being negative and reprimanding her child in the therapy session may be tempted to tell the mother not to do that, and in that way reprimand the mother. The supervisor, observing the therapist and the family, may call the therapist, point out this error, and tell him or her to put the mother down by reprimanding her. Thus, the mother's "negative" behavior toward the child has precipitated the therapist's negative behavior toward the mother and, in turn, the supervisor's negative behavior toward the therapist. If the supervisor reprimands the therapist, the therapist is more likely to reprimand the mother, who is then more likely to reprimand the child. What is necessary in this instance is for the supervisor to intervene less directly. One possibility would be for the supervisor to call the therapist and assign a task that will change the focus in the room, without explaining the reason for doing so at that time. The reason can be explained later, when reviewing a videotape. Generally, the milder the problem, the more democratically the supervisor can behave. The more emergent and crisis-oriented the case, the more authoritarian the supervisor, and consequently the therapist, must be. This authoritarian stance by the supervisor will strengthen the therapist and help to steer the family through a crisis.

UTILIZATION OF SKILLS

The skills to develop as a strategic therapist—the supervisory strategies as well as the psychotherapeutic strategies—derive from hypnosis.[1] Well trained strategic therapists also think how best to utilize client behavior and motivation quickly and courteously. Just as this is a therapy of courtesy (Haley, 1976), so the supervision is a supervision of courtesy. Each therapist brings with him or her certain strengths, a philosophy, and particular life experiences. It is the task of the strategic supervisor to design a plan by which those strengths and experiences can best be used in relation to building a framework for the therapist that allows more effective treatment of clients. During live supervision, the supervisory interventions are individually designed for a particular therapist in the context of treating a particular client.

Clearly, some therapists will be more difficult to train than others. The supervisor should be ready to accept the therapist's presenting behaviors and to design a way of building on the therapist's abilities. The supervisor should initially strive to develop a good rapport in order to have a working relationship with the therapist. It is not necessary that the supervisor be "liked" by the trainee, but that the trainee learn from the supervisor. The supervisor who thinks the most important dimension in training the therapist is to be liked by the therapist might limit the range of interventions in the supervision.

One supervisor was having great difficulty with a trainee. Whatever was asked of this particular therapist resulted in an argument. The supervisor was puzzled and concerned that the therapist was not making good use of the training. The therapist, an older man, was quite experienced in his private practice but was having a difficult time understanding the strategic model. The supervisor's supervisor suggested that the supervisor begin each supervisory session by asking the therapist what he had planned for the session. The supervisor was to inquire politely into the therapist's hypotheses about the case and the rationale for each planned intervention. The supervisor was to maintain a benevolent and courteous attitude toward the therapist, but was not to offer any suggestions unless explicitly requested by the therapist. After the supervisor adopted this strategy, the arguments ceased and the therapist began to ask the supervisor's advice during the sessions. This supervision strategy allowed both supervisor and therapist to win. In the event that the therapist did not need supervision, he would succeed by successfully carrying out the therapy. In the event that he did have difficulty and asked for supervision, he would win again. In the event that the therapist did need the supervision but would not accept a plan directly from the supervisor, he had the opportunity to engage in a more collegial discussion. It is not recommended that this strategy be used with every argumentative trainee, any more than a particular technique should be used with every argumentative family! A strategy that is appropriate for one therapist may not be appropriate for another.

Sometimes a supervisor might think of an intervention that is appropriate for a particular client but that the therapist cannot carry out. One therapist had a rather narrow range and had been working unsuccessfully with a couple for about six months. As the couple appeared grim and hopeless, it was important to lighten the session as a way of indicating that change was possible. One possible directive depended on the therapist's willingness to be a bit flirtatious with the husband and say: "I can tell by the twinkle in your eye that you are a man with a good sense of humor. It has been my experience that men with a good sense of humor are able to. . . ." For the therapist to be light and humorous in the session, it would be useful for the supervisor to be light and humorous with the therapist. Because of the newness of the supervisory relationship, as well as the therapist's anxiety and lack of humor, it was clear that the therapist would not give the directive in a way that would lighten the session. The husband most likely would have argued with the therapist about his sense of humor! The supervisor changed her plan. The actual directives used concentrated on tactics familiar to the therapist and utilized the therapist's directive style and serious nature.

Another example of designing an individual strategy for a therapist is seen in the case of a psychoanalytically trained psychiatrist. In his analytic training, this psychiatrist had learned to comment cleverly on and interpret metaphor. Although he reported success with his individual analytic patients, it was not a successful strategy with the family he was curently treating. The identified patient, a schizophrenic young man, thought that werewolves were going to kill his wife. Whenever the psychiatrist would comment on a metaphoric communication, the family would verbally attack and attempt to disqualify him. Because of the intensity and depth of this therapist's previous training, he persisted in making interpretations despite the supervisor's instructions to the contrary. The supervisor stopped advising him directly. Sometimes she would let the family successfully attack him. Other times she deflected the attack with a directive designed to interrupt the sequence. After some weeks employing this strategy, the therapist stopped commenting on the family's metaphors; he had realized that making analytic interpretations was inappropriate with this family.

Haley (1976) says that metaphoric communication is a language of courtesy and should be received by the therapist as courteously as it was given:

> It is assumed that . . . they do not lack understanding but a way to resolve the problem. To force them to concede . . . is discourteous. Accepting their way of presenting the problem and offering a change within that framework shows respect for them. The crucial difference in point of view centers on whether the therapist thinks that patients need education and understanding. If the patient already understands, what he needs is a graceful way out of the problem. (p. 212)

Interpretation violates the nature of the communication by being too direct, and is therefore discourteous. Attempts to interpret metaphor will oversimplify a complex analogic communication in the same way that describing a painting will oversimplify that art form. The therapist who wishes to respond properly will do so in the same form the patient did, that is, metaphorically. Responding in metaphor is an advanced therapeutic skill. Most beginning therapists are better off to listen respectfully, to treat the information communicated as a gift, and use the information in designing a strategy.

VARIOUS TECHNIQUES OF INDIRECT TRAINING

The use of indirect forms of suggestion in therapy was pioneered by Milton Erickson. The most significant characteristic of indirect suggestion is that the "subject's own unique repertory of associations and behavioral potentials can be activated in the response" (Erickson & Rossi, 1980). Indirect supervision strategies should enable a therapist to generate more strategies than a supervision that, by being totally direct, ignores many of the resources a therapist possesses. Using indirect techniques also allows the supervisor a greater range of supervision strategies needed when training a variety of therapists.

When a strategic supervisor is working within a context that produces change in a therapist, paradoxical techniques are powerful tools. For a paradox to be successful, it must be executed within a context. Haley (1963) points out that the very nature of therapy is paradoxical. The therapist may direct the client to spontaneously behave differently when he or she is not in the therapist's presence. Likewise, a supervisor may direct a therapist to spontaneously design interventions for other clients after the supervision has ended.

An example of a paradoxical intervention from a therapy case may clarify the advantages of a benevolent framework. A therapist had been struggling with a difficult and chronic problem. The therapy had not been going well, no significant change was being made, and the therapist was becoming discouraged. A new strategy was needed. Supervisor and therapist implemented a restraining intervention in which the benefits of not solving the problem were carefully described to the client. The paradox was that, within this context of seeking change (the client came to the therapist for help), when no change was prescribed (because of the described "benefits" of the symptom), the only position left to the client was to prove that he could change. Haley (1963, p. 54) notes that "when a hypnotist encourages a subject to resist him after asking for cooperation, the subject is in a peculiar situation. If he resists he is doing as asked, and if he cooperates he is doing as asked." If the client continues to display the symptom, it is now under the therapist's direction. The only way that this patient could be "one up" was to prove the therapist's directive of no change ineffective. When change occurred, the therapist acted slightly puzzled, surprised, and confused as to how and why there was a change. If the therapist were to say gleefully, "I knew that if I told you not to change you would change!" the intervention would be ruined. Likewise, when implementing a paradoxical supervision strategy, the reaction of the supervisor to the therapist's new success is crucial.

When a supervisor has identified a clear supervisory problem, and the therapist has been unable to correct the error easily, the supervisor may consider the advantages of paradoxically prescribing the therapist's error. Like all symptom prescriptions, the hypothesis is that if the therapist can control the error by increasing its frequency, he can also decrease or eliminate it. Madanes (1984) relates a supervision strategy used by Haley:

> Haley . . . tells about his approach to a very shy student, who was terrified of Haley's supervision behind the one way mirror. He instructed her to go into the therapy room to interview a family and to be sure to properly make three mistakes. Two of these mistakes would be obvious, and one mistake would be one that would not be evident to Haley. The student conducted the interview and after a while came out of the room to discuss the problem with Haley. He asked, "Did you make the three mistakes correctly?" She answered, "Screw you!" and was no longer overconcerned about his opinion. (pp. 130–131)

It should be noted how important a benevolent framework is when working in this way. If this therapist had thought that Haley wanted her to fail and look foolish, she might have become more nervous than before. As Madanes pointed out, she was after all in a context of learning to do therapy properly; to be asked to make three mistakes by her supervisor is incongruous. Most paradoxes have a benevolent framework and are constructed with incongruities.

Another therapist being supervised, whose native tongue was not English, often needed to rephrase several times the directives she gave as interventions. But each time she repeated a directive, the meaning would be altered in a way that was clear to a native English speaker, but unclear to her. Thus, the family (and the supervisor) would be faced with a barrage of statements, each similar to the last, but each with a slightly different meaning. The therapist was therefore told that she should concentrate on saying each statement three times, that each time the directive should resemble the last, and that the meaning should change very slightly. She was to concentrate on doing this in the first 20 minutes of the interview. The therapist couldn't understand the reason for doing this. She was told that it would serve to confuse the family and that they would appreciate her clarity and be more likely to follow her directives later in the interview. She became so preoccupied with devising ways of revising her comments that when the 20 minutes were up she gladly said each directive just once. She subsequently said that the first 20 minutes had been very hard work, and that she did not want to repeat the experience. The supervisor talked about the advantages of this technique and very reluctantly agreed to let her discontinue the repetitions.

A restraining intervention that has been successful with therapists who need to be motivated further in their work is to increase frustration through the "You're not ready yet" technique. Telling a therapist that he or she is not ready to implement a particularly interesting intervention can be done in a straigthforward manner with therapists who are uncertain and shy. It allows them to take the time to observe more skillful colleagues, study videotapes, and concentrate on their reading. At the other extreme are the "blasé expert" therapists who assume that they know more than they do. Use of this strategy with these therapists may generate some anger toward the supervisor. The supervisor should be prepared to specify how the therapist might become ready. When the frustration becomes high enough, the therapist will be more curious, accepting of the current training, and ready to put aside previous learning. The supervisor who finds it necessary to increase the therapist's frustration further can pay more attention to therapists who are ready. When working hypnotically, the supervisor can further increase frustration by using dangling phrases and incomplete sentences. The therapist will pay greatest attention to the sentences and directives that are complete.

Having the opportunity to work with groups of therapists presents the supervisor with the possibility of using teaching anecdotes about other therapists as a training tool. Erickson was a master in his use of anecdotes or teaching tales. Anecdotes can be used in a variety of ways. They can be used to embed directives in a particular therapist or group of therapists, who can listen to problems other therapists have, how those problems were solved, their struggles with particular clients, and new interventions and techniques. Anecdotes assist the therapist both in understanding issues that are common to other therapists, and in having hope for future improvement of skills. The therapist listening to an anecdote can apply the relevant parts of that anecdote on one level and absorb other aspects on a different level. Discussing problems that therapists encounter from a new perspective (i.e., the vantage point of a story) allows the therapist to respond to the supervisor in a new way. Some stories may promote uncertainty and allow a therapist to ask for help less directly. When telling stories about therapists, the supervisor should give the therapist's error some positive connotation. This allows the therapist the opportunity to describe future errors to the supervisor and ask for advice. Therapists tend to re-member these anecdotes clearly. Sometimes, months later, a therapist will say, "Re-member the therapist you were talking about who . . . ," and then describe an analogous situation.

Another technique is using a directive for the family that is an indirect communica-tion to the therapist. For example, the supervisor can call the therapist and say, "Tell the father *he will have more success* the more *clearly he tells him* [referring to the father's son] *what to do.*" Here the supervisor is indirectly telling the therapist that if he (the therapist) will be more clear with the father, he will have greater success. An advanced supervisor can work at metaphoric levels designing interventions for both the therapist and the family.

A well known supervisor was observing a female therapist who was quite rigid. The case she had was one in which a young man was having difficulty separating from his parents and developing relationships with women, and was afraid of being considered effeminate. A problem for both the supervision and the therapy was that when the female therapist told this young man what to do, it weakened his position in relation to other young women. The supervisor had the therapist act helpless and naive, asking the young man questions as if she were somewhat bewildered. When he complained that he didn't know how to behave on a date, the therapist responded by saying, "You think men have a hard time, let me tell you about the position of a young woman on a date. If the man makes a pass, she thinks that he doesn't respect her. If he doesn't make a pass, then she thinks that she is ugly and unattractive!" The therapist continued in this manner, using herself as a metaphor for an anxious young woman. A short time later, the young man found a girlfriend. Now the therapist became more flexible and kindly, and began dressing in a more feminine manner. The supervisory directives regarding a more feminine position produced a change in both client and therapist.

In another example, the same supervisor was observing a young, intense, and very determined male therapist. He was working with an alcoholic who was considerably older than he was. The harder the earnest young therapist worked, the more passive and sullen the client became. The supervisor changed strategies and told the therapist to begin each statement by saying, "I'm not going to tell you that you should . . . respect you wife . . . love your children . . . stop drinking . . ." and so forth. The supervisor told the therapist that the rationale for the intervention was to allow an older man to save face by not accepting advice given directly by a younger man. However, the intervention also had the covert effect of helping the therapist to be more detached and relaxed in the session.

Another well known supervisor sometimes gives a nonverbal task to therapists who usually concentrate only on what people say. For example, he will call such a therapist and say, "This interview will be a success if by the end of the hour the couple is sitting with their legs crossed toward each other." The therapist cannot achieve this through verbalization alone. It requires a change in body posture and close attention to nonverbal communication. Likewise, this supervisor will direct a change in the seating arrangement in the room as a metaphor for a structural shift in the family or as a metaphor for the desired position of the therapist.

A supervisor may find it useful to use Erickson's confusional approach when dealing with sophisticated therapists who have basic strategies and tactics clearly in mind. Beginning therapists generally do not benefit from directives that are given in a confusing or obscure way. The guidelines for using this technique with an advanced therapist are the same as Erickson described in his paper entitled "The Confusion Technique in Hypnosis." Dr. Erickson described the technique (Haley, 1967) as involving the

> consistent maintenance of a general casual but definitely interested attitude, and speaking in a gravely earnest and intent manner expressive of certain, utterly complete, expectations of their understanding of what is being said or done together with an extremely careful shifting of the tenses employed. Also of great importance is a ready flow of language, rapid for the fast thinker, slower for the slower-minded, but always being careful to give a little time for a response but never quite sufficient . . . the whole process is repeated with a continued development of a state of inhibition, leading to confusion and a growing need to receive a clear-cut comprehensible communication to which they can make a ready and full response. (p. 130)

This technique is best employed when the therapist comes out of the therapy room and behind the mirror, but not over the supervision phone. Assuming that the therapist is advanced, but having difficulty with the particular session, the supervisor may begin talking in the way that Erickson described. The therapist should not be given time to speak on entering the observation room. The supervisor's intervention stuns the therapist into silence. The first clear supervisory directive will be followed immediately by the therapist. For example, one supervisor called a therapist out of the room and talked in a most hypnotic fashion, with dangling sentences, a change in tenses, and at a pace that was different from normal speech. After a short while, she said to the therapist who had been having trouble with the interventions called over the phone, "Now (pause), take this pad of paper and write down what you are to do when you go back into the room." The therapist immediately took the pad of paper and pen and wrote down what the supervisor indicated. He did not have any difficulty with the rest of the session.

This technique would be contraindicated for a therapist who is generally in a state of confusion. It would be better for this therapist to be given instructions clearly, simply, and with short statements. The use of confusion as a supervision tool is indicated only for advanced supervisors. It is important that a supervisor clearly know what he or she wants the therapist to do before using this technique. Just as the strategic therapist takes responsibility for designing an intervention to solve the clients' problems, so the strategic supervisor takes responsibility for designing interventions to expand and broaden the therapist's range and success with cases.

Having therapists imagine that they are someone else is another technique that derives from hypnosis. A young therapist was struggling with a family in which the parents were much older than he. The therapist was close in age to the identified patient. Because of the therapist's youth and lack of experience, he had difficulty conducting himself in a way that truly convinced the parents that he was an expert. The supervisor noticed that the therapist was talking too quickly (due to anxiety) and was sitting forward in a nervous fashion. The therapist was called out of the therapy room and asked to behave as if he were his grandfather. He was to talk at the pace that his grandfather talked, sit as his grandfather would sit, and generally carry himself as his grandfather would carry himself. The therapist went back into the therapy room. The change was quite remarkable. Indeed, the pacing of his words changed, his body posture changed, and the reaction of the parents of the identified patient changed. They took him more seriously, as if by changing his nonverbal behavior he had entered their generation.

A supervisor skilled in hypnosis can place the therapist into a trance in order to capture and focus the therapist's attention on the supervision. The new focus will be communicated to the family when the therapist goes back into the therapy room. Through the use of hypnosis, the supervisor can suspend what is ordinary, can more easily introduce the absurd, and can fix the dynamics of the case more clearly in the therapist's mind.

Madanes (1981) has worked most successfully with similar interventions involving "pretending." In those interventions, the changes are obtained when family members are asked to step into another way of behaving, and consciously choose to behave in that different way. Changes can also be obtained in a therapist who is "pretending" to behave in a different way.

In another indirect teaching technique that derives from both Erickson and Haley, the supervisor provides a "worse" alternative for the therapist. For example, a new therapist was very nervous about being supervised in front of the mirror for the first time by a well known supervisor. The therapist confessed his nervousness. The supervisor told the therapist (who was about to have a first interview with a difficult heroin addict) that the family was *so* difficult and would give the therapist *such* a hard time that he wouldn't have an opportunity to be nervous about the mirror! The therapist later reported that each supervisory intervention was most comforting because the family was so difficult. The supervisor had provided the alternative that the family would be more difficult than the supervision.

Throughout the training day, the strategic supervisor can be seeding ideas for therapists to develop at a later point. In his work, Dr. Erickson would begin with an idea, drop it for a while, and come back to it later after it had had time to take effect. This is an excellent indirect strategy for supervision as well; supervisors can seed ideas about the proper way to present cases, how to diagram a case, the importance of reading, what more advanced therapists know, how to begin advancing oneself, and so on.

A supervisory strategy that derives directly from the idea of "pacing" in hypnosis is for the supervisor to anticipate a therapist's reaction to a directive. This is useful with the therapist who tends to disagree with whatever the supervisor is suggesting. The supervisor could say, "This may sound crazy, but I know that it will work . . . ," or, "I have a plan that will definitely work and that you will be sure to disagree with." This preempts the therapist's opportunity to disagree with the supervisor.

From time to time, it is important to allow the therapist the privilege of learning from his or her mistakes, and to let the therapist fail. The supervisor should not let the session fail, but allow the trainee to make some errors. The dilemma in the live supervision situation is that the supervisor assumes a rather direct responsibility for the case. Thus, a supervisor who thinks that a particular therapist could benefit from making mistakes must be careful that the errors are not ethically compromising to anyone involved. There is a rather delicate balance that must be struck between the responsibility for training the therapist and that of helping the family. This dilemma is even more acute when therapy is provided at a training institute as opposed to a clinic. Haley suggests that second-year students should do the first interview of their second training year without supervision calls. Supervisors are expected to come from behind the mirror if there is a problem, but it is diagnostically important for these therapists to try to conduct a session without input from the supervisor. This is especially useful for therapists who work in isolated settings. The supervisor should observe the errors therapists make in that situation, and how they rescue themselves. That diagnostic information can be the basis for supervisory strategies.

TYPES OF THERAPISTS

There are obviously as many different therapists as there are families. At the risk of oversimplification, I will proceed to characterize eight types of therapists frequently found in training institutes, and discuss possible supervisory strategies for each.

The Overly Eager Therapist

This therapist comes to the training having read everything by Haley and Madanes. He or she cannot wait to begin, and is impatient, wanting a case quickly, perhaps wanting to show off in front of colleagues, or to demonstrate how well read he or she is. Often this therapist is more dogmatic and orthodox than the authors he or she is emulating. The first step for the strategic supervisor is to understand what problem this therapist is demonstrating. The therapist may have a veneer of competence, so that the supervisor may think that there is little or nothing to teach. As the goal of strategic supervision is to increase range and flexibility, one issue for the supervisor is how to instruct in a way that allows this therapist to maneuver successfully without thinking the maneuvers are written in stone. It is important that the therapist's behavior does not provoke the supervisor to take an even more expert (and sometimes dogmatic) position. The therapist's enthusiasm should be utilized during the supervision. This therapist will generally complete given tasks thoroughly and well. The strategic supervisor should not hesitate to ask this therapist to complete written assignments and case studies. One possible intervention is to have this therapist review videotapes, re-read case materials, and observe the variety of ways a particular therapeutic objective can be achieved. For example, the therapist could write 20 ways of increasing the father's position in the hierarchy, or describe 15 ways to decrease the identified patient's power. The supervisory objective would be to help this therapist remain flexible and become less dogmatic while maintaining enthusiasm and goodwill.

The Totally Passive Therapist

"I'm in your hands now." This therapist doesn't generate ideas, but waits for the supervisor to phone directives before making a move. This therapist has not learned enough of a conceptual framework to generalize from one case to the next, and may be petrified of making a mistake, or assume that none of his ideas will be worthy. Unlike the therapist in the previous example, the supervisor needs to provoke this therapist to action. It is important for the supervisor to check that the required reading has been done and to determine whether the lack of initiative is due to ignorance, modesty, or fear. The supervisor should inquire carefully before each session what plan the therapist has generated. This should be done in a kindly manner and will, with repetition, help the therapist to understand that he or she should have a plan before each session. The supervisor should be clear that this therapist understands the structure of the family he or she is working with, and the theoretical rationale for various interventions. The therapist should be praised for anything initiated during the session. In addition to these interventions, the supervisor may use techniques that produce mild frustration, such as the "you're not ready yet" technique. Any interventions for the family that require action on the part of the therapist are useful. Having the therapist move people's position in the room indirectly provokes some action on the part of the therapist. Telling stories about other therapists in the beginning of training, how they become more active and directive, may help as well. The supervisor can ask this therapist's opinion as to what another therapist should do next.

The Blasé Expert

"I've done this all before, I've been trained at the Ackerman Institute, the Mental Research Institute, The Philadelphia Child Guidance Center, The Milan Group," etc. This therapist may be comparing the current work unfavorably with other places he or she has trained (and may have done the same thing at each of the other training institutes). There is a sense that the therapist is engaging in the training just to say that he or she has done it, rather than to broaden the repertoire. It is important that this therapist be challenged to shed previous trainings and concentrate on this way of working. One possibility is to utilize the interest in various models of training by encouragement to study this one in as "pure" a way as possible during the brief time available. It would be easy for the strategic supervisor to become caught in "selling" the strategic model as superior to others. It is much better if the supervisor can maintain a courteous attitude and arouse the curiosity of the therapist as to the interventions being employed. Use of confusion may quiet a particularly aggressive therapist, as he or she will not want to appear ignorant. Indirect techniques are generally best. Telling the group stories about therapists who came to the training and did not leave with more than they arrived with can be useful. The supervisor may want to take a modest position and to help the therapist focus on the client's problems rather than on the theoretical model. In extreme cases, the supervisor may permit the therapist to make a few errors and ask for advice. If the supervisor does not imply that a "revolution" is underway, and that only those who sincerely wish to learn can be taught, the "blasé expert" may back down.

The Nonpracticing Dabbler

This therapist is interested in the therapy on some theoretical level. For instance, such a therapist may hold an academic position at a university and be in charge of training graduate students in psychotherapy. One of the supervisory issues is that this therapist thinks he knows more than he does about therapy. This therapist is often well read, but has little actual experience. Because this therapist may have status outside the training facility, it is important he or she not be embarrassed. In the beginning, the supervisor may suggest the therapist approach the interview as a beginning therapist. A face-saving rationale should be given for this. One possibility is to say that it would enhance the teaching of beginning therapists to place oneself in the position of one. Thus, the therapist can be asked to step out of character and pretend to be a novice. The supervisor could also ask that this be done for the sake of the other students who are observing. The notion would be to prepare for training graduate students. The supervisor must be especially careful if this therapist is considerably older than the supervisor is. The therapist may have dabbled in many different approaches over many years; these experiences should be respected and appreciated. It is important that the supervisor maintain the hierarchical position in regard to this therapist, and find ways of blocking should the therapist begin to lecture the group behind the mirror. In addition to using indirect techniques, the supervisor should encourage the therapist to begin a private practice or provide volunteer clinical services outside the training facility.

The Digital-Compulsive Note-taker

This therapist always asks the supervisor to repeat directives, and copies them verbatim, but never seems to integrate ideas or to generate new ones. This therapist will often have an encyclopedia of interventions and notes, but will generally appear helpless in front of the supervisor. This therapist might report a much better performance at the regular workplace, and appears to be aware of the deficiencies in the supervised session. This trainee is generally compliant in following directives; the primary lack is in generating new ones. This therapist needs to utilize notes more appropriately, and has a tendency to intervene without understanding the consequences or rationale for each intervention. The therapist might select a particular intervention because it was used with a similar presenting problem, even though the context of the therapy might have been totally different. One strategy is for the supervisor to ask the therapist to diagram anticipated changes if various interventions are implemented. This therapist may be required to submit a written plan prior to the session, and shown how to make use of the notes. Sometimes giving this therapist a schema for analyzing a case in a structured way will utilize the note-taking behavior. Other useful interventions include prescribing errors, seeding ideas, and using directives for the family that are indirect communications to the therapist. Anecdotes relating to spontaneity and creativity are useful as well.

The Analogic-Impulsive Therapist

This therapist does not think that a plan is needed before the session begins. Seeing himself or herself as eclectic, which gives a rationale for doing whatever he or she wants, the therapist may not follow directives. In a peculiar way, he or she is often "anti-intellectual" and thinks that the development of technical skills in therapy is counterproductive. The therapist may rationalize this behavior in a session by saying that it "felt right." This therapist can best be organized by designing interventions for the benefit of the clients that result in the therapist's organization. For example, this therapist could hold a discussion with the family about a typical day. This task will force the therapist to structure the session. It is especially useful to have this therapist review the videotapes and discuss the notion of hierarchy. One supervisory goal is to help this therapist overcome the idea that it is more important to be "liked" by the family than to get the job done.

The Anxious Therapist

This therapist forgets the plan made before the session, can't remember directives called over the phone, has problems joining the family, and is usually passive during the session. This therapist may report that he or she does not have the same problem in the workplace. This therapist may also report that despite much time preparing for the session, the heart pounds or the voice cracks, and that he or she literally "blanks out" when in front of the one-way mirror. The strategic supervisor should give the anxious therapist small goals that utilize skills he or she already has. For example, the therapist could be told just to get to know the family during the first interview. The supervisor should try to keep phone calls to the therapist to a minimum, and if the therapist appears to be extremely anxious, to call him or her out of the room for a "break." Once the therapist accepts the notion that the supervisor will be more supportive than critical, he or she may calm down. A clear plan should be made before the session, the therapist should be encouraged to take notes into the session, and the supervisor should alter the plan the minimum amount necessary to complete the interview. It is best if any changes in the strategy are discussed with the therapist behind the mirror rather than over the telephone. It is useful for the supervisor to find some attribute of the therapist to build on. For example, the supervisor could say, "I saw how you took an interest in "x" today, let's use that in the session in this way. . . ." Case selection is also important. A case should be selected that will require some clear organizational tasks. The same courtesy and respect asked of the therapist toward the family should be offered from the supervisor to the therapist.

The Disqualifier

This therapist plays the devil's advocate, and disagrees with whatever the supervisor suggests. Most supervisors will find this particular therapist troublesome. The least troublesome aspect of this therapist's style is that he or she is fairly predictable. This therapist should be led to think that he or she is in charge of planning the session. The supervisor should try to get this therapist to take a position on issues before the supervisor does. The supervisor should keep language as indirect as possible, and consider the use of paradox only if able to establish rapport with the therapist. The use of anecdotes and seeding ideas can be very useful here, and indirect communications should be skillfully embedded. This therapist responds to retraining. For example, the supervisor could begin the supervision by saying that there is a limited amount of time in which to work. The supervisor could then anticipate the therapist's disagreement by noting he or she will probably not agree with the plan in mind, because this plan is generally used with very advanced therapists. The supervisor's demeanor must be very sincere when using this intervention. If the therapist thinks the supervisor is being sarcastic or demeaning, he or she will be extremely difficult to work with. It is best if the supervisor does not reveal the plan until the therapist has demonstrated readiness to carry it out exactly as described. The supervisor can direct this therapist to read, study videotapes, and observe more advanced colleagues as a way of preparing for this intervention. This therapist will often disagree with these tasks and protest that he or she is ready now. Eventually, the only way this therapist can demonstrate readiness to implement the intervention is to agree with the supervisor. It is best if the supervisor continues the restraint until this therapist is clearly asking for supervision.

USE OF DIRECT TECHNIQUES

It should be pointed out that although the emphasis in this chapter is on the use of in-direct techniques there is no reason for a trainer of therapists to abandon the use of direct techniques in teaching. There are bodies of literature and research on the design of curriculum and on the advantages of identifying goals and objectives, and of giving feedback directly (Barnes, 1978; Reinhartz, 1978). It is not necessary or particularly useful to teach using only indirect techniques. Educational research indicates that teaching by identifying skills and building a competency-based system is very effective (Greenhill, 1982). Most indirect techniques are used after training expectations are made clear. Training objectives set a framework for the development of technical skills. These technical skills, useful only in context, help define basic interventions. For example, a first-year therapist should be able to make structural changes in a family and understand the rationale and consequence for each intervention. By the end of the second year, a therapist is expected to be able to generate a number of strategies to solve a specific problem. This occurs only when the therapist has truly understood the model and has a different way to approach problems.

One direct intervention is the *identification of specific skills*. Haley developed a list for trainees entitled "How to Do and What to Know" (Haley, 1977). Based on this work, Ortiz (1980) developed a self-paced guide for therapists. It is broadly divided into categories such as (1) what to know about situations and interventions, (2) skills needed to introduce a change, and (3) skills needed to assume various postures. There are many other skills not subsumed under these categories, including knowing how to do a final interview or follow-up, and engaging absent family members through phone calls. These training objectives are each to be broken down into smaller steps. Each therapist can perform a self-evaluation as to whether he or she has minimally, partially, or fully accomplished each item. Many supervisors discuss training objectives that are specific to that therapist.

Live supervision calls have a direct component; a supervisor may tell a trainee to use specific words in a particular way. Specifying directives in this way is most often reserved for beginning therapists.

A supervisor should be prepared to notice and amplify small changes for each therapist. Amplifying small changes builds on a therapist's strength in a constructive fashion. The therapist may have learned how to clarify a problem or when to change the seating in the room. A supervisor might say, "Since you were able to move the father's seat so he could talk more easily to his wife, now you can ask him to reach agreement with his wife on expectations for his son."

Another way to build on existing skills is for the supervisor to emphasize the positive aspects of the therapist's work. This relaxes the therapist and allows him or her to be more spontaneous in the session. The therapist who thinks that every call will be a reminder of a mistake may become anxious, defensive, or passive and immobile. If the therapist does make a mistake, the supervisor could comment, "I wouldn't do it that way," as opposed to saying, "That was an error." This positive emphasis is also important when debriefing a session or reviewing a videotape. That is, the supervisor should not ignore errors, but should discuss them in a positive context.

Clearly, there is a place in a training program for the use of both direct and indirect techniques. There are times when it is more advantageous to use one or the other. When the therapist is very confused or disorganized it would be best for the supervisor to set clear expectations and establish a structure. It is assumed that the way in which the supervisor treats the therapist affects the way in which the therapist treats the family. Thus, if the supervisor is clear with the therapist there is a higher probability that a confused therapist will be clear with the family.

Is it important for the therapist to have insight regarding his or her skill level? Generally, the therapist's insight about this will most naturally follow changes in ability, and would not be a direct result of a supervisor's evaluation.

The use of indirect techniques in training is an advanced supervisory skill. It is important that "indirection" not be used as a cover-up for lack of direction. A supervisor should be simple and direct, or do nothing and let the therapist follow his or her own instincts. It would be unfortunate if, at that moment of decision regarding use of indirection, the supervisor purposely acted in a confusing manner. A supervisor has an obligation to approach the supervisory situation with the same dedication as a therapist approaches a therapy session. It is my hope that supervisors in the future will become as inventive in designing a strategic supervision as strategic therapists have become in designing a strategic therapy.

Acknowledgment

Appreciation is expressed to Jay Haley and Cloé Madanes, Directors of the Family Therapy Institute of Washington, D.C., who provided the supervision opportunities while the author was Clinical Director, resulting in the ideas expressed in this chapter.

Note

1. Hypnotic strategies rest on the incorporation of the clients' individual characteristics in the therapy. The hypnotherapist learns to use these characteristics, behaviors, thoughts, and responses to produce trance and influence change.

References

Barnes, H. (1978). Senior medical students teaching the basic skills of history and physical examination. *Journal of Medical Education, 53*(5), 432–434.

Erickson, M. H., & Rossi, E. L. (1980). The indirect forms of suggestion. In E. L. Rossi (Ed.), *The collected papers of Milton H. Erickson* (Vol. 1, pp. 452–476). New York: Irvington Press.

Greenhill, M. (1982). Formulation and assessment of public administration educational objectives to optimize learning in adults and other "non-traditional" students. *Higher Education, 11*(3), 261–268.

Haley, J. (1963). *Strategies of psychotherapy*. New York: Grune & Stratton.

Haley, J. (Ed.) (1967). *Advanced techniques of hypnosis and therapy: Selected papers of Milton H. Erickson, MD* (p. 130). New York: Grune & Stratton.

Haley, J. (1976). *Problem solving therapy*. San Francisco: Jossey-Bass.

Haley, J. (1977). *How to do and what to Know*. Unpublished manuscript.

Madanes, C. (1981). *Strategic family therapy*. San Francisco: Jossey-Bass.

Madanes, C. (1984). *Behind the one-way mirror: Advances in the practice of strategic therapy*. San Francisco: Jossey-Bass.

Ortiz, M. (1981). *Self-paced guide for therapists*. Unpublished manuscript.

Reinhartz, J. (1978). Improving teacher instructional effectiveness. *Action in Teacher Education, 1*(1), 30–70.

7

An Integrative Psychodynamic and Systems Approach

WILLIAM C. NICHOLS
Tallahassee, Florida

EDUCATIONAL/TRAINING PHILOSOPHY

I have some discomfort with the concept of *training* family therapists, and it seems worthwhile to address the issue at the outset of this chapter. The approach to the preparation of family therapists that I have followed for two decades has been one in which preparation has been construed more broadly than the term "training" implies.[1] Training in dictionary terms means to subject someone to certain actions or exercises in order to bring about a desired condition—to train a surgeon's hand to make it steady—or to instruct so as to make someone proficient or qualified—to train nurses at a hospital. A trainee is a person undergoing vocational, military, or similar training.

Training also implies that one is involved in acquiring skills, particularly expertise involving the use of the hands or the application of techniques. While training in this sense is essential for becoming a family therapist, it is only a part of the process. My concern is to turn out family therapists who are more than technicians, even highly skilled technicians. Hence, my intent is not to indoctrinate developing family therapists in a sectarian fasion but to help them to become students (persons who study and integrate) and practitioners (persons qualified to practice a profession).

Preparation of individuals to practice a profession involves providing them with a solid grounding in the substantive knowledge and theoretical underpinnings on which the practice is based, as well as training in the applied aspects of the knowledge base. Hence, I shall use the term "student" or "student–trainee" to emphasize that the approach to preparation most desirable to me is one in which the student becomes an individual who studies and investigates human behavior, as well as one who applies certain techniques and skills to the treatment of human beings and to intervention in family systems. Learning family therapy ideally embodies the mastery of a knowledge base that constitutes the foundation for an ongoing and interactive learning process in which substantive materials and theory are continually refined by clinical experience and research and fed back into the clinical practice in a relatively open-systems fashion.

The concept of preparation that best fits such an understanding for me is one in which "education" is used in its basic sense of the Latin term *educere*, meaning to lead out, to infer from data. While there are times when students need to be taught specific content and particular techniques, and to conform to program expectations, the focus throughout remains primarily on encouraging students to apply their knowledge and skills in the most appropriate ways they can. There is much room for idiosyncratic personality factors and for doing therapy according to one's own style.

Underlying systemic education is the amalgam of a student's life experiences within one's family of origin, extended family, and other social systems. Those experiences and their residue, along with the effects of present involvement in individual and family life cycles, form a mosaic against which theory and current therapeutic involvement with families are perceived and interpreted during the student's clinical work.

The career-development perspective is very important in preparing family therapists. That is, the knowledge and skill training given by the supervisor depends on the student's career stage and degree of personal development. Different backgrounds and abilities are expected of postdoctoral students with several years of work experience than are expected in beginning master's students. The teacher starts with students where they are and takes them as far as possible during that particular educational/training program; subsequent educational/training efforts build on what has been done at the earlier stage.

Model of Therapy

The Family Therapy Glossary (AAMFT, 1984) has defined psychodynamic family therapy as "A general term covering a multitude of approaches in which the history of family members is considered critical and may be based on the theory of object relations. The goal of the approach is insight into the past with the hope of avoiding repeating past roles in families." I am not writing about psychodynamic family therapy in that sense, but about a combination–integration of psychodynamic and systemic approaches.

The integrative model of psychodynamic/systems theory discussed here has been and is an evolving model. The early stages were shaped more strongly by psychodynamic perspectives than by systemic outlooks. The term psychodynamic is used in a broad sense because of my early exposure to the interpersonal theory of Harry Stack Sullivan (1953, 1954), with its systemic emphases, and also because I perceived that classical psychoanalytic theory has limited uses and severe limitations. The psychodynamic model used here certainly does retain an appreciation of the role of unconscious dynamics in individual and family life.

The integrative approach accepts the idea that intrapsychic conflicts may exist for the individual, but seeks to determine how relevant these conflicts may be for the functioning of the individual, for the work of the therapist, and to effect change. As such the approach does not retain the primacy of psychic determinism found in classical psychoanalysis. As Framo (1970) has pointed out, symptoms may be understood from a family-transactional viewpoint, and the family may be considered the context of assessment and treatment, because of the unique and powerful effects that it has on the life of human beings. Treatment concepts thus are broadened beyond the individual to include efforts to alter contexts.

This approach involves a strong developmental element, and emphasizes that historical factors constitute a major part of human personality and family systems that must be addressed in certain situations for the most effective interventions to occur. Students are taught the concepts of family, marital, and individual life cycles, as well as the cogwheeling, interlocking nature of the various cycles. These cycles and their interaction have implications for the present functioning of the family and its relevant subsystems; hence, interventions take a developmental perspective into account.

A subsidiary assumption is that the marital subsystem, which serves as the nexus of the family, deserves particular attention. Much family therapy eventually takes the marital subsystem into consideration and works directly with it. Students learn the nature of the attachment between spouses, as well as between the individual mates and their respective families of origin. Knowledge about mate selection, including cultural and ethnic factors, and object relations theory, especially the work of Fairbairn (1952), are considered essential. Models of relating learned by the spouses in their respective families of origin, and the degree and nature of differentiation they have achieved from their families, also are important for integrative family therapy.

The understanding of family systems used here is, in most respects, consistent with that held by many other family therapists. Concepts about relatively open systems, feedback, boundaries, rules, structure, process, family myths and secrets, and other matters are considered basic. Change in the family system is both a desired goal and a method for achieving additional change in the family's dysfunctional patterns. Integrative family therapy, however, does place more reliance on family members' awareness of dysfunctional elements and behaviors, and the direct enlistment of their cooperation in efforts to produce change, than do therapies that rely almost entirely on the use of indirect approaches. Indirect approaches, including paradox, are part of the integrative approach, but they are used sparingly.

The broad goal of integrative family therapy is to deal with the family's complaints and relevant problems to secure necessary and desired change. More specific goals include the removal or amelioration of symptoms and the restoration or establishment of functioning that is "as good as is possible" at the time. These goals may work together; that is, the removal of dysfunction may allow for normal growth and development patterns of the family, marriage, and individuals.

Zuk's (1975) metaphor of dipping into a flowing river to influence its course is an apt representation of what is to be hoped for in many instances with families. As he notes, the goals in some cases should be appropriately modest, not grandiose. As would be the case with other therapies, one seeks to achieve short-range or process goals as well as outcome goals. A short-range goal might be the temporary alleviation of particular family tensions or the achievement of more effective communication among family members. Either of these also could contribute to broader and related systemic changes, but such changes do not lead automatically in any simple or linear fashion to ultimate outcome changes.

I attempt to help trainees make critical decisions about change on a case-by-case basis by helping them assess the possibilities that a family will change in response to the therapist's interventions. What I do is similar to Nathan Ackerman's (1958) "tickling the defenses" of the family. Does the family change? Is the family satisfied with the changes that have occurred? Whitaker's idea that one reschedules with a family each session, on the basis of the family's decision as to whether or not it wishes to reschedule, is a part of this process. Always, I try to help students recognize that one cannot go beyond the point that the family wishes to move to in its alterations. Only the passage of a large amount of time will determine the amount and kind of change that has occurred. We have to live with the decisions of the families, and with a significant degree of ambiguity regarding what actually has transpired.

Assessment consists of a combination of interview and observation of the family. Relevant familial subsystems may be seen separately; however, the family is always considered as a unit and, whenever observed, is watched for the patterns of interaction that occur among all the members (Reiss, 1980). Data may be collected from other sources besides the family, including other professionals or members of other systems such as schools.

The therapist in my approach to family therapy is an expert in the field of human relations and human interaction after the model of Sullivan (1954). Change in the family is basically the responsibility of the family, with the assistance of the therapist. The therapist essentially occupies the role of participant–observer with the family; a detached observer in some ways, but a participant in other ways, whose presence affects the behaviors and functioning of the family. Realistically, even though we talk of joining families, therapists are at most "in but not of" the families with which they work.

Ideally, the therapist is an enabler who facilitates change. Although we may talk of "therapeutic personalities," none of us heals. If we are reasonably successful in helping to bring about positive change, we do so by aiding the processes of nature and of the familial systems and subsystems in healing or attaining better functioning. The therapist in the integrative approach seeks to be an assistant, and not an engineer who tinkers or mechanically manipulates the family and/or situations he or she faces with the family. One implication of the foregoing is that the therapist is respectful of the family, of its right of self-determination, and of its integrity. He or she is called in as a helper, as a kind of consultant, not as the final decision maker into whose hands the total destiny of the family is placed.

I consider it exceedingly helpful for the therapist to understand experientially the feelings clients undergo when they come to therapy. Not only experiencing therapy for themselves, but also going through the intake procedures as if they are clients at the clinic where training is conducted, aids therapists in understanding the impact of the clinic and their own actions and attitudes on the families with whom they are working. Not infrequently such experiences help therapists to recast their role—to become less rigid, authoritarian, and "professional," and to be more flexible, open, and "human" in their dealings with families.

The techniques associated with an integrative psychodynamic/systemic approach to family therapy are many and varied. The frequency of use of various techniques depends partly on what the therapist finds through initial and continuing assessment and the therapist's own preference for particular techniques. Fortunately, equifinality (AAMFT, 1984) prevails and there are many ways of performing therapeutic tasks and reaching treatment goals.

Among the general techniques used are the following: exploration of both present and past, particularly to elucidate the family's patterns of living (Sullivan, 1954) and to establish the possibilities of change; persuasion of family members to take action; modeling and self-disclosure by the therapist; family skill development, such as the improvement of communication and the establishment of patterns of negotiation and compromise. Specific techniques would include reframing or refocusing, detriangulation, and others.

Students should be exposed to at least three different supervisors in order to learn the value of different approaches and the use of diverse techniques. The practical result from such an approach is that students must struggle to integrate various viewpoints and approaches from supervisors.

Basic Presuppositions of the Educational/Training Process

SIX ASSUMPTIONS REGARDING EDUCATION TRAINING

1. Exposure to certain amounts and kinds of theoretical content and substantive materials on families should precede active clinical involvement with families. When inexperienced individuals are thrust into a complex clinical situation without adequate content preparation, the resultant anxiety may not be conducive to effective learning. One is reminded of the "fraternity initiation" type of introduction to mental patients in which students/interns were sent into hospital wards on their own to learn and intervene as best they could. Such an approach doubtless provided some learning, but one has to question the cost–benefit ratio of the method. The teacher–supervisor in such instances can either let the student-trainee "sink or swim," or move to supervise and intervene actively, providing a rescue if necessary but perhaps at a cost of fostering heavy dependency or unproductive resentment and rebellion. Such an approach contrasts sharply with one in which students are adequately prepared and gradually introduced into clinical work so their unproductive anxiety is at a minimum, and they can be expected to provide a reasonable rationale for the interventions that they are making. Students can be brought into clinical situations with families on a step-by-step, graduated basis that prepares them for appropriate and responsible functioning without coddling them or stunting their professional development.

Students in doctoral programs, or other programs where they enroll with clinical experience, can be introduced into treatment situations relatively early in the program. With students at all levels the gradual approach can involve observation of clinical work by others, particularly by other students, and monitoring of case staffings that deal with intake (initial assessment), ongoing case review, and termination. Students should witness the functioning of students rather than that of faculty and supervisory staff. Such an approach enhances the ability of students to build a belief in their own capacities to learn and to develop as they observe their peers.

2. The educational/training program is intended to serve as a learning experience rather than as an obstacle course. Cooperation promotes learning more effectively than competition does. Cooperation is sought among students as well as between faculty and students, and efforts are made to eliminate unnecessary elements that cause distress to students. Following Selye's (1966) familiar distinction, education/training provides sufficient stress—which it is to be hoped students experience as helpful stress or "eustress"— to temper and mature students without creating a competitive and unnecessarily painful and distressful situation for them.

3. A hierarchical structure with regard to authority is desirable. Just as tests are administered by faculty in academic courses, so supervision is provided by faculty/

supervisors in clinical settings. Students should not be subjected to grading, evaluation, or criticism of their work by peers.

4. Clinical training and supervision should approximate the kinds of clinical settings and circumstances that students can expect to encounter in the real world of practice. That is, students are given close supervision and didactic instruction in the use of techniques during the early phases of their clinical training, but move steadily toward a stage in which they assume responsibility for a case and use a supervisor more as a consultant than as a closely functioning supervisor. The student is assumed to be a developing professional, and not an apprentice to a particular teacher, supervisor, or mentor.

5. The educational/training program needs take precedence over the service needs of the case. Clients need to be informed that they are being provided service in a training setting, so that they are handled ethically through the provision of "truth in packaging" and have the options of accepting therapy with a student/trainee, requesting an experienced therapist, or going elsewhere for assistance. Giving the student/trainee responsibility for case handling means that the supervisor does not interfere in the treatment directly as long as the clients are not being harmed. If the student's behavior or case handling is harmful or irresponsible, ethical and perhaps legal considerations do require active intervention by the supervisor. Continued lack of improvement in a case because of demonstrable and identifiable ineptness on the part of the student/trainee similarly signals the need for intervention and perhaps reassignment of the case.

6. Educational/training programs are not designed to serve therapeutic purposes for students. While personal psychotherapy or family therapy for the student is helpful as part of the preparation of the family therapist (Kaslow, 1984), and can be coordinated with education/training (Nichols, 1968), therapy should be considered adjunctive to the educational/training process.

Students who do enter therapy are assigned a therapist on the basis of availability and the perceived "fit" between therapist and student. The therapists do not supervise the students they treat (Nichols, 1968). Students work on general personality issues; interpersonal conflicts; the process of differentiation from family of origin; and their struggles with the educational/training program, including problems with supervisors. Information from therapy is not available to supervisors and program administrators, but therapists and supervisors can discuss student needs and functioning in general terms. The evidence has been clear over the years that students' problems with clients (and with others in their program) are ameliorated through the use of personal psychotherapy.

Basic Mission of Education/Training. The basic mission of education/training is threefold: first, to provide students with an adequate basis for performing family therapy according to their best abilities, level of development, and maturity; second, to provide a basis for learning how to acquire additional knowledge and skill; and third, to integrate such acquisitions with their current orientation and abilities. A "main stream and tributaries" metaphor helps to depict the idea that education/training provides the student with a fundamental theoretical and substantive and practical orientation to the field and practice of family therapy. As students from each educational level move through their careers, they should be able to add to their knowledge and skills through various "tributaries" that reach or pour into the main stream of knowledge and skill that furnishes the basis for their practical work. They are prepared for the present, but they also "learn to learn," so that they can add to what they know and can do so in a reasonable and responsible way long after they have left the educational/training program.

The ongoing part of this process requires that students be equipped to learn from clinical experience and observation, and from their consumption of relevant research into family therapy. The ability to think critically—to weigh the factors observed in a dispassionate manner and reach reasoned conclusions—is one of the best tools available for gaining new information and skills. At the master's level, students should be equipped to search out, assess, and interpret research studies against the body of knowledge on which the field is based. Doctoral students, of course, should be prepared to do research in family therapy, as well as to comprehend the meanings and significance of research in relevant areas. Such a foundation of knowledge and ability protects practitioners from dropping behind the ongoing developments in the field, or naively accepting as valid the multitude of new writings and clinical demonstrations that flood the field. Students cannot be equipped once for all time—an impossibility—and should not be left to rely on the authority of others without being able to make their own informed and discriminatory observations and decisions.

Individuals accepted into postdegree programs should be screened in order to ascertain whether they possess an adequate foundation of substantive knowledge and theory in a psychodynamic/systemic approach, as well as whether they have developed appropriate critical abilities. Experience and observation indicate that it is exceedingly difficult to accomplish the kind of mission described here within the confines of an internship year, for example, unless such knowledge and ability are already present in the students. Potential postdegree students can be required to fill in missing portions of substantive knowledge as a prerequisite to entering the program. The absence of critical abilities constitutes a larger problem, which when serious enough would disqualify applicants for postdegree training programs.

Organizing Concepts. Learning objectives are dealt with in a flexible manner using a broad framework and the philosophy of "establishing a structure, then stretching it as necessary." How objectives are implemented varies, depending on the particular strengths and needs of the student and the peculiarities of the educational and especially the clinical situations emerging in the program. This model does not employ learning objectives in terms of specific lists of items that can be closely measured, sequenced, and programmed, as in the case of computerized educational and vocational efforts. Many client problems may be dealt with adequately by several different approaches, any of which may be judged acceptable when evaluated by a reasonable standard. The choice of solution often involves a degree of educated judgment for which there exists no baseline standards by which to determine which course is most desirable.

Among the major objectives of the program are competency in the following abilities:

1. To demonstrate knowledge of the substantive materials on which family therapy is based and to integrate such material with appropriate and defensible approaches to assessment and clinical interventions with families.

2. To think and to intervene systemically, while retaining or manifesting an ability to remember that systems contain individuals.
3. To "stay in the room with a family" physically, emotionally, and intellectually.
4. To attend adequately to the functioning and manifestation of the dynamics of the family system or subsystems.
5. To assess adequately the problems manifested by the family, as well as the strengths of the system. The students should be able to describe adequately both the structure and processes of the family system and the relevant subsystems.
6. To plan and implement treatment plans consistent with the initial and ongoing assessments of family strengths and problems.
7. To continue assessing adequately, and to change strategies flexibly as indicated as a result of ineffectiveness of the strategies that have been attempted or other indications of a need for alteration in strategies.

Along with these broadly stated abilities, the student's work is observed to determine whether more specific abilities are evidenced. For example, how well does the student handle "beginning struggles with families" (Napier, 1976), deal with questions of "resistance," use supervision, and so on?

Theory of Learning and Change. Students/trainees are expected to learn conceptually and experientially, that is, cognitively, consciously, and by identification. Not only the professional identity, but also the personal identity, of the student undergoes alteration during the period and processes covered by the educational/training program.

The acquisition of concepts and sharpening of skills tend to lessen anxiety and to increase confidence in the student's ability to function as a family therapist. Less frequently, increased exposure to family therapy, and heightened pressure for the student to change, may bring about fairly serious identity conflicts and crises. Those students accustomed to regarding clients from an individual perspective may struggle with the idea of viewing clients in contextual family terms. For them, the idea that dysfunction ultimately results from intrapsychic conflict, and that "real therapy" is not being performed unless one is probing for unconscious meanings, may be too deeply rooted. Others may become caught in a loyalty struggle between the pull to adhere to theories and mentors from earlier in their careers and the acceptance of new theories, taught in a different educational setting by faculty and requiring involvement with new family therapy groups and organizations.

The total structure of the program is used in shaping students, and aiding them to learn. Treatment of students as professionals by the faculty and staff, and the maintenance of professional demeanor in all public contacts and gatherings, is part of the effort to enhance the formation of the professional identity and the manifestation of professional behavior on the part of students. An important factor is the faculty's maintenance of a high level of ethical concern and sense of responsibility for dealing with clients and students.

Learning by identification involves more than identification with a teacher/supervisor. Students are also provided opportunities to observe, interact with, and model after advanced students in the program. Efforts are made to encourage identification with a "generalized other," which is somewhat analagous to identification with models of relationship in one's family of origin, and involves attaching oneself to, and incorporating aspects of, the educational/training program as a whole, and the field of family therapy.

The things I specifically ask and encourage students to copy and imitate are the approaches to learning and to dealing with clients that we attempt to manifest in the program. That involves approaching clients and learning as responsibly as possible. Expressed in personal terms, my approach may be stated as follows: "To the best of my knowledge and understanding of myself, I don't need for you to do things the way that I do them. I don't need disciples or any more dependents. I do ask that you do your best to know what you are doing when you approach clients, that you have as sound a rationale as possible for what you are doing, that you not act impulsively or do something simply because you saw somebody do it in a workshop or read about it, that when you don't know something you become able to say, 'I don't know,' and do the best you can, and that in all instances that you keep trying to learn."

Students are helped to make sense out of what they are encountering, to deal with data against the background of theory and substantive knowledge about families and family functioning that they possess, as well as against the mosaic of their earlier personal and family experiences. Students are urged to take up questions and problems of dealing with families in their individual and group supervision. Out of this process emerges an interesting mixture of change in the students. They not only have the experience, but also acquire awareness of what their new encounters and experiences mean. The combination of confidence and excitement that emerges in students/trainees at all levels is contagious and tends to spread among members of the group.

Feedback is provided to students in both the academic and clinical portions of the program. Encouragement is provided by faculty in as much of a "let's learn" atmosphere as is possible. The formation of study groups among students preparing for comprehensive examinations is promoted and facilitated, so that students may teach each other and thus maximize their own individual learning. The point is made both subtly and overtly that students are not judged against one another in either their academic or their clinical work, but against the levels of ability that the faculty deems appropriate in any given area. This "hard but fair" atmosphere also provides students with a sense of achievement when they overcome the necessary hurdles and attain the goals that they have sought. Finally, efforts are made to provide them with support and morale enhancement through the provision of attractive physical surroundings.

THE EDUCATIONAL/TRAINING CONTEXT

Setting

My teaching and supervision of family therapy has been done at postdoctoral, doctoral, masters, and postdegree (masters and doctoral practitioners) levels, and in free-standing institutes, degree programs, and consultative arrangements with individuals and groups from clinics or independent practice bases. Initially I worked with postdoctoral fellows during the "glory days" of the pioneering Merrill Palmer Institute in Detroit during the

1960s and at another free-standing institute. Those experiences were followed by an opportunity to translate the evolving integrative model and a well informed educational and pedagogical model into a doctoral program at Florida State University. Following a move back into private practice, I worked on an adjunct basis with students at a Michigan university, teaching and providing supervision.

Currently I provide case consultation on family therapy with mental health practitioners who are working in outpatient psychiatric clinics. Family therapy training is perceived as a need by those clinicians, rather than by the administrators of their agencies. Motivation of these students is high.

Use of the integrative model in various forms in the several settings in which I have worked has resulted in satisfactory training outcomes. The common factor in all but one setting was that family therapy had a sole or at least a high priority rating, and that the teachers/supervisors occupied a correspondingly high position of power and influence in the program. The one exception providing a decided contrast was a university program in which I served as the lone family therapist with an adjunct faculty position in a psychology doctoral program that was strongly and conservatively psychoanalytic in orientation. The differences in paradigms between family therapy even of a psychodynamic/systemic variety and a psychoanalytic orientation created too much dissonance for students and too little satisfaction for me.

Teachers/Trainers

The years that I have been involved in preparing family therapists reflect the evolution of the credentials required to teach and train in our field. My earliest experience involved working with a faculty that had gained its own graduate education and doctoral degrees in such varied areas as clinical psychology, psychology, and marriage and family. Most were self-taught in family therapy and emerged mainly from a child-guidance background. They had extensive experience in a variety of mental health settings. My later experiences included teaching where at least some of the faculty members had earned their doctoral degrees in marital and family areas. Individuals currently being hired for such positions in academic settings are required to hold doctoral degrees in family therapy.

While there was a core of commonly held ideas and commitments among the faculty, there also was considerable variation in their orientation and diversity in their supervisory methods. Nobody moved in lockstep, and the variety was considered a positive aspect of the program and a plus for the students. In retrospect, the amount of tension generated among students by the intensity of the program sometimes seemed to result in less than optimal learning conditions.

In subsequent settings I have considered it desirable to have a mixture of commonality and diversity among the faculty. Commonality is important concerning the substantive and theoretical orientations held by the faculty. Diversity of approaches to supervision and case handling, given a sound core of common assumptions, values, attitudes, and goals, is more workable than wide diversity in substantive and theoretical foundations. Using various paths to get to the same goal appears to be more possible than working together from widely diverse assumptions, values, attitudes, and goals. In other words, some diversity is helpful, but too much, including unnecessary hurdles, conflicts, and barriers, is counterproductive and even harmful to the education/training of students.

Students/Trainees

Students accepted into postdoctoral and doctoral programs meet some similar and some different requirements. All are expected to be available for full-time study and clinical practice in the program.

Students accepted for postdegree education/training on a consultative or supervisory basis must work in "a legitimate practice setting" where they are carrying a full caseload under a bona fide organizational structure that assumes administrative responsibility for them. The major focus for postdegree students is on families selected from their caseload that will be followed through the course of treatment. General issues in family therapy that emerge from this work are closely considered as well. Generally, postdegree students are seen in small groups.

Candidates for graduate programs are screened through paper credentials such as transcripts and letters of recommendation, and through interviews with faculty members. Intellectual brightness, indications of ethical awareness, and manifestations of kindness are major characteristics that are sought in candidates, along with the demonstrated ability to work hard.

Our expectation is that postdoctoral and doctoral students have several years of "real-world" clinical experience before being accepted into a program. We also desire that students be at least 30 years of age and have completed the typical developmental tasks of young adulthood. The difficulties of retraining motivated older students who have come from an orientation other than family therapy and have acquired a significant amount of clinical experience and personal maturity generally are not as great as those of attempting to make family therapists out of students who are in their 20s.

Previous or current therapy for students, whatever their age, is seen as highly desirable, provided that the relationship with their therapist does not produce conflict with the educational/training program. Family-of-origin work by students appears to be essential to the development of the kind of therapist who can work with families using an integrative psychodynamic/systemic model.

Resources

Students are expected to learn to work with a wide range of families from different socioeconomic backgrounds, and with a range of value systems, problems, and resources. In most settings there is a skewing of cases toward the middle-class and upper-middle-class levels. Such skewing is not considered totally undesirable because most students will be working primarily with middle-class clientele following completion of their educational/training programs. Students are acquainted with the sociocultural elements that shape various ethnic groups, and taught to ask families to help them understand what they do not comprehend about a family.

Securing cases is the responsibility of the faculty and program administration. A wide range of problems—marital, child, total family—with a number of common diagnostic entities—depressive reactions, anxiety reactions, and others—are sought for students. When doctoral students are placed in outpatient mental health clinics, they are under the administration of that clinic and function as members of its staff, but are under the clinical supervision of a faculty member of other designated supervisor who holds adjunct faculty status and participates in the educational institution's program.

All clinical training facilities contain interviewing rooms, some of which have one-way mirrors, and audiotaping capacity. Videotaping capacity is considered desirable, if the taping can be done from outside the interviewing rooms and with a minimum of obtrusiveness. Knowing that clients form attachments to the clinical setting as well as to the therapist has led to deliberate efforts to "treat by the structures" and to "train by the structures." This means that formal relationships are maintained in public, that physical facilities for both students and clients are decorated aesthetically and comfortably and kept neat, and that in a variety of ways professional demeanors and behaviors are maintained.

EDUCATIONAL/TRAINING METHODS AND CONTENT

Format

METHODS OF TEACHING THEORETICAL CONTENT

The core of basic education for the family therapist is similar for students at all levels, but advanced students are expected to master more difficult and extensive materials.

Solid grounding in the following areas should precede actual clinical work in the program: *human development* in both its normal and abnormal expressions, including individual and group studies and human sexuality; *marital and family studies*, including family development, mate selection, and studies of families in various sociocultural settings and times; *marital and family therapy*, including diverse orientations to family therapy and a thorough acquaintance with family systems concepts; and *professional studies*, including the history of the field, legal issues, and ethical issues. Some content course work and clinical training will, of course, be handled by the student simultaneously.

Education and training in research can be done simultaneously with clinical training. Some repetition, updating, and expansion of substantive material from the areas mentioned above provide opportunities for learning and integration when done simultaneously with clinical training. My experience in teaching at the graduate level is that the faculty-led courses are superior to seminars for the systematic coverage of essential materials. Seminars and readings are more helpful for students who have already gained most if not all of the desired basic education for family therapy.

Observation of abnormal behavior and dysfunction, as well as normal family and individual processes, is important. With beginning graduate students, discussions of role plays and videotaped materials may be used, but I prefer actual clinical experiences. Probably this is a function of my own personality, being "a game player rather than a practice player," meaning that while I perceive some value in discussing things in an abstract, noninvolved fashion, I do not find it to be the same as dealing with an actual situation in which one is actively involved and has to make responses that count.

METHODS OF CONVEYING AND TEACHING THERAPEUTIC SKILLS

The methods used in conveying and teaching the skills of an integrative approach depend in part on the level of the program. For purposes of brevity, I shall concentrate on doctoral-level graduate programs and postdegree programs. Entering students with several years of work experience are expected to possess basic interviewing and intervention skills, at least for dealing with individuals and in many instances groups of non-kin individuals. Most students have had some experience with families, frequently as an adjunct to therapy with a child. Hence, the major focus in the program is on helping the students learn how to assess and to deal effectively with family systems.

Most of the teaching of therapeutic skills is done through clinical supervision. Other information about techniques is conveyed through observation and reading. Students start by observing case conferences in which advanced students and faculty discuss cases treated by the advanced students and, frequently, by observing advanced students doing clinical work. After starting with cases and with individual supervision, the beginning students typically move into group supervision. This move permits them to generate generic issues that provide a bridge to an accompanying seminar where the issues can be discussed. A considerable amount of discussion in the seminar is on techniques and modes of intervention, including the rationale for making the interventions, as well as the methods of doing so.

Individual supervision focuses on retrospective discussion of cases and videotape playback of therapy sessions. I have not used "live" supervision since the late 1960s. I believe that the case belongs to the student/trainee and that the focus on his or her growth and development as a responsible therapist takes precedence over all concerns, except harm to the clients. Observation of actual treatment in progress may be used, although in reality it provides little for the supervisor that videotape viewing does not. Observation of ongoing sessions thus is used sparingly and prescriptively in order to provide immediate feedback to a student.

The kind of live supervision popular in the field today meets the needs of the case or the supervisor more than it does the growth needs of the student. My experience was that one could get quick change in the actions of the trainee by modeling or intervening into the therapeutic work of the trainee. If, however, one looked carefully at the development of the student a year or so later, it generally turned out that the student had tended either to rebel against the stance taken by the supervisor or to slavishly follow the mentor's actions. In either instance, the student had not progressed in his or her own growth in the way that was possible when the supervisor/teacher was absent. There are examples of the need of students to "unpack the training bag" and find their own way of doing treatment to be found in the literature (e.g., Sugarman, 1987). My personal hope is that the field of family therapy will eventually gain the maturity to scrutinize carefully the results of using "live" supervision, and not merely the quick changes in student behaviors that are so readily observable.

A systemic approach to teaching therapeutic skills is used in the program. Students are helped to work with several broad phases of treatment, and to use appropriate techniques and modes of intervention. A considerable amount of time may be given in case conferences, individual supervision, and group supervision to the techniques of joining a family and making an initial assessment, to defining the problems, and to recasting or reframing the family's perceptions of their difficulties. Once therapy is past the initial phase and into the middle and main treatment period, students are helped to learn how to (1) involve relevant subsystems, (2) use multigenerational approaches, (3) aid the family in learning to communicate better, (4) take "I" positions, (5) help family members rearrange their emotional relationships, (6) recognize and restructure emotional triangles, (7) "midwive" relationships, (8) help family members differentiate themselves, (9) learn to use side-taking and other interventive roles, and (10) use other techniques as appropriate. Finally, where possible, students are helped to work out planned terminations. They also are taught to deal with matters of confidentiality, to use resources and reports from outside agencies, and to cope with various other issues.

The actual processes of individual supervision may vary from time to time, depending on the stage of the case, the dynamics of the family, the needs of the student, and other considerations (including, on occasion, the supervisor's desire for variety). For example, supervisor and supervisee may watch a tape, monitoring processes and stopping when either wishes to discuss something. On occasion the supervisee may bring in marked spots on which he or she wishes to focus. One time the concern may be with family dynamics, another time on interventions made by the trainee, and in still another instance the focus may be on general case management issues. Sometimes the discussion may swing to the kinds of issues that are emerging in the case or cases that provide roadblocks for the student/trainee. My preference is to keep the sessions varied and to reinforce in reasonable ways the fact that it is the supervisee's case to treat, using the principle of *educere* as much as possible.

As students move into clinical work, theory becomes a less explicit concern, fading more into the background and becoming a kind of backdrop against which decisions are made and interventions are undertaken. In other words, students become more knowledgeable and more certain of what they are seeing and doing. Consequently, they become less mechanical, smoother with their interventions, and clearer about why they are making them. Interventions are carried out without the need for the student to stop and think through slowly and perhaps laboriously all of the potential issues before acting.

Learning Goals/Objectives and Evaluation

LEVELS OF SOPHISTICATION EXPECTED

Students are expected to complete graduate programs with a working integration of the major concepts of family system and psychodynamic theory. Such concepts have to do with structure, function, motivation, and related concepts. Object relations and multigenerational perspectives, including transgenerational dynamics, are considered particularly important. Other learning objectives mentioned earlier include the ability to continue learning, and knowing how to build on the knowledge basis that students have obtained during their graduate education.

Students are expected to achieve an acceptable level of therapeutic skill in three broad areas. First, they should demonstrate an ability to relate to families in ways that enable families to trust them and work with them in a productive manner. This is an existential element of therapeutic work.

Second, they should be able to assess families adequately and appropriately. This includes the ability to assess the family while standing both equidistant from family members and next to them simultaneously and serially as dictated by the needs of the therapeutic situation. The need at such times is not to be objective, but to be impartial and equitable as one relates, assesses, and also fulfills the third task.

This third ability, of course, is that of intervening effectively and appropriately. Under the rubric of intervention can be listed a number of skills, of which the following are but examples: assisting the parental, and perhaps the grandparental, generation in the differentiation work of teenagers and young adults, as well as helping adult children to resume their incomplete differentiation from their parents; helping clients to advance their own best interests and to be willing to give and to risk—pain, loss, embarrassment, for example—through persuasion and sometimes behavioral techniques; using the therapeutic relationship, in both present real-life relationship terms and through exploitation of transference factors that may affect present relationships and behaviors, in order to help clients move in desired directions; and assisting clients to develop appropriate and effective communication and negotiation skills where such are needed.

EVALUATION

This is an ongoing part of the preparation process. The personal qualities sought in graduates are, of course, the same as those that are looked for at the time of initial screening for entry into the program. Briefly, graduates are expected not only to be intellectually bright, but also, at the point of graduation, to have demonstrated effective use of their intellectual abilities through the comprehension of relevant concepts and mastery of techniques. Additionally, they are expected to demonstrate kindness and sensitivity in dealing with clients, to be ethical in their behaviors and relationships, to manifest a commitment to work and to behaving responsibly toward people and obligations.

Academic portions of the program are evaluated through the usual academic testing and grading procedures. Faculty members also appraise students' abilities to use such knowledge in practical situations. Clinical and professional behaviors are evaluated on an ongoing basis by the supervisors and faculty. Written and/or oral evaluations are provided to students on a systematic basis, and the perspectives of both faculty members and the students being evaluated are discussed at such times. In some cases students are asked to provide written evaluations of their own performance, using the same outline employed by faculty members and supervisors.

A significant part of the evaluation assesses the kind of positions and settings in which graduates are equipped to function, such as in clinical settings or in academic roles. Doctoral graduates have a large amount of choice open to them. Those who wish to pursue an academic career at some time are counseled to consider going directly into the academic world, the rationale being that such a move may be easiest at graduation. During the final evaluation, the kinds of cases that students are considered capable of handling and those with which they may need help are explored with students. Most graduates can be expected to handle all types of cases that are appropriate for family therapy.

Students who are not ready to function as family therapists or family therapy educators at graduation are given guidance to move into another occupation or to complete additional work to address deficiencies. Such a student might be guided into clinical work in a postdoctoral setting, for example.

Teacher–Student Relationship

HIERARCHY

The relationship between teacher and student, or trainer and trainee, is by its very nature hierarchical. One does not go to a peer who is no more knowledgeable or experienced than oneself in order to learn. This does not mean that the student may not be a peer of the teacher in some respects. Postdoctoral fellows in the Merrill-Palmer program, for example, sometimes were older than some faculty members and held comparable professional positions in other institutions. Hierarchy means that the teacher is an expert in the area in which he or she is teaching and that the student is not a peer in that area of expertise. In graduate programs the hierarchical nature of the relationship is highlighted by the presence of faculty ranks and by the fact that the student is seeking a degree at or below that held by the teacher.

During the process of supervision the teacher occupies the role of an expert but certainly can try to function in a cordial and collegial manner. Whether a teacher uses a strong degree of directiveness or suggestiveness in dealing with case matters depends on the issues involved. My preference is to stay with suggestion in regard to a student's work with an actual family as much as seems practical and appropriate. Directiveness tends to be used only when it is needed to "rescue" either therapist or family. A rescue can be used when a student cannot get himself or herself started and committed to a course of action. A typical rescue would offer an alternative approach to the student, using language such as, "Have you thought about . . . ?" or "What do you think about trying . . . ?" Occasionally there may be a direct suggestion to "Give it a try and let's see."

Just as supervision tends to move with the passage of time from a "tight" supervisory control pattern to one resembling consultation, so also do other aspects of the teaching relationship. The teacher is always in the evaluating position but can continue to underline the developing competence and professionalism of students and their movement toward colleague status.

RESISTANCE ISSUES

Manifestations of lack of desire to change old approaches to doing things, and otherwise to learn in the program generally, are regarded as stemming from anxiety on the part of the student. On occasion they may come from the presence of negative transference-countertransference attitudes on the part of student and teacher. At some point reality may be harming the ability of the student to learn. A common manifestation of resistance is in struggles with supervisors over clinical work.

Resistance generally is handled in a straightforward manner, with both faculty and students examining the issues, facing up to the problems, and making whatever changes are possible. Strong efforts are made to deal with such issues in a responsible manner. At times students may be shifted from a case, or other moves may be made, but typically the solution involves helping all parties to stay with the issues and work out an acceptable pattern for proceeding. Sometimes it is necessary to help students face the fact that their resistance is a manifestation of personal problems that require therapeutic assistance for them.

CURRENT AND FUTURE DIRECTIONS

The major wish that I have for education/training in the family therapy field is that we may soon witness the passing of an "apprenticeship" and "school" era in which charisma and enthusiasm can very easily obscure the need to have education/training based on substantive knowledge about families. There are a few glimmers of light to support the hope that the concern with personalities and techniques may be giving way here and there to a recognition that more is needed than anointment by a mentor and the passing on of techniques. For example, discovery of the family life cycle concept, and the recent emphasis on ethnicity, both present indications that content issues are coming to be regarded as significant. Whether there will soon or ever be a general recognition that the basis for family therapy is knowledge about families and family processes, that the appropriate grounding for family therapy is family and not psychotherapy as such, is something that cannot be predicted with any degree of certainty.

My hope is that the content and the learner will be the focus of education/training in family therapy much more in the future than has been the case in the early decades of the family therapy movement. My hope also is that research and practice will be wedded much more widely and generally than has been the case in recent years. Again, there are some indications that research holds a strong interest for many adherents of family therapy, as witnessed in the rapid growth of the research institute associated with the American Association for Marriage and Family Therapy. With regard to the wedding and integration of theory, research, and practice, my hope is that education/training will become much more established in university graduate programs, at the same time that free-standing institutes continue to be hale and hearty, and that the better contributions of each domain will be brought together in creative ferment and productive ways.

Note

1. "We" could be used in this chapter instead of "I" primarily because much of what is discussed here belongs in part to other colleagues with whom it has been shared and from whom parts have been borrowed over the years. The elements of invention and synthesis are only partly the work of the author.

References

Ackerman, N. W. (1958). *The psychodynamics of family life.* New York: Basic Books.
American Association for Marriage and Family Therapy. (1984). *Family therapy glossary.* Washington, DC: Author.
Fairbairn, W. R. D. (1952). *Psychoanalytic studies of the personality.* London: Routledge & Kegan Paul.
Framo, J. L. (1970). Symptoms from a family transactional viewpoint. In N. W. Ackerman (Ed.), *Family therapy in transition* (pp. 125–171). Boston: Little, Brown and Company.

Kaslow, F. W. (Ed.). (1984). *Psychotherapy with psychotherapists.* New York: Haworth Press.

Napier, A. Y. (1976). Beginning struggles with families. *Journal of Marriage and Family Counseling, 2,* 3–12.

Nichols, W. C. (1968). Personal therapy for the marital therapist. *Family Coordinator, 17,* 83–88.

Reiss, D. (1980). Pathways to assessing the family: Some choice points and a sample route. In C. K. Hofling & J. M. Lewis (Eds.), *The family: Evaluation and treatment* (pp. 86–121). New York: Brunner/Mazel.

Selye, H. (1966). *The stress of life.* New York: McGraw-Hill.

Sugarman, S. (1987). Teaching symbolic-experiential family therapy: The personhood of the teacher. *Contemporary Family Therapy, 9,* 138–145.

Sullivan, H. S. (1953). *The interpersonal theory of psychiatry.* New York: W. W. Norton.

Sullivan, H. S. (1954). *The psychiatric interview.* New York: W. W. Norton.

Zuk, G. H. (1975). *Process and practice in family therapy.* Haverford, PA: Psychiatry and Behavioral Science Books.

8

Functional Family Therapy: Basic Concepts and Training Program

LEONARD J. HAAS
JAMES F. ALEXANDER
C. HAYDEE MAS
University of Utah

MODEL OF THERAPY

Functional Family Therapy (FFT) both influences and is influenced by its context. Thus a description of the FFT model in its present form would fail to capture the contextual influences (time-specific, institution-specific, and person-specific) that have shaped and continue to shape its development. This introduction will therefore provide a brief review of the origins of FFT, allowing us to present the basic assumptions and to define characteristics of the model as reflections of an interactive and evolutionary process, rather than as a final state.

FFT Origins and Contributors

Functional Family Therapy had its origins in the mid-1960s when the second author (J.F.A.), then a graduate student, experienced a major shift in intervention philosophy. Prior to this shift he had received excellent training in psychodynamic and relationship approaches to intervention that left him with a deep appreciation for the critical role of individuals' affective, cognitive, and perceptual processes in the etiology and modification of clinical problems. His training had also left him with a similar appreciation of the critical, subtle, and complex nature of of therapist characteristics and the therapeutic relationship (Alexander, 1967; Alexander & Abeles, 1968, 1969).

The shift in intervention philosophy was prompted when Alexander moved from a university-based counseling center to an urban psychology clinic and a rural community mental health center. In conjunction with changing training sites, he also began treating a younger population. In this process he encountered different treatment problems, which raised questions about the utility of an individually oriented intervention model that was poorly suited to the powerful environmental factors that seemed to have a dramatic influence on the nature and course of intervention. Under the guidance (and sometimes the forceful urging!) of mentors, Alexander sought out alternative models that could formally and systematically include extrapersonal influences (such as systemic or environmental) as well as intrapersonal influences on behavior.

This search led to an interest in two concurrently emerging alternatives to traditional therapeutic interventions: the "new" systems approaches that were exemplified in Haley's (1963) classic work, and the "new" behaviorism exemplified by the classic book by Ullmann & Krasner (1965). These models had considerable appeal because each conceptualized ways in which the environment influenced individual behavior. The appeal of both of these models, particularly the systems model at the conceptual level and the behavioral model at the technical level, contributed to an early form of the FFT model of intervention which was formally described as "systems–behavioral" (Alexander & Parsons, 1973). Other factors also enhanced the appeal of these two models. First, both models emphasized accountability and empirical support. From the systems perspective, accountability was raised regarding the appropriateness of treatment and consideration of the context in which treatment occurred. While objective outcome data were not initially characteristic of this approach, considerable creativity and attention were reflected in early translations of systems and communication principles into specific research designs (e.g., Haley, 1962, 1964, 1967).

From the behavioral perspective emerged a strong emphasis on formally identifying and measuring attainment levels of the targets of intervention. Also, from the social learning variant of the behavioral model came the concept of reciprocity and coercion (Patterson & Reid, 1970). This concept demonstrated the interlocking and mutually reinforcing nature of what appeared to be sometimes very unpleasant family sequences. In the context of convention presentations and discussions, Alexander had the advantage of observing these theorists as they struggled to carefully operationalize family interaction. This observation had considerable impact on the early formulations of FFT, an impact that continues to this day.

Another strong influence on the developing FFT model was found in the conceptualization by structurally oriented models of how behavior serves both to reflect, and at the same time to maintain, relationship properties, such as hierarchies (Haley, 1967) and boundaries and coalitions (Minuchin, 1974). It is from this early influence that the concept of "function" evolved: function meaning each individual's preferred psychological distance from another individual in a relationship (Morris, Alexander, & Waldron, in press). Just as individuals work to maintain relationship hierarchy (e.g., complementarity versus symmetry—see Haley, 1967) and coalitions (see Minuchin, 1974), according to the FFT model individuals also work to maintain certain levels of psychological distance, or functions. The ways that people attempt to create functions in a relationship, and the "fit" of participants' mutual creations, determine whether or not relationships become problematic (Morton, Alexander, & Altman, 1976). In conceptualizing functions as individual maneuvers in a relationship context, FFT simultaneously considers both systemic and intraindividual processes. Thus the FFT model researches not only how system processes (such as the reciprocity of defensiveness) relate to deviant behavior (e.g., Alexander, 1973; Barton, Alexander, Waldron, Warburton, & Turner, 1983), and how changes in systems processes relate to clinical improvement (e.g., Alexander, Barton, Schiavo, & Parsons, 1976; Alexander & Parsons, 1973; Parsons & Alexander, 1973), but also defines functions as properties of individuals (Morris, Alexander, & Waldron, in press). In this way the model maintains an individual perspective at the same time it conceptualizes systemic effects. For example, unlike concepts that identify relationship properties of *the entire family*, such as enmeshment–disengagement (Minuchin, 1974) or cohesion–adaptability (Olson *et al.*, 1983), FFT believes each individual, and each relationship, may vary considerably in terms of desired and achieved psychological distance and closeness with another. FFT thus argues that general concepts applied to the entire family will miss variations within families, for example, the kind of situation in which certain dyadic relationships are quite close, but others are quite distant. FFT argues that by identifying each of the relationship patterns, family treatment strategies can be more individualized for each family configuration.

FFT also retains an individual perspective by virtue of examining how individual family members' attributions influence problematic system processes (Barton *et al.*, 1983), and how changing these individual attributional frameworks can facilitate change in the larger system (Morris *et al.*, in press). Thus FFT represents an attempt to develop a true transactional model that integrates both individual effects and systemic effects on behavior. Of course, the utility of this integration must be evaluated in the future. At present, trainers and trainees of FFT enjoy the excitement resulting from being clinical "consumers" of a range of research and clinical models.

The Training Context and Its Influence on the Model

The training context, a university psychology department, also provided a number of factors that influenced the development of FFT. First, because the model evolved in a "publish-or-perish" type psychology department, progenitors needed to develop a model that was pragmatic, researchable, and included a strong empirical component. Second, because of many competing demands on trainees, such as dissertations, course work, preliminary exams, and the academic quarter system (i.e., 10 weeks at a time), the model needed to be learnable and "do-able" in a short time period. Third, because referrals generally consisted of families with marginal motivation at best, the model had to attend formally to issues of motivation and resistance as a relevant issue of family therapy process, not a characteristic of families or people. In particular, referrals to FFT often included juvenile-court-referred families who were urged (but not required) to attend treatment. In response to other treatment approaches, these families were notorious for high dropout rates, considerable resistance, and uneven (or no) attendance by one or more family members. Fourth, because trainees came to the program from a variety of backgrounds, their value systems were often quite different from those of many of the referred families (half of whom belonged to the conservative and highly value-oriented Mormon culture). Because of this discrepancy, as well as value differences within many of the families, the FFT needed to develop a set of intervention techniques that allowed therapists to be effective in a context of divergent value systems. Fifth, because the model evolved within a larger clinical psychology training program, FFT trainers had little selection authority over participants in the FFT prepractica and practica. Further, departmental goals required that students be trained in a wide range of interventional methods and theoretical frameworks, sometimes within the same time period. As a result, FFT trainers have always had to be particularly sensitive to "paradigm clashes" that occur, and to recognize that sometimes the systemic perspective is seen by trainees as inconsistent with the models to which their major advisors adhere. Though creating difficulties from time to time, this contextual influence has also helped FFT trainers to remain open to the potential contributions of alternative frameworks.

Basic Principles of FFT

CAREFUL SPECIFICATION OF PHASES AND COMPONENTS OF INTERVENTION

Because of the need for a model that could be researched and reliably transmitted, FFT has paid particular attention to identifying the different phases that constitute family therapy (Alexander, Barton, Waldron, & Mas, 1983; Warburton & Alexander, 1985). The phases that have been identified include acquaintance–impression, assessment, induction–therapy, treatment–education, and generalization–termination. Each of these phases has unique goals, depends on a unique set of therapist characteristics and abilities, and is characterized by a unique set of activities. By virtue of identifying these phases, and creating clear descriptions for the activities in each, FFT has attempted to reduce the magical aura that can surround family therapy.

ATTENTION TO THE THERAPIST'S MODEL-BASED REALITY AND
THE FAMILY'S PHENOMENOLOGICAL REALITY OF FEELINGS AND COGNITIONS

FFT makes a major distinction between the "reality" that the family experiences and the "reality" that the therapist uses to interpret the family's behavior. This latter reality is based on the conceptual model used by the therapist, and often includes concepts and phrases that are quite different from what the family members think they are experiencing. According to FFT, both realities must be incorporated in a successful change program: the therapist's reality because we bring to families an alternative view of their problem with specific techniques to help; the family's reality because they must be motivated to change, continue to engage in the intervention process, and be able to carry out the solutions we offer.

These two realities receive special attention in two of the major phases of intervention. The family's reality is addressed during the induction–therapy phase, where cognitive restructuring techniques, such as *relabeling* and *developing a relationship focus*, are designed to influence the way family members think and feel about one another. Rather than pointing out all of the family dynamics as they see them, during this phase therapists attempt to create alternative realities for the family that will be conducive to change. The special emphasis on a nonblaming approach to this process enhances positive rather than negative affect (Alexander & Parsons, 1982; Morris *et al.*, in press).

In contrast to these techniques that target the family's phenomenological reality as a focus of intervention during the induction–therapy phase of intervention, during treatment–education the focus changes to effecting specific interaction patterns. At the outset of intervention, these patterns are identified as problematic by the therapist, but not necessarily by the family. Thus therapists target and attempt to change specific patterns of interaction that, according to their model of pathology and change, they see as necessary to help the family become a happier and more adaptive unit. This component of intervention utilizes such specific techniques as communication training, a variety of technical aids (e.g., notes and reminder cards), and specifically assigned interpersonal tasks that facilitate the development of new interaction patterns.

In order to develop a model that is effective (Alexander & Parsons, 1973; Barton *et al.*, 1983; Klein, Alexander, & Parsons, 1976) and also short-term, FFT has developed a set of goals that are both realistic and appropriate to the families we see. A *matching-to-sample* philosophy is used, wherein the goals of intervention are derived not from some ideal theory of human functioning, but instead from an identification of the wide variety of patterns that characterize "normal, happy, adaptive" families (Alexander, 1973; Parsons & Alexander, 1973). This has allowed FFT to work toward a larger range of desired outcomes that include variations produced by alternative family structures, subcultural orientations, and the like.

As part of this philosophy, FFT is designed to change specific patterns of behavior, thoughts, and feelings, but *not* to change basic value structures, which include political and religious orientations, ethnic orientations, and interpersonal functions. As described earlier, interpersonal functions represent the psychological distance that each family member prefers in relation to each other family member. Family members may or may not be "aware" of these values and functions, just as they may or may not be aware of the grammar that governs their language behavior. Nevertheless, they behave in characteristic ways that we identify as functions—for example, they consistently elicit attention and control, they consistently elicit distance by withdrawing, or they consistently send both "come here" and "go away" messages. As mentioned above, these patterns are often dyad-specific—for instance, a child and mother may coalesce through mutual closeness, while at the same time the mother and child each attempt to create distance from the father. People are not necessarily uniform in their preference for closeness or distance in all their relationships.

Changing deep value structures and functions is difficult, time-consuming, and perhaps even ethically questionable. FFT works to allow each family member to maintain his or her basic value structures and functions, but works at the same time to change the ways in which family members express and maintain these values and functions. By maintaining the values and functions, and changing only their modes of expression, resistance is considerably reduced and treatment shortened.

Resistance represents not just a natural process experienced by individuals and families when they change. It is also a feedback mechanism with respect to intervention. During each phase of intervention, resistance reflects a specific reaction, which may represent different things in different phases. In the initial phase (introduction–impression) resistance occurs when clients do not see the therapist and/or treatment agency as credible resources. During the induction–therapy phase, resistance signals a "technical" error on the part of the therapist, resulting most often from a failure to "join" the family effectively, or from adopting a blaming or an individual focus. In the treatment–education phase, resistance occurs because family members experience the specific change attempts by the therapist as inconsistent with their deep value structure and/or functions (Barton & Alexander, 1980). While Functional Family therapists have an extremely wide range of change techniques potentially available, only a subset can be used with a given family because of that family's unique blend of values and functions that are responsive only to certain techniques.

INDIVIDUALIZING INTERVENTIONS
FFT pays careful attention to individualizing interventions during the assessment and treatment planning process. Rather than adopting a general view of pathology, wherein the entire family is seen as experiencing a generalized maladaptive process, each dyadic relationship is evaluated in terms of the "fit" of values, functions, and the way family members attain them. Dyadic relationships are then viewed in the context of larger (triadic) relationships involving coalitions, triangulations, and so on. Because each person in each relationship is considered, specific change attempts are individualized so they "fit" each individual and each combination of the individuals.

TRAINING IN FFT

Components of the Training Process

In order to develop trainees' abilities and knowledge to implement the phases of FFT, training emphasizes four broad components: conceptual, emotional, technical, and relational. Much of the conceptual component of training is didactic and involves education in the theories and concepts of FFT. Elements that are emphasized in training include the systemic view of family processes, the relational view of psychopathology, and the notion that therapy or change is most efficiently accomplished in a context that legitimizes family members. The emotional component of training primarily involves trainees' ability to work with real families who have real concerns. Trainees must possess (or develop) the affective "strength" or resiliency necessary to cope with the intensity of family interaction. This aspect of training includes developing the trainees' ability to develop an adequate working relationship with families that differ widely in their preferred modes of interacting with therapists. The technical components of FFT primarily involve the procedures making up assessment, therapy, and education. Technical skills are emphasized in the experiential and practical phase of FFT training. The relational component of training, as used in this context, concerns the development of an adequate working relationship with supervisors.

In addition, training in FFT consists of two distinct stages, described in detail below: the didactic and the practicum. The didactic stage emphasizes exposure to conceptual bases of the FFT model. The practicum stage emphasizes coaching in the application of the model to actual cases.

Organizing Concepts

There are two organizing concepts in FFT training above and beyond those elaborated in the model itself: responsibility and comprehension. Responsibility concerns the obligations of both trainees and of trainers, while comprehension involves understanding the impact of one's actions on the family and understanding the point reached by the family–therapist–trainer system in the overall training/therapy process.

RESPONSIBILITY

In the FFT model, the family's motivation for therapy is largely the responsibility of the therapist. Of course, the family must have a presenting problem or reason for attending, but the therapist is responsible for instilling the hope that if they persist in the process they will benefit. Stated differently, the therapist cannot evade responsibility by labeling the family as "unmotivated." Rather, issues of motivation are seen largely as technical problems, focused on the therapist's ability to offer the family a possibility of change from which they will all benefit, and through which none of them will be blamed. In addition to this primary responsibility, FFT trainees are also responsible for using the training context to develop their skills to the fullest extent. The responsibility for trainees' motivation, in turn, falls largely on trainers. That is, trainers cannot simply categorize trainees as motivated or unmotivated, but must actively show trainees the potential of FFT for enhancing their clinical skills. In addition, trainers must show trainees the areas in which they possess or are developing strengths, and use this evidence to enhance trainees' interests in becoming competent FFT therapists. Finally, as members of therapy "teams," trainers are deeply involved in the treatment of each family, and are responsible for ensuring that the families actually are helped.

COMPREHENSION

Trainees must understand the sequence of intervention, and also understand the phase they are at with a given family. Because FFT is so stage-specific, it is vital that therapists not try to do everything at once. The therapist skills appropriate for one phase are very different from those required in another phase (Alexander *et al.*, 1983). Thus trainees must be helped to learn to adapt their styles and choice of intervention strategy to the current phase of the intervention process. Failing to do this may confuse the family or, at worst, drive them out of treatment. Conversely, trainees' understanding of where they are in the process of doing and learning FFT helps to allay some of the inevitable anxiety and discouragement that accompanies the realization that doing therapy is different from talking about it or watching it. These issues typically arise in the transition from the didactic to the practical phases of training.

Theory of Trainee Learning and Change

The FFT theory of training, learning, and change is both cognitive–developmental and operant. It is cognitive–developmental in that trainees incrementally learn to perceive family behavioral and emotional patterns from a systemic perspective. This process begins with a formal presentation of systems principles, followed by didactic presentations of systems-based family therapy principles. Finally, trainees are helped to interpret and conceptualize videotaped and live family interaction from this systems perspective. This process rests on cognitive–developmental theory in that the exposure to new information, and the learning of new frameworks into which this information may be processed, produces discontinuous accommodations or shifts in trainees' information-processing capabilities. Although a detailed discussion of cognitive–developmental theory is beyond the scope of this chapter, it may be useful to point out that FFT trainers assume that by teaching trainees the concepts of FFT, they produce an increased "perceptual readiness" to make sense of events in the family from a systemic viewpoint.

The operant aspect of the FFT theory of trainee change focuses on the application phase of training. In the process of supervised experience in the delivery of FFT, it is assumed that the trainee will change his or her style partly in response to what "works." That is, trainees observe the effects of their interventions, and presumably will be inclined to repeat those interventions that result in decreased negative affect, increased effective problem solving, a broader range of family members' functioning, and so on. It is also assumed that trainer feedback functions as an important reinforcer of trainee behavior. Thus, even though the impact of a particular intervention may not be immediately apparent, the supervisor may provide the trainee with feedback in order to reinforce the trainee's use of that particular tactic. Clearly, these two hypothesized mechanisms work reciprocally as the trainee becomes a more effective FFT therapist. That is, the trainee is able to perceive the interactional, systemic aspects of a particular event in the family, the more options for intervention will be open to the trainee, and the more likely it is that a positive result will be produced for the family.

In some respects, trainee change is similar to the changes that family members experience, but in other important respects a different process takes place. With family members, several factors contribute to learning and change; the therapist, a credible source who has no obvious stake in siding with particular members, points out a different way of viewing events. Further, family members' blaming of each other is reduced, and later on the family members are given explicit instructions to practice something new within the family. Family members are motivated for this process by being shown that it is possible for them to have more positive experiences within the family.

In the case of trainees, the context is similar; a credible expert points out a different way of viewing events, and the therapist is given explicit instructions to practice something new with the family in the context where the therapist believes that, if instructions are followed, a benefit will result. However, it is also assumed that trainee change will be affected by observational learning, cognitive restructuring, and evaluative feedback. The therapy team approach (described more fully below) provides many opportunities to observe fellow trainees working with families. Cognitive restructuring occurs when the trainer suggests new ways of viewing the family and persistently shapes trainees' ideas about family functioning into terms consistent with the FFT model. Constructive feedback is thought to be a powerful motivator in changing trainees who desire to help families effectively.

Three further assumptions bear mentioning at this point. First, it is assumed that trainers must encourage and reassure trainees through the inevitable periods of discouragement and artificiality that accompany learning such a nonintuitive system of therapy.

Second, trainees must be given a cognitive map of the phases and stages of development that are part of conducting FFT and part of learning the model. In other words, trainees must be made aware of the acquaintance–impression, assessment, induction–therapy, treatment–education, and generalization–termination phases of FFT, as well as of the didactic, early practical, middle practical, and advanced practical stages of

FFT training. A corollary of this point is that supervisory style should be tailored to a trainee's particular stage of training. For example, in the didactic stage of training, the trainer might be more likely to emphasize the theory behind a given maneuver being observed on a videotape of a therapy session, while in the practical stage the trainer might be more likely to role play variations on the intervention. Similarly, as will be noted in more detail below, with trainees in the later stages of training, the trainer might become more Socratic in postsession feedback sessions, since the trainee must soon function as a more independent therapist and must begin to generate ideas for effective change independently.

Third, trainees are encouraged to expand their own range of functioning or to resolve personal concerns, but to seek such growth outside of the training setting. In cases in which individual trainees wish to work on particular personal issues they are often referred to practitioners in the community who are willing to treat graduate students for a reduced fee, or they are directed to the university counseling center. As a corollary of this point, it is underscored that family therapy training is different from family therapy; among other reasons for this, the therapist–family system is seen as temporary and voluntary. That is, unlike family members who often cannot (except by quite costly means) terminate from their families, therapists can terminate treatment or refer their families elsewhere (and families can do the same). Family members "enroll" in treatment in order to change a painful existing situation; trainees, on the other hand, enroll in training to build competencies (of course FFT should have the effect of building competencies in families as well, but the context of change is different). There are certainly outcomes of FFT training that are "therapy-like" for trainees (such as the ability to see their personal relationships in functional terms, and the ability to relabel events in less negative terms), and that increase trainees' competencies and comfort as persons, but these are not the explicit focus of the training program. As a relatively short-term, intensive training experience designed to teach a short-term, problem-focused model of intervention, the major focus of FFT training is on the ability of trainees to perceive functional aspects of family events and to intervene effectively in changing maladaptive aspects of family functioning.

These differences between therapy and training lead trainers to be more evaluative when considering trainee behavior than therapists would when considering the family members' actions. Since FFT trainers are often held responsible for the actions of their trainees (or at least they feel responsible—after all, it is they who grant the "stamp of approval" to trainees after they have finished training), there is strong interest in seeing that the FFT trainees become competent at assessing and intervening in families. Thus, while therapists work very hard to fit goals and techniques to the family reality, training often forces trainees to fit their concepts and techniques to the reality of the model—not vice versa.

Training Context

This section describes the three major contexts in which FFT training is typically delivered, and briefly outlines the human and physical resources that constitute those contexts.

TRAINING SETTINGS

FFT training has typically occurred in one of three settings: university training, in-service training for professionals, and institute-based training. University-based training is part of the clinical psychology training program at the University of Utah. A majority of the trainees are clinical psychology graduate students, although trainees are also drawn from graduate programs in counseling psychology, social work, and psychiatric nursing. All the training, from didactic phase through practical phase, occurs on campus. In-service training typically occurs at the worksites in the community, and such training is usually compressed into a smaller number of intensive training days. The sequence of training is similar to that of campus-based training, although the intensity and length of time is different. FFT training is also delivered through the provision of training placements at a free-standing private nonprofit family therapy institute.

TRAINERS

Training faculty for the FFT training settings noted above are typically mental health professionals with MSW or PhD degrees. All have had graduate training in family therapy, and almost all have had direct experience in the ongoing development of the FFT model. A core of trainers, the "primary faculty," has advanced degrees and several years of experience in model development, as well as in service delivery and training delivery. A secondary group, "trainers in training," also possess advanced degrees in a mental health profession and have had extensive training in FFT. Thus, FFT trainers are committed to the model, well versed in its application, and, ideally, experienced in a wide variety of clinical problems.

TRAINEES

As noted above, most FFT trainees are either graduate students in one of the mental health disciplines or already working in the mental health or human service field. These trainees have included bachelor's degree–level and paraprofessional workers in youth corrections, family services, welfare, child protection, and the like. For the didactic phase of FFT training, trainees are most often self-selected by their interest in the model. In some cases, typically of the in-service sort, the agency director has found the FFT model compelling and has involved relevant staff. Thus trainees may be selected by the amount of contact they have with cases the director thinks are amenable to a FFT approach. In the practical phase of FFT training, trainees are selected by successful completion of the didactic phase.

RESOURCES

The families seen in FFT training settings range from upper-middle-class to lower-class in socioeconomic status. Presenting problems span a large range, from transient situational disturbances to major psychopathology. The majority of the cases, however, have involved the problems of early and middle adolescence. Compared to traditional outpatient caseloads, a substantial portion of the families seen by FFT trainees would be considered unmotivated and largely lacking in resources.

The full range of technical resources is available to FFT trainers and trainees. Video cassette recorders are routinely used in recording and supervising FFT. A videotape library is available that illustrates sessions conducted both by FFT trainers and by FFT trainees. The clinic used by the FFT on-campus training program includes a suite of therapy rooms with one-way glass and both video and audio tape-recording facilities. In-service training most typically employs portable video and audio tape-recording.

TRAINING METHODS AND CONTENT

Format

Training occurs in two phases. The first phase involves 30 hours of didactic training (in the campus-based training, a 10-week "prepracticum" course). Didactic training focuses on both theoretical material and therapeutic skills, but involves no direct treatment of families. Practical, supervised experience follows the didactic training and emphasizes the learning of therapeutic skills mainly through direct therapy experience. Although the focus of the didactic phase is primarily theory, and the focus of the practicum phase technique, in fact theory and technique are interwoven in both phases. For example, role plays and observation of videotape demonstrate techniques during the didactic phase, while group discussion and additional reading often direct trainees' attention to theory during the practicum phase.

DIDACTIC TRAINING PHASE

Academic didactic training starts with a "core course" in interactional theory. This course uses readings, lectures, videotapes, and discussions to review the major principles of general systems theory, and descriptions of various therapy models and their conceptualization of a variety of referral problems. The prepracticum portion of the didactic phase focuses on the FFT proper and its consistency with a systems approach to mental illness; the matching-to-sample notion, the phases and domains of change, and the model's empirical base are introduced at this time. Lectures and readings are emphasized in the first few weeks of training, since some trainees are unfamiliar with systems theory and family therapy models. Once trainees have been provided with a solid base of knowledge in this area, discussions and videotapes become the primary method of teaching theory. Videotapes and discussion allow the trainees to see and question how general and sometimes vague concepts are translated into more concrete, practical applications.

Therapeutic skills become a primary focus later in the didactic phase. Discussions, videotapes, and role plays quickly supplement lectures, and enable trainees to observe, practice, and ask questions about specific FFT techniques. All trainees are required to participate in role play situations in order to experience roles of therapist and family members. Immediately following each role play, the instructor and other trainees provide feedback to the role players describing the processes they observed between "family members" and the ways in which the "therapist" was able to affect family members. The timing and types of procedures used to convey both theoretical and more technical therapy skills are similar; both parts of the didactic phase initially focus on lectures and readings, which are then quickly followed by more specific, concrete examples in which trainees participate directly.

PRACTICUM PHASE

Practicum experience follows the didactic training, and consists of 80 to 100 hours of supervised experience with families in the clinic. Therapy sessions are audiotaped and videotaped so that trainees can review these tapes between sessions. Discussions and role plays are also continued in the practicum at weekly meetings where cases are reviewed and specific intervention styles are discussed.

Trainees are assigned a supervisor, a fellow trainee, and one to two cases at the beginning of the practicum experience. Each trainee's family therapy session is observed through a one-way mirror by a supervisor and the trainee's partner. The therapy team of therapist, partner, and supervisor are involved in the entire course of family therapy for each case. This system functions to provide the therapist-in-training with reliable support and ideas for intervention strategies. Each trainee, therefore, has a number of families that he or she follows. The trainees observe their partners doing therapy with several families. Since trainees are both therapists and observers, they are exposed to the application of FFT techniques with a variety of family styles and referral problems. Trainees learn not only from direct experience, but also from observing and modeling themselves after their partner in therapy. Furthermore, they are exposed to the subtle interaction of therapy techniques and therapists' skills with different families.

The trainees' use of their partners and trainers as consultants is critical because FFT has numerous goals for any one session and emphasizes short-term therapy (10 to 12 weeks). The therapy team also serves a purpose similar to that of a cotherapist: the team can help to reduce the intensity of therapy, assist in providing intervention strategies, and help the trainee in conceptualizing the family in FFT terms. FFT does not use cotherapists, primarily because of the structured and complex nature of the assessment and therapy phases. Combining these techniques in supervision behind a one-way mirror while having one therapist present them in therapy yields more effective and integrated interventions.

Supervision occurs in a variety of formats and focuses on various training issues, with an emphasis on technical and conceptual components. Supervision can focus on immediate or postsession feedback. Immediate feedback usually occurs during the session, behind a one-way mirror. The therapist can leave the therapy room to talk with the team; thus at any time trainers and partners can provide trainees with brief feedback and answer questions. This type of interchange is initiated by either the supervisor or the trainee and is typically quite brief. Both the trainers and the trainee's partner are involved in providing feedback to the trainee; there are no *a priori* restrictions on the partner's freedom to give feedback. However, if the trainer observes that the partner's feedback is excessively individual-oriented, or disposition-focused, the trainer will attempt a sort of "meta-supervision" in order to reorient the feedback along FFT lines.

An additional option open to supervisors is that of direct involvement in the session. If the situation seems to call for it, the supervisor may enter the therapy room and demonstrate specific intervention techniques for the trainee. This intervention is used sparingly, primarily on occasions when the therapist appears to be paralyzed by the family's interaction style or when the family is sending out critical cues that the therapist continues to ignore, even after feedback. Initially, these difficulties are dealt with by calling the therapist into the observation room for feedback. If this is ineffective, the supervisor may consider going directly into the session. However, the supervisor must recognize the risks of this action. These risks can include loss of trainee credibility in the family's eyes and loss of self-confidence and self-efficacy for the trainee.

Postsession supervision occurs immediately after the therapy session, and also involves the therapy team. This type of supervision usually lasts about 30 minutes. Feedback may cover technical issues as well as conceptual and affective components of training. These sessions appear to have impact because theoretical constructs and therapy techniques can be quickly supplemented with examples from previous sessions.

Trainees receive further training at weekly group supervision meetings. The group includes all the trainees and supervisors involved in the practicum. FFT's general concepts are reviewed and creative applications of FFT techniques are frequently discussed in the group context. Furthermore, trainees periodically bring the group up to date regarding each of their cases. In addition, trainees complete forms concerning their own behavior and that of various family members between therapy sessions. The behaviors include such variables as talking rate, number of attempted relabels, apparent role assignments within the family, and so forth. Other trainees, not necessarily their partners, and other supervisors are available between sessions for further consultation regarding specific family issues, therapist characteristics, and application of FFT techniques.

Learning Goals and Objectives

The overall program goal, as noted previously, is to develop the most effective family therapists possible. Effective FFT therapists are defined as trainees who understand the FFT model, who have the emotional resilience to cope with the impact of a wide variety of family problems, who can use the techniques of FFT with families, and who can develop beneficial working relationships with supervisors. These goals translate into specific objectives in each of the stages of training, as summarized in Table 8-1.

FFT training, in part because it is embedded in a clinical psychology training program, aims to produce competent FFT therapists who are also well trained clinical psychologists. Early in the FFT training process, trainees need to have enough understanding of nonfamilial models of pathology and treatment to communicate adequately with other professionals (or family members convinced by other professionals) who adopt such models. Trainees must also understand nonfamilial models well enough to know what they imply about change and improvement that is different from FFT. This focus is emphasized during the didactic phase. Most often, if trainees do not bring to their FFT training a reasonable level of awareness of nonfamilial models, it is recommended that they do outside reading.

For many of the trainees, FFT is their only exposure to a systemic model. Partly in keeping with the training program philosophy of providing some generalist training, FFT training provides a brief overview of other family systems models. Understanding other family therapy models is necessary to know how and why FFT is different. It is also helpful in enabling therapists to develop alternatives and to realize that other perspectives are possible. Other family therapy models are also discussed, at least briefly, in the early portion of the didactic phase of training.

TABLE 8-1. Goals of FFT Training (By Stage of Training)

I. Didactic stage:
  Knowledge of:
    basics of systems theory;
    basics of FFT; functions, AIM, relabels;
    basics of intervention sequence;
    beginning awareness of own therapist characteristics.
II. Beginning practical stage:
  The ability to:
    identify sequences of behavior, affect and/or cognition:
    employ general relabels ("concern," "help," "loss," "worry," etc.);
    identify functions, with assistance;
    keep family members in treatment;
    give constructive feedback from FFT perspective to teammates;
    recognize when therapy phase of FFT has been accomplished.
III. Middle and later practical stage:
  The ability to:
    generate creative relabels;
    easily and comfortably form relationship with families;
    employ own characteristics effectively in establishing credibility;
    generate useful homework assignments;
    articulate one's general intervention strategy with a given family;
    plan and carry out the education phase of FFT;
    deal with intense resistance from family members.
IV. Advanced stages:
  The ability to:
    conduct FFT with fragments of families;
    supervise beginning FFT therapists;
    fit concepts from other frameworks into FFT appropriately, as needed;
    use FFT even in settings (e.g., busy outpatient clinics) that present logistical/political obstacles to its
      most effective use;
    identify own difficulties and seek consultation when appropriate.

With trainees who have considerable talent, the program goal is to produce superior therapists. An equally important goal is to work with trainees of average talent to produce competent FFT therapists who have maximized their talent, who are flexible, and who know how to develop alternative resources in areas that represent weakness for them.

It is a goal of the program that successful trainees can create, within many different agencies or institutions, a structure that allows the flexibility to conduct FFT in the most efficient manner, and that supports evaluative research on the model. This program goal is attempted most typically in the consultative relationship characteristic of advanced FFT training.

An important program goal is to provide clear feedback to trainees regarding their progress. This is accomplished primarily through use of evaluative instruments, and feedback during supervision. The primary evaluative intrument is the "Therapist Characteristics Checklist" shown in Table 8-2.

Additional rating sheets that monitor family progress have also been designed for each of the three training contexts. In addition to the use of written evaluation instru-

TABLE 8-2. Therapist Characteristics Checklist

		Rating	Good example on tape	Poor example on tape
Relationship skills	"Linking" Humor Warmth Nonblaming Self-disclosure			
Structuring skills	Clarity Self-confidence Directiveness			
Therapy skills	Creative relabeling Integrative interpretation			
Process skills	Equivalent talk time Drawing out "the quiet one" Slowing down "the chatty one" Successful interruptions Generating effective family communication between members			
Meeting "between session" plans or goals	Progress in "sequences of intervention" Completion of "understanding and treating family members"			
Education skills	Protecting *functions* with education "Packaging" education Dealing with resistance Identifying/reinforcing progress			

ments, feedback from supervisors is ongoing. In the case of trainees who are not accomplishing minimal goals in the training program, more specific evaluative feedback is necessary. At the minimum, trainees experiencing prolonged difficulty are given clear feedback on their weaknesses, and sometimes directed to additional training opportunities. They may also be counseled out of FFT into some more suitable area.

Trainer–Trainee Relationship

The relationship between trainer and trainee is typically that of expert and novice. This fact has costs and benefits. On the positive side, the fact that the trainees can adopt a lower-status learning role gives them "permission to fail." That is, the burden of having to be a perfect mental health professional can be (temporarily) dropped, and the risk of making mistakes taken in a supportive environment with team assistance. On the other hand, for beginning graduate students who are already experiencing a number of opportunities to fail, and for established mental health professionals who already have reputations as competent practitioners in other areas of practice, the adoption of the learner/subordinate role can be quite stressful. Thus, most often the FFT trainer tries to minimize activities that emphasize hierarchy (e.g., going into the therapy room to accomplish only a specific intervention task) and attempts to use somewhat more "tentative" approaches to providing feedback (e.g., "Did you think about trying X?" versus "You should have tried X"). As trainees become more accomplished as therapists (and as they demonstrate their willingness to seek out and use feedback), the amount of authoritative behavior from the supervisor decreases correspondingly.

The trainer–trainee relationship is not that of therapist–client. In most cases the trainer keeps the feedback and guidance on the technical and conceptual level. The training context is not seen as a domain that emphasizes therapists' meeting their own needs (except needs for efficacy). Of course, if it becomes necessary, the trainer can help the trainees to locate appropriate sources of therapeutic help outside the training context. It also occasionally occurs in supervision that the trainer helps the therapist to identify sources of difficulty arising from personal experience (e.g., a trainee realized with his supervisor's help that his prolonged blaming of a particular mother stemmed from her resemblance to his own mother). Nonetheless, working through such issues typically occurs outside the training context (e.g., in the trainee's own therapy).

In cases where trainees actively seek therapeutic help from the supervisor (typically without asking for it directly) the supervisor gently redirects the issue to the trainees' work in FFT. For example, a trainee might ask why he or she is so critical of himself or herself, and the trainer might respond with, "What in the family you are treating is leading you to hold yourself to such high standards?" He or she might also respond with, "Oh, so now you have some sense of how the kids in this family feel; let's see if we can use that, in a nonblaming way, to show Mom. . . ."

The trainer typically gives more directives early in the training process; as the trainee develops a grasp of the fundamentals of FFT and needs guidance primarily with specific techniques, the trainer shifts to contingent directiveness. As this process continues, the status differences between the participants decrease; trainers may use more self-disclosure and may discuss the relationship between other facets of trainees' activities and FFT approaches.

Trainee Problems

The difficulties experienced by a trainee may be conceptualized as stemming from (1) demand characteristics of the training setting, (2) aspects of the trainee's style, (3) features of the FFT model, or (4) characteristics of the trainer–trainee relationship.

In practice, the trainers work through a sort of "decision tree" to identify sources of difficulty (Table 8-3). The trainer focuses first on those aspects of training that are somewhat simpler to remedy, and works through to the more complex issues if the earlier ones seem not to be the source of the resistance or difficulty. For example, if a trainee has extreme difficulty initiating therapeutic maneuvers, the trainer will intervene and point out the difficulty. If the problem persists, the trainer will question (privately, and with the trainee) the trainee's understanding of the FFT model. If the trainer is satisfied that the

TABLE 8-3. The FFT Trainer Decision-making Process in Schematic Form

Source of difficulty (in terms of components of FFT training)	Supervisor question	Supervisor action

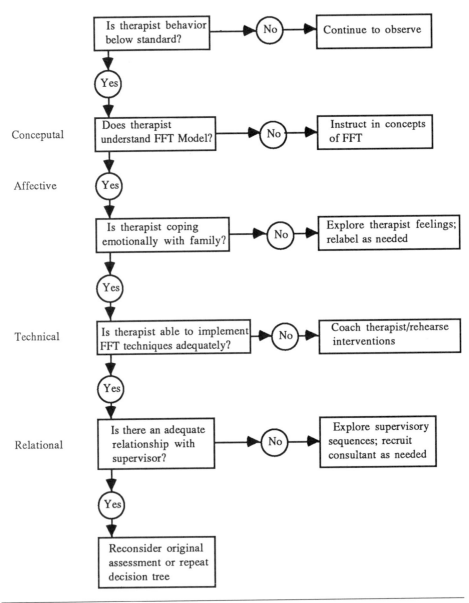

trainee understands the model, the question of the family's emotional impact on the trainee will be raised. If it is clear that the trainee is not experiencing an emotional response to the familiy that prevents the effective application of FFT, the question of the trainee's ability to adopt a relabeling frame of mind will be considered. If this too seems not to be the root of the problem, the trainer must investigate his or her relationship with the trainee.

The setting of the training (primarily the on-campus one) may be the primary source of difficulty. Typical issues include fear of evaluation, competitiveness with peers, loss of status as one attempts to adopt a new model of treatment, and unrealistic wishes that the techniques will solve one's own problems.

Problems may stem, secondarily, from the trainee's emotional response to the family. For example, a trainee's rate of activity during sessions may be inappropriately low, or a trainee may be persistently critical of and blaming of one or more family members. If it is clear that the trainee has grasped the essential features of the model, it is assumed that attention needs to be directed to the emotional impact the family is having on the trainee. Certain therapists may be especially vulnerable to this sort of difficulty in beginning phases of practical training. Trainees who work in quasi-legal settings (such as child welfare workers or drug abuse workers) may also, because of their training in controlling harmful deviance, be lured into nontherapeutic stances by their reactions to family members. The emotional reactions of the trainee, or the trainee's self-concept ("detective," "avenger of injustice") may contribute to difficulties in conducting or learning FFT.

Adoption of the FFT model itself may pose problems for some therapists. First, FFT is a short-term directive therapy that involves perceived changes in the role of therapist from "understanding helper" to "manipulator." Second, difficulty in relabeling is the "common cold" of FFT trainees. Some trainees simply do not have the type of cognitive capacity needed to relabel. This does not imply a lack of intelligence, nor is it necessarily the result of failure to understand the FFT model, or of a paralyzing emotional response to the family. Rather, it is something akin to having difficulty in developing a sense of humor; that is, "getting" a joke depends on something beyond "understanding" it, and telling a joke (or seeing something as being funny enough to be told as a joke) depends on something beyond intelligence and ability to notice details. In addition, it is clear that sequence, timing, delivery, and context are all crucial in successful joke telling, and in the attribution by others that one has a sense of humor. So it is with relabeling; some of our trainees (fortunately a minority) seem simply unable to develop the slightly absurdist mental set necessary to relabel. In such cases, trainees are helped to develop a pool of behavior/feeling/cognition descriptions known as "stock" or "generic" relabels; for example, these might involve recasting *criticism* as *concern, anger* as *intense involvement,* or *depression* as *overconsideration of others' needs.*

If no other source of resistance can be identified, it may be the case that resentment of the supervisor, excessive dependence on the supervisor, or inability to understand supervisory direction is handicapping the trainee. Clearly, each of these difficulties may be described equally well as the trainer's overdirectiveness, the trainer's need for control, or the trainer's communication problems, respectively. In short, there may be problems of hostility, dependence, or poor communication in the relationship. These sorts of problems may be best addressed by involving a consultant who may either discuss the issues with the trainer alone, or meet (in very difficult cases) with the trainer–trainee pair.

CONCLUSIONS

Functional Family Therapy is a dynamic model that can be noted as much for its growth as a conceptual framework as it can for its basic principles. Trainers and trainees alike have experienced the reciprocal benefits of research and training; both activities represent a mandate of the program in which FFT is embedded. In this unique context faculty have the dual roles of training students in the conceptual and technical aspects of providing family therapy, while at the same time teaching the same trainees principles of scientific methodology and appropriate scientific skepticism. Thus the FFT model has been under constant research scrutiny, undergoing modification as research data accrue and conceptual frameworks expand. In keeping with a desired result of this type of training, a substantial proportion of trainees graduate to positions as scientist/professionals in clinical psychology training programs.

Because of this, FFT qualifies less as a "school" of family therapy than do other models. FFT training does not involve formal certification (as an FFT specialist per se), public workshops, or advertised clerkships/internships in which trainees accrue senior status. Instead, the FFT training program is part of a larger training program that aims to produce professionals who can further develop the knowledge base in the field of clinical psychology. As indicated above, this context has influenced both conceptual and technical components of FFT. At least as exciting, however, is the fact that in a true systems manner FFT has also, in turn, influenced its context. It represents the basis for a required psychology department core course for clinical and clinical child/family psychology students. Thus, unlike its early days, the model no longer represents an "adjunct" to other conceptual models and intervention approaches. Instead, it is now a basic component of training in its own right, and provides a delightful context for spawning even greater advances in the conceptual underpinnings and the technical applications of the model.

References

Alexander, J. F. (1967). The therapist as a model—and as himself. *Psychotherapy, Theory, Research and Practice, 4*, 164–165.

Alexander, J. F. (1973). Defensive and supportive communications in normal and deviant families. *Journal of Consulting and Clinical Psychology, 40*(2), 223–231.

Alexander, J. F., & Abeles, N. (1968). Dependency changes in psychotherapy as related to interpersonal relationships. *Journal of Consulting and Clinical Psychology, 32*(6), 685–689.

Alexander, J. F., & Abeles, N. (1969). Psychotherapy process: Sex differences and dependency. *Journal of Counseling Psychology, 16*(3), 191–196.

Alexander, J. F., Barton, C., Schiavo, R. S., & Parsons, B. V. (1976). Behavioral intervention with families of delinquents: Therapist characteristics and outcome. *Journal of Consulting and Clinical Psychology, 44*(4), 656–664.

Alexander, J. F., Barton, C., Waldron, H., & Mas, C. H. (1983). Beyond the technology of family therapy: The anatomy of intervention model. In K. D. Craig & R. J. McMahon (Eds.), *Advances in clinical behavior therapy.* New York: Brunner/Mazel.

Alexander, J. F., & Parsons, B. V. (1973). Short term behavioral intervention with delinquent families: Impact on family process and recidivism. *Journal of Abnormal Psychology, 81*(3), 219–225.

Alexander, J. F., & Parsons, B. V. (1982). *Functional family therapy: Principles and procedures.* Carmel, CA: Brooks/Cole.

Barton, C., & Alexander, J. F. (1980). Functional family therapy. In A. S. Gurman & D. P. Kniskern (Eds.), *Handbook of family therapy*. New York: Brunner/Mazel.

Barton, C., Alexander, J. F., Waldron, H., Warburton, J., & Turner, C. W., (1983, December). *Family intervention, alternatives, and seriously delinquent youth: A program evaluation study*. Poster session presented at the World Congress on Behavior Therapy/1983 AABT Convention, Washington, DC.

Haley, J. (1962). Family experiments: A new type of experimentation. *Family Process, 1*, 265–293.

Haley, J. (1963). *Strategies of psychotherapy*. New York: Grune & Stratton.

Haley, J. (1964). Research on family patterns: An instrument measurement. *Family Process, 3*, 41–65.

Haley, J. (1967). Speech sequences of normal and abnormal families with two children present. *Family Process, 6*, 81–97.

Klein, N. C., Alexander, J. F., & Parsons, B. V. (1976). Impact of family systems intervention on recidivism and sibling delinquency: A model of primary prevention and program evaluation. *Journal of Consulting and Clinical Psychology, 45*(3), 467–474.

Minuchin, S. (1974). *Families and family therapy*. Cambridge, MA: Harvard University Press.

Morris, S., Alexander, J. F., & Waldron, H. (in press). Functional family therapy: Issues in clinical practice. In I. R. H. Falloon (Ed.), *Handbook of behavioral family therapy*. New York: Guilford Press.

Morton, T. L., Alexander, J. F., & Altman, I. (1976). Communication and relationship definition. In G. R. Miller (Ed.), *Annual reviews of communication research: Volume 5. Interpersonal communication*. Beverly Hills, CA: Sage Publications.

Olson, D. H., McCubbin, H. I., Barnes, H., Larsen, A., Muxen, M., & Wilson, M. (1983). *Families: What makes them work*. Beverly Hills, CA: Sage Publications.

Parsons, B. V., & Alexander, J. F. (1973). Short term family intervention: A therapy outcome study. *Journal of Consulting and Clinical Psychology, 41*(2), 195–201.

Patterson, G. R., & Reid, J. (1970). Reciprocity and coercion: Two facets of social systems. In C. Neuringer & J. Michael (Eds.), *Behavioral modification in clinical psychology*. New York: Appleton-Century-Crofts.

Ullmann, L. P., & Krasner, L., (Eds.). (1965). *Case studies in behavior modification*. New York: Holt, Rinehart & Winston.

Warburton, J. R., & Alexander, J. F. (1985). The family therapist: A forgotten aspect of change? In L. L'Abate (Ed.), *The handbook of family psychology*. Homewood, IL: Dow Jones–Irwin.

SECTION THREE

PRAGMATICS OF SUPERVISION

Introduction

The evolutionary paths of both family therapy supervision and family therapy practice models have, not surprisingly, strong similarities. These parallels are distinctive in at least three ways: the public nature of both endeavors, their emphasis on the interactive process, and their flexibility and creativity.

Family therapy broke traditional rules about the individual patient's confidentiality by inviting family members to participate in the therapy. Once defined as a public event, it was an easy next step for family therapy to be observed by others, initially for research and later for team approaches to therapy and supervision. This public nature helped create the most popular forms of family therapy supervision, live and videotape.

Family therapy's emphasis on the interactive process also required a method of supervision capable of accessing this process. Therapist recall, process notes, and even audiotapes could not capture the richness and complexity of interaction of a family therapy session; consequently, means of direct observation evolved, culminating, for now at least, in the methods of live and videotape supervision.

Live and videotape supervision are not, however, the only methods used by family therapy supervisors. In fact, just as family therapists are able to generate an endless supply of creative interventions, so also supervisors continue to produce creative approaches to supervision that involve novel uses of the team, phone-ins, role play, and so on.

For the past decade, the editors of this volume, and their associates, have devoted much of their time to the development of family therapy supervision methods, examining the process surrounding this development, and analyzing the impact these methods have on the supervisor–supervisee relationship. Four of the chapters in Section Three describe these efforts. Also, because supervision methods are only as good as the supervisors providing them, we felt this volume should include a chapter devoted to the important issue of training supervisors.

9

Systemic Supervision: Conceptual Overlays and Pragmatic Guidelines

HOWARD A. LIDDLE
University of California, San Francisco

> *A journey of a thousand miles must begin with a single step.*
> —Chinese Proverb

ON THE IMPORTANCE OF STARTING SUPERVISION WELL

With most things in life, starting well helps. It is commonly asserted that an effective start in therapy greatly enhances the probability that it will end in success (Haley, 1976). This is as true in supervision as it is in therapy; the failure to begin the supervisory process on at least a partially successful note can make this creative and exciting endeavor tedious, if not tortuous. Furthermore, supervision that has lost, or never gained, focus, and that spins off track, can be notoriously difficult to realign with one's training objectives.

Although supervision can be defined narrowly as the process of teaching a clinician how to conduct therapy, it frequently affects many aspects of a therapist's professional and personal development. Effective supervision prepares trainees for their career and, further, upgrades the profession and advances the field. It can help therapists to launch their professional lives toward the highest possible trajectory of confidence, given their maturity, training, and experience. Alternatively, inferior supervision by inexperienced or inept supervisors, or by those who have lost the generative spirit inherent in a vital supervisory situation, does not merely affect a group of unlucky trainees, it also influences the entire field. Therapists who repeatedly have inadequate supervisors are at increased risk for providing poor service to their clients, and tarnishing their own and their profession's standing in the community and society. Additionally, after demoralizing and debilitating training experiences, clinicians who are at formative stages of their professional development may become discouraged and cynical about the psychotherapy profession as well as their career choice. Unfortunately, at this early stage it is not uncommon for therapists to doubt themselves and the wisdom of remaining on a clinical career path rather than question mediocre or incompetent supervisors.

Supervision thus involves significantly more than the mere transmission of techni-

cal information or clinical skills: it challenges participants both personally and intellectually in a context in which the best and worst of a supervisor's or therapist's individual
style can emerge. For instance, the supervisory situation provokes anxiety for trainees and
supervisors alike. Fear of exposing one's personal, interpersonal, cognitive, and professional inadequacies; performance anxiety; competitiveness with colleagues; and, for
therapists, resentment about finding oneself in the learner role, are the most obvious and
intensely felt concomitants of being supervised and conducting supervision. The ways in
which this intimate, task-focused relationship influences the personal and professional
development of both therapist and supervisor has been the subject of serious inquiry in
the psychotherapy supervision literature for some time (Matarazzo & Patterson, 1986)
and has recently received attention in the family therapy field (Draper, 1982; Duhl, 1983;
Hess, 1987; Liddle, in press; Liddle & Halpin, 1978; Schwartz, Chapter 10, this volume;
Whiffen & Byng-Hall, 1982).

A complex subsystem in the training domain, supervision is both a whole entity—
with mutually influencing cognitive-, affective-, and behavioral-shaping properties—and
a part, a multifaceted piece of a broader fabric constituting the training system. It is a
context that has reciprocally influencing domains of conceptualization and action. Since
complexity can be defined as the hallmark of a training context (Breunlin, Liddle, &
Schwartz, Chapter 13, this volume; Liddle & Schwartz, 1983) this setting demands careful
attention to a multitude of factors and processes.

This chapter serves as a companion piece to a previous paper (Liddle, 1982b) that
was designed to offer therapists a rationale and a suggestion for clarifying their clinical
epistemology. The present work offers clinical supervisors a series of conceptual overlays
and pragmatic, skill-focused guidelines, with particular emphasis on beginning the
supervision process. It details what the supervisor needs to keep in mind before and
during supervision, and articulates how a supervisor can proceed at the outset of and
throughout supervision, to prevent unnecessary problems and to keep supervision on
track. These guidelines are based on our overall supervision paradigm (Liddle & Saba, in
press), research conducted on the outcomes of supervision (Liddle, Davidson, & Barrett,
Chapter 25, this volume), and previous analyses of the family therapy training and
supervision field (Liddle, 1982a, 1985a, 1985b, in press; Liddle & Halpin, 1978).

THE SUPERVISOR'S CONCEPTUAL LIFE: KEY OVERLAYS

In a national survey of family therapy trainers, the majority of respondents wanted
additional substantive work on models of training and theories of supervision (Saba &
Liddle, 1986). In particular, these supervisors asked for superordinate models to guide
their training. What follows is an attempt to address these expressed needs: we examine
the elemental domains of thinking and action that can guide a supervisor's work.

The Isomorphic Nature of Training and Therapy

This principle has been the foundation of our conceptualization of the complex,
multilevel processes of training and therapy. We have thought of it as a cognitively
orienting and action-suggesting template for supervisors.[1] It has served as the "overlay of

overlays"—a framework under which all other elements of the training process can be subsumed.

Recently, however, the use of this term to refer to the interconnectedness of therapy and training has been criticized. Some authors (Everett & Koerpel, 1986) have preferred the term "parallel processes," coined by the psychodynamically oriented writers on supervision in the 1950s and 1960s. This term has been employed to refer to those interactional patterns that replicate themselves and are transferred from the treatment to the training domains (or from the training to the treatment domain). Whereas both "isomorphism" and "parallel process" can be used to label a process in which a family's discouragement or despair can be "caught" by the therapist and then passed on and unwittingly incorporated by the supervisor watching behind the mirror, "parallel process" does not adequately capture what we might term the *action potential.* Parallel process refers only to, or primarily to, a process-level *description* of interaction between subsystems. In this, its most common usage, there is no inherent intervention potential, no action or intentionality inferred in the supervisor's observation of the parallel interactions. Here parallel processes are phenomena that are meaningful only or primarily in a perceptual or assessment sense. Hence, the author prefers the term "isomorphism" over the less technical term "parallel processes" because its inferences are both more comprehensive and more precise, given the intervention-ability of the supervisor.

Isomorphism in its present usage is a broad, more inclusive and pragmatic concept. The isomorphic nature of training and therapy not only refers to this pattern of sequence replicability across subsystem boundaries, but also contains other aspects. This term not only implies that the parallel processes are interactional processes to be charted in the training and therapy systems, but also includes the notion that these interactions are capable as well of being altered and shaped—that they are subject to intentional supervisory intervention and change. The replication of certain processes across system boundaries can be detrimental to the therapeutic and supervisory systems. Using the isomorphism perspective, the supervisor can transform this replication into an intervention, redirecting a therapist's behavior and thereby influencing interactions at various levels of the system.

The isomorphic nature of therapy and training is thus a principle that exists not only in the domains of observation and description, but also *in the domain of supervisory intervention.* Isomorphism does not simply refer to patterns that exist in an assessment-only sense: the replicating interactions are information that can be reshaped. They are realities that can be altered; thus, assessment and intervention become blurred. With forethought and intentionality, the supervisor uses the interactional information (i.e., the way in which problematic patterns replicate themselves in the training and therapy domains) to redirect the co-created course of the training–therapy system. Supervisors are not passive observers of pattern replication, but intervenors and intentional shapers of the misdirected sequences they perceive, participate in, and co-create.

Another useful aspect of the isomorphism concept refers to the interconnection and interdependence of the principles that organize therapy and training—the assumptions consistently driving a therapist's and supervisor's work. This perspective on isomorphism assumes that *one's guiding premises about how systems are organized* (e.g., hierarchical structure, subsystem interdependence), *evolve* (e.g., thinking in terms of developmental stages and life cycle), *and change* (e.g., principles about the mechanisms of learning and change) *in one domain* (e.g., therapy) *are applicable as guides in the other interconnected and complementary domain* (e.g., training). Briefly stated, one's principles about the goals, methods, and means of evaluation in therapy can be utilized as an aid to conceptualization and action in training. The process of articulating one's assumptions about the nature of therapeutic change and the role of the therapist, previously described as making an epistemologic declaration (Liddle, 1982b), can help supervisors build a training framework with clear guiding premises (Liddle & Saba, in press). This personal framework, with both idiosyncratic and generic aspects, is indispensable in the organization of the supervision context.

Formation of the Supervisory System

This section defines the preeminent factors constituting and influencing the successful formation of the supervisory system.[2]

SUPERVISOR VARIABLES

The premises about therapy and change that a supervisor brings to the training situation are crucial determinants of that training system and its formation. These assumptions invariably influence the supervisor's orientation toward supervision and supervisees.

The supervisor's level of clinical skill in the observational, perceptual, conceptual, and communication realms is also important. Yet it is not necessary to have expert clinical skills in order to be an expert supervisor.[3] The capacity to *conduct* therapy skillfully does not necessarily transfer to the behaviors required for expert supervision. Many virtuoso clinicians cannot articulate or translate their skills into the arena of teaching and training; and it is also possible to be an excellent teacher of therapy and do average clinical work. Effective supervisors, however, are experts about the nuances of therapy and therapists. They have a fund of knowledge and experience to draw on, are adept communicators of this knowledge, can successfully access and translate their knowledge in a clinical context, and understand the complexities of the teaching/learning situation (see Liddle, Davidson, & Barett, Chapter 25, this volume).

Supervisor's Role Development

In the successful articulation of one's training epistemology, role definition is another area that requires attention, particularly in the early stages of one's career as a supervisor. Although it is well recognized that the supervisor's essential role is to help therapists gain skills so they can then help their clients, this fact is nonetheless often forgotten, especialy by beginning supervisors. For example, supervisors who think like therapists rather than supervisors may be inclined to bypass the trainee level of the training system.

Often supervisors think how *they* would, and not how the therapist should, intervene with the family. As a result, the supervisor will fail to conceptualize the *therapist plus family* as the primary unit to be supervised (i.e., how can I *help this therapist* do what I think needs to be done?). The supervisor is thus distracted from the essential challenge: how to help the therapist implement an intervention or strategy, given the therapist's idiosyncrasies and level of competency, and the particulars of the case and supervisory method.

A second issue of role development concerns how supervisors view their professional role and their profession. Supervisors have varying degrees of enthusiasm for their work. Is supervising students a dreaded chore, something that comes with senior status in an agency, or is the designation *supervisor* something to be worked toward energetically, and cherished and nourished once it is achieved? In short, as with other walks of life, the *attitude* supervisors bring to their task—their enjoyment, expectations for fulfillment, and enthusiasm for the work—influence the formation of the supervisory system. Supervisors who are dedicated to, and willing to work at, their craft are powerful role models to their trainees. Formal training in supervision can instill beneficial attitudinal as well as skill sets in clinicians interested in becoming supervisors.

A final issue of supervisory role development concerns the training environment. In a setting in which there are other supervisors with whom to discuss one's work, there is a likelihood of meaningful and enriching interchange about training and supervision issues. Being the only systems-oriented supervisor in an agency or academic setting can be ultimately enriching, but may also be a limiting, isolating, or professionally disabling experience (Lebow, 1987; Ribordy, 1987; Saba & Liddle, 1986).

ARTICULATING A SUPERVISION FRAMEWORK

The transition from therapist to supervisor is often a difficult one, especially since few conceptual guidelines are available to the new supervisor. Just as therapists are aided by specifying and exploring their guiding premises about the basics of therapy (e.g., theory of change, the role of the therapist) (Liddle, 1982b), supervisors too should clarify their training presuppositions—those principles that guide their daily work. Referred to as a "supervisor's epistemological declaration," this process consists of formulating and posing to oneself the essential questions of training and supervision, thereby establishing the underlying rationale for a supervisor's every action. This activity, ongoing in nature and occurring over a supervisor's career, is designed to help formulate one's identity and assumptions about the processes and mechanisms of change in training and supervision, and in therapy.

As noted above, there will be an isomorphism between one's ideas about change in families and about change in trainees, but the correspondence may not be exact. A supervisor's views of change in therapy are related to, but not identical with, ideas about change in training. Although these views will be isomorphic to each other (i.e., have a similarity with respect to the structure or process of change), the specific content of change in therapy and supervision, naturally, will be different. In order to clarify one's beliefs about the conditions under which therapeutic change occurs, principles or assumptions about processes of change in general must be constructed, distilled, adapted, and translated into the therapy domain. Supervisors must take the additional step of adapting and defining these beliefs about change as they pertain to training.

The following are some questions designed to help supervisors construct a clear training epistemology.[4]

1. What are my beliefs about how change occurs in both families and trainees?
2. What are the crucial variables in a training situation?

3. What are my criteria for success in supervision?

4. What do I do to increase the likelihood that success will occur?

5. To what extent should I use specific training or learning objectives?

6. What forms of feedback or corrective learning will I provide the trainee?

7. Has the model I am intending to teach been sufficiently articulated, and am I sufficiently knowledgeable about the specifics of the approach?

8. What are the personal qualities I define as positive in therapists?

9. More basically, does the concept of a therapist's personal qualities have value to my work?

10. Along these lines, to what degree do I believe therapists are born and not made, and, conversely, to what extent do I subscribe to the notion of the trainability and expandable capacities of *any* therapist in training?

11. What are my values and attitudes about training therapists of different genders, and various racial, ethnic, social class, and cultural backgrounds? How do these inclinations and preferences shape my supervision?

12. What should I consider my "golden rule" of training?

TRAINEE VARIABLES

Many trainee variables that given trainees bring to the supervision experience are similar to those of the supervisor. The trainee's explicit or implicit theories of therapy, change, and human nature (ill formed as they might be at this stage of a therapist's development), previous training in systems- and non-systems-oriented models, present work setting, conception of how the present training situation fits with current and future aspirations, and developmental stage and personality variables, all have their part in shaping the therapist's expectations and contributions to the training process.

The trainee's work setting, outside of the training context, is a major influence on the trainee's learning capacities in a formal program or in supervision. For example, therapists might be trainees in one setting, while being supervisory staff at their primary work site. They could have one supervisor in their training program and another in their agency, creating competing loyalties and conceptual confusion. Additionally, clinicians' recollections of critical incidents in their development as therapists; their current conceptions of themselves, shaped by their work setting, daily interactions with colleagues, and feedback from clients; and their projections of themselves as continuing (or choosing not to continue) on the career path of a clinician, all have a strong impact on a clinician's everyday behavior.

With the foregoing discussion or construction[5] of the predominant variables brought forth by supervisor and trainee in the training setting, it could be noted that one's assessment of a training situation in light of this analysis might seem a simple matter. This is not the case, however. Mapping the interaction between supervisor, trainee, family, and context is difficult at best, and on some occasions is more akin to reading tea leaves than pursuing a logical, objective inquiry. Clashes of interpretation of reality and expectations often occur in the newly formed training system. Different stages of professional development, motivation, interest, commitment, and energy, in addition to difficulties in the relationship of supervisor and supervisee, can all be formidable obstacles to the formation of a working supervisory alliance and contract.

The supervisor's capacity to remember that patterns between training and therapeutic systems are parts of a wider nexus of influence (that is, that supervision is both a whole and a part, and that the training system is, similarly, both whole and part) is another important dimension of training and supervision. Just as isomorphism exists between therapy and training domains, isomorphism also exists between the training system and the systems with which it interacts. The supervisor's ability to think dynamically in expandable and contractible concentric circles[6] of systems organization is crucial to the design (Liddle, Breunlin, Schwartz, & Constantine, 1984; Wright & Coppersmith, 1983) and implementation of training programs, especially those conducting live supervision on a regular basis (Berger & Dammann, 1982; Breunlin, Liddle, & Schwartz, Chapter 13, this volume).

The surrounding institution's economics, mission, stage of development, and history, as well as its perceptions about its future, staff, and other trainees, all interact with and can affect, positively or adversely, the training program and supervision being conducted (Framo, 1976; Haley, 1975; Liddle, 1978; Meyerstein, 1977; Morrison *et al.*, 1979; Sluzki, 1974). Further, the characteristics of the training program serve as powerful influences on the training system's formation and maintenance. For instance, the structure, characteristics (such as a degree-granting program, or a free-standing institute), location, facilities, financial base and solvency, developmental level, staff characteristics, service and training balance, embeddedness and legitimacy of training in the setting, administrative or community support and connectedness, are all variables that affect the shape of the training program and the experience of training. Just as a trend exists in the clinical domain of family therapy to attend to the contextual variables in the delivery of therapy (Coppersmith, 1983; Liddle, 1985a; Minuchin, 1985; Schwartzman, 1985), the same message must now be made to supervisors (Liddle, 1985b). Family therapy supervisors must transfer their skills in systems assessment (if not intervention) from the clinical to the training domain. Failure to do so will result in a curious inability to operationalize, in training, the systems framework we hold so dear in our clinical work. The usefulness of the systemic framework (which, of course, includes the isomorphism notion) with its organizing and intervention-suggesting potential is no less essential in training than in therapy.

Stages of Training: A Useful, Constructed Truth

Thinking in stages has been a useful metaphor that has become a practical organizing scheme in the family therapy field (Breunlin, 1986; Haley, 1976, 1980; Solomon, 1973). Haley contends that it is best if a therapist assumes that "change should occur in stages" and that it is not wise to "jump from the problem stage to the cure stage in one leap but [to] have other stages in between" (Haley, 1976, p. 131). One way to think about stages is through the life cycle paradigm (Carter & McGoldrick, 1981; Falicov, Chapter 21, this volume; Haley, 1973; Liddle, 1983). Although not without its potential difficulties in conceptualization and implementation (Holloway, 1987; Liddle & Saba, 1983a), the family life cycle has helped theorists, practitioners, and researchers view people's lives in a way that has facilitated change. Recasting intrapsychic and negatively attributed problems as understandable and expectable difficulties associated with a certain stage of a family's development has also provided a more hopeful perspective for many families, reversing their previous demoralization.

Applying the concept of stages to family systems teaching (Liddle, 1980; Liddle & Saba, 1982), supervision (Tucker, Hart, & Liddle, 1976; Tucker & Liddle, 1978), and training (Liddle, 1988; Liddle & Saba, 1983), as well as to analyses of the training and supervision field as a whole (Liddle, 1982a, 1985a, 1985b; in press) has been an important part of our developing training model. Therapists-in-training as well as seasoned supervisors have perceived the concept of stages of therapy and training to be useful in their work (Liddle, Davidson, & Barrett, Chapter 25, this volume; Saba & Liddle, 1986). In training, the concept of stages has applicability in a number of ways. For example, planning and evaluating therapeutic goals according to the phase of therapy, the change in trainee and supervisor (as individuals and as a dyadic subsystem), and the developmental aspects of the training group, are all obvious ways in which thinking in stages can be helpful. While useful at broad, metaphoric levels, the concept of stages is often not specified sufficiently at operational levels. The intent of this section is to do so.

THE INITIAL PHASE: ESTABLISHING THE FOUNDATION FOR SUPERVISION

Perhaps the most critical developmental task of the initial stage of supervision is the formation of a stable working relationship between the supervisor and the trainee. The information that is transmitted between supervisor and trainee will have the greatest effect if it exists in the context of a strong relationship that supports and gains access to each member's existing competencies, while challenging their continued development. A relationship that encourages trainees to become increasingly invested and involved in the learning process is an essential training objective. Such a relationship permits their preferred interpersonal and conceptual style to become apparent, allowing the supervisor access to important aspects of the trainee. Just as the therapist seeks to arrange situations in the therapy room to elicit the family's preferred interactional pattern, the supervisor has a similar goal with the trainee. Therapists' preferred conceptual and interpersonal styles are valuable, indeed essential, supervisory information, upon which generic training goals are modified idiosyncratically.

In addition to supporting the crucial nature of the supervisory relationship, the literature also indicates that establishing a clear contract—which includes trainee and supervisor expectations, scope and nature of the training, methods of supervision, means of assessing progress, and evaluation—is another primary initial task of training and supervision (Liddle, in press).

Trainees often complain that their primary work setting does not support the thinking and methods of their systems-oriented training. Supervisors must, of course, deal with these matters as they arise, but a missionary spirit on the beginning therapist's part should not be encouraged. Competence and confidence must be cultivated first. Indeed, during the early stages of training, if the supervisor encourages anything at all it should be a noninterventive stance on the therapist's part in relation to outside, unsympathetic agencies. Beginning trainees should not be distracted with the political struggles within an agency; they should instead be encouraged simply to do their clinical work.[7]

ENDING THE INITIAL STAGE

Certain goals should be accomplished at this stage of the training process: the contract between supervisor and supervisee should be clearly established (e.g., logistics of video-taping, tape review, expectations regarding trainee's preparation for supervision sessions), negotiated within the limits of the necessary and inevitable hierarchy of the training relationship, and accepted.

Typically at this stage there will be a growing sense of togetherness, a collaboration toward a shared purpose. A common culture will have been formed. It will have its own history, rules, language, the beginnings of a jointly held vision of human problems, and clear expectations regarding the nature of the work ahead. By this point, there will have been challenges to the flexibility, if not the viability, of the training system. For instance, the trainee might challenge the authority or expertise of the supervisor (which is more likely with an advanced trainee), and likewise the supervisor might challenge the thinking or personal style of the therapist. These challenges do not have to threaten unduly the successfully forming relationship in the training system. For the most part, to use Whitaker's familiar phrase, "the battle for structure" is over (Whitaker & Keith, 1981). Of course, this is not to say that there are no longer any relationship struggles, but rather that the conclusion of the first phase of training is characterized by an absence of overt conflict and disagreement, and the presence of a shared feeling that although hard work lies ahead, the journey will be a positive one.

A "getting-down-to-business" atmosphere pervades the supervisory system at this time. The supervisor is clear about the way in which this particular trainee thinks about people, problem formation, change, and supervision. The supervisor will have made an assessment of the trainee based on his or her impressions from conversations with the trainee, and from observations of the trainee with other therapists, with cases, or on videotape. The supervisor will have developed a *therapist profile* of each trainee—completing one's personalized assessment schema of desirable clinician thinking and behavior. This formulation is, like all assessments, flexible, tentative, subject to alteration in response to new feedback, and generous in its inclusion of therapist resources and strengths. The supervisor's assessment is not necessarily shared in its unabridged form with the therapist, but again, as with all assessments, it is shaped into workable, goal-focused statements that lead to alternatives. Dead-end confrontations or interpretations are out of place in this approach. The goals emanating from this assessment of the trainee are juxtaposed to the supervisor's generic goals for clinicians (those objectives that apply to all trainees), yielding a complex, universally *and* idiosyncratically derived set of objectives.

By this point as well, one of the basic goals of the first stage of supervision—articulating the therapy model being taught—will have been accomplished. Obviously, the supervisor's capacity to teach therapists in an ongoing seminar, in which readings are required and videotapes are regularly analyzed, concurrently with clinical supervision greatly facilitates meeting this objective. Trainees should have learned the rudiments of the model on both intellectual and experiential levels.

The supervisor too has had some experiential learning with the trainee to incorporate into the therapist profile. In making "mistakes" therapists provide invaluable information about their natural conceptual and behavioral tendencies. It is the supervisor's task not only to process cognitively oriented, verbal data from the trainee, but also to access and, indeed, to provoke (as one does with a family) a glimpse of the trainee's predominant patterns and current style and model of therapy. This snapshot of a therapist's style provides an assessment of the trainee's current level of ability with the new model, as well as a sample of his or her previous ways of thinking and working. At this point, it is particularly important for the supervisor to maintain the contextual, benevolent, and resource-focused view of trainee behavior. For instance, the supervisor can understand the behavior of the therapist as, in part, a result of the multifaceted stresses of the training setting. This is a context in which therapists are caught, temporarily at least, between comfortable previous ways of thinking and responding, and a novel, perhaps exciting, but still unfamiliar territory of a new therapeutic model, supervisor, and professional peer group.

The shift from the initial phase of supervision can be a declared (acknowledged by the supervisor and the therapist) or undeclared one. As in therapy, this degree of overt distinction drawing depends on the goals and circumstances of the particular training system and trainee. With respect to a training relationship that has begun poorly, it might be best for the supervisor to announce the need for a fresh start, a new beginning now that the crisis is over and has been handled in the best possible way. Another situation might be one in which the trainee has done very well, exceeding the demands and expectations of the supervisor (and perhaps of himself or herself as well). In this second scenario, the supervisor, perhaps taking the cue from the trainee, might declare that what has gone on before has been a good beginning, but that more will be required from the trainee in terms of personal flexibility. The supervisor might indicate that the therapist needs to be more active in generating alternative interventions, and so the supervisor will be expecting more of the therapist in this regard. In this way, the supervisor and trainee both co-create a clear, goal-oriented transition point in the training process, thereby providing focus, motivation, and positive anticipation for new challenges in thinking and behavior.

THE MIDDLE STAGES: INCORPORATING AND WORKING THE MODEL

By this stage the awkwardness and many of the difficulties characteristic of the formation phase of the supervisory relationship will have been resolved; the contrast has been clarified and a working alliance has been established. A feeling of collaboration, and an evolving mutual trust, characterize the new supervisor–therapist unit. Feedback to the trainee, and often to the supervisor from the therapist, becomes more direct and personal. This phase is distinguished by an increasing capacity to identify and work on idiosyncratic elements of therapist style—those personal mannerisms and ways of acting and thinking that hinder successful adoption of the approach being taught. Therapist self-consciousness will decrease as a newfound spirit of experimentation and risk taking takes hold, pushing the therapist into new and unfamiliar therapeutic territories (see Breunlin, Karrer, McGuire, & Cimmarusti, Chapter 12, this volume).

Initially, therapists are eager to please their supervisors, intent on demonstrating that they can "do the model." Prior to this, there is the struggle to understand the new approach, since many of its underlying assumptions (e.g., searching for strengths) and fundamental methods (e.g., enactment) can be quite foreign. The middle phases of supervision, however, are practice-oriented. The therapy model is worked and reworked in an attempt to gain familiarity with the approach and, naturally, to help the clients at the same time. Here, training is marked by a philosophy of *"learning by doing, and doing again."*

In the context of a solid supervisory relationship (Schwartz, Chapter 10, this volume; Schwartz, Liddle, & Breunlin, Chapter 11, this volume) and an increase in the trainee's number of clinical hours, therapist self-consciousness, obvious and intrusive in the early stages, becomes less of a supervisory obstacle. In one sense, there is no longer time to be self-conscious. At this stage therapists are (it is hoped) seeing a number of cases, watching the sessions of other therapists-in-training, participating in the supervisor's analysis of their own and others' videotaped interviews, and completing directed readings that relate to specific cases. Rereading previously studied articles or books through the lens of new experience can be particularly beneficial at this point. Therapists often report that they derived new and more personally significant meaning from a specific article or text after seeing a case in which issues in the readings were highlighted (Liddle *et al.*, Chapter 25, this volume). The *"readiness-to-learn"* concept might very well be operational here. That is, after acquiring an experiential knowledge of a particular family phenomenon or intervention, therapists might be able to see and hear in new ways. Learning is thus facilitated, in part at least, by the sometimes planned but often fortuitous sequence of exposure to ideas and experience. Readiness to learn can be defined in a contextual way (Kagan, 1984). It can be understood as a simultaneous report on and comment about the context and timing of learning. Taken in this way, readiness to learn becomes a more useful and systemic concept. It is therefore expanded beyond its usual meaning as an individual trait or aspect of personality and is more inclusive of the context in which such "readiness" is fostered or retarded.

Training tapes of expert clinicians can also be valuable at this point in the supervision. Less grandiose attributions are given to these training materials as therapists now have an informed experiential base with which to judge what they see. During this phase, therapists are also able to incorporate learning from these training tapes into their own work. Therapists increasingly develop the capacity to differentiate those aspects of the other clinicians' styles that are and are not consonant with their own stylistic goals. More basically, clinicians are able at this point to draw distinctions between the elements of a particular approach and the style in which those elements or techniques are being delivered. As a result, therapists are likely to produce their own personal interpretation and improvisation of the therapy model being taught. Formation of the long-term goal of developing a personal, evolving model of therapy (Liddle, 1985) begins at this stage.

During the middle phases a different type of stress appears for supervisor and trainee alike, and is especially apparent in live supervision. Here the pressure on the supervisor to be helpful to the therapist in the moment he or she really needs it—during a session—is increased. Nowhere are supervisor inadequacies more apparent than during live supervision: it is a context of therapy and learning in which both trainer and therapist are on the line. Therapists have higher expectations of their supervisor, and, similarly, supervisors have higher expectations of therapists in live supervision. In this context, there can be an intense focus on the outcome of any particular session. In live supervision, one's limitations as a supervisor and a therapist have obvious, immediate reverberations. The therapy either goes well or not. Therapists soon realize that they are the instrument of the model and, as such, are a key ingredient in week-to-week outcome. This aspect of supervision is often underemphasized by supervisors in an effort to ease the pressure on developing trainees. Monitoring therapy outcome in a realistic way (Ryder, 1987) is a major focus of and, indeed, one criterion of effective supervision (Kniskern & Gurman, Chapter 23, this volume).

In the context of this new, yet normative pressure for therapeutic results, the therapist is helped to take more risks, pushing past previous personal limits and establishing new beachheads of self-confidence and skill. As the freedom to experiment and take risks becomes available, therapists alter their former ways of thinking and acting. Alternatives are experienced as less alien, more natural, as therapists discover and tolerate previously unavailable affect, cognitions, and behaviors in the conduct of therapy.

THE END STAGES: CONSOLIDATING THE CHANGES

Demarcating the end stages of training is a misnomer; there is, of course, no end to the process of training. The ideal is that we continue to evolve as both individuals and clinicians. The final phases of the contracted training period, then, should be an assessment of the degree to which this lifelong or career-long learning and development value has been embraced by the therapist. Since the hierarchical structure of the relationship is less obviously operational, it is an opportune time for supervisors to share with trainees some of their personal travails along the path of career development. Discussions with the therapists—projecting them into the future—can help in this regard. Discussion of career goals and the possibilities of job shifts are all appropriate and potentially valuable at this juncture.[8]

The so-called end stages, then, are characterized by processes of consolidation. The therapist's acquired knowledge and skill have largely been incorporated into a new and more effective way of thinking and working. The supervisor and trainees have reviewed what has transpired throughout the training, what has been accomplished, and what the therapists need to do next to continue their professional development. It is a time of identifying the nature of the changes, personal and therapeutic, and charting a future course. In the end-stage, the individual issues of therapist style identified in the middle phases need to be addressed further by supervisor and therapist. Progress in this area is frequently more limited until a repertoire of basic clinical skills is mastered. Gradually, broadly stated goals relating to therapist style have been transformed into individualized objectives. These are carefully monitored by the supervisor and, if necessary, revised. Such fine tuning is possible with a careful reading and incorporation of feedback emanating from the therapist's practice with the new behaviors.

As therapists must deal with termination with their families in therapy, supervisors, too, must address the issue of launching their trainees. Addressing autonomy, of course, is not entirely new to the supervisor, since in the middle phases of training the effective supervisor has been sensitive to the increasing need to permit the therapists more autonomy. A lack of supervisor flexibility in this regard is especially obvious in a live supervision context in which an overintrusive supervisor constantly phones in or walks into the therapy room, thereby demonstrating a failure to appreciate the importance of therapist autonomy.

At the later stages of training, supervisors should permit supervisees to arrive at conclusions, generate strategy and interventions, and evaluate their work on their own.[9] As has been noted, when supervisors become aware of therapists' capacity to generate sound clinical alternatives—strategies that may be different from their own preferences—the hierarchical dimension (at least in terms of how it previously existed) of the relationship is less necessary, apparent, or existent. Thus, with a skilled therapist, the supervisor functions more as a consultant than an instructor, serving to fine tune, shape, and provide feedback on the therapist's well formulated plan. As in the therapeutic setting, the challenge for the supervisor in the training setting is often to *stay out of the way* to allow trainees to develop their competencies further.

The end phase is a time of sealing, generalizing, and transferring the therapist's changes. The supervisor should demarcate the changes in therapist thinking and action by reminding therapists where they started and what they have accomplished. Reviewing with trainees a tape of one of their early sessions is a useful difference-demonstrating activity. The supervisor should be generous with support and encouragement, highlighting, indeed celebrating, the acquired skills and changes. In this phase the nature of supervisory challenges should appear in the form of expecting creativity on the trainees' part; for example, can they go beyond their previous way of working a particular operation in a session, or can they generate several alternatives to handle a given clinical situation? The supervisor can address issues of generalization and transfer of learning by discussing cases from the trainees' other work contexts.

Faculty in a variety of training programs have observed that in the later phases of training trainees often report that they are too frustrated with their current jobs to remain at them, and feel they must seek new employment in a setting in which they can practice a family systems orientation. In the concluding stages of training, with supervisors in a consultant role, therapists often confer with supervisors about concrete strategies to deal with their work site (other than seeking a new job). As is the case with their therapeutic skills, however, therapists at this point often need minimal guidance in generating an assessment and appropriate plan. It is at this phase that trainees often report clarity about the principle of the isomorphic nature of training and therapy as they apply their systemic therapy principles to their work settings. For trainees engaged in these kind of activities, the leap of understanding to the interconnection of therapy and training is not difficult. Sometimes selected readings on what have been referred to as the emotional and political hazards of teaching and learning family systems therapy (Liddle, 1978) can help students plan solutions to work-related problems, or may simply support and validate their difficult experiences (see Appendix, this volume).

CONCLUSIONS: NOTES FROM THE SUPERVISORY FRONT

Our beginnings as supervisors are often marked, or shall we say marred, by simplistic thinking or the scrambling for technological panaceas to sooth our nerves about the composite drama known as supervision. Audiotapes, videotapes, live supervision, and use of the team have made supervision, as well as our thinking about it, more effective and sophisticated. These useful advances, however, are tools—not, in and of themselves, supervisory solutions; crucial organizational, conceptual, and technical skills (Liddle & Schwartz, 1983) alone will not yield the desired results in training and supervision. Thus, in our enthusiasm for effective methods and powerful results, we must not neglect the all-important *basics of supervision*. What follows is a list of these basics; they can serve as orienting guideposts in a supervisor's complex work.

Supervisors Supervise

Remember the simple, obvious, but often forgotten principle that you are the supervisor and not the therapist. The preferable unit of analysis and intervention is the therapeutic system (i.e., therapist plus family). As supervisors we generally influence the family system indirectly through our trainee. Supervisors touch the therapeutic situation through the therapist, who provides a means to achieve an end of good therapeutic outcome, and whose training is an end in and of itself. Thus we directly try to influence the therapist and, in this process, indirectly affect the therapeutic system. Thinking clearly about and preserving the boundaries between the supervisory and therapy systems is a simple but powerful way to improve one's supervision rapidly. When we misuse influential techniques such as live supervision and supervisor walk-ins, for example, we violate a powerful rule of supervision: supervisors supervise. Therefore, in these circumstances we must be particularly cognizant, indeed accepting, of our role as a once-removed influencer of therapeutic change.

Utopian Expectations in Supervision

In therapy there are few magical or quick cures; in supervision there are fewer still. Dealing simultaneously with the supervisory (supervisor, therapist, plus observing group) and thera-peutic (therapist plus family) systems necessitates superior conceptual, information-process-ing, and interpersonal skills. Developing this repertoire requires commitment, diligence, and time. Appealing as they might be, shortcuts are naive and ultimately defeating.

Organizational Skills

The difficulty of organizing a sound and flexible context for therapist learning and risk taking should not be underestimated. Effectiveness is learned, produced, and reproduced in contexts with certain characteristics. The supervisor's capacity to understand and work with the components and processes of a given training environment (setting characteris-tics and constraints, therapist style and values, family ethnicity, presenting problem, and composition) is key to facilitating maximal learning.

Relationship Factors and Interpersonal Skills

This dimension is frequently taken for granted in the success or failure of both therapy and training. Yet being taken for granted does not necessarily imply that interpersonal skills are successfully utilized in a training context; sometimes being taken for granted means being ignored or neglected. Thus we need to remind ourselves of the necessity of monitoring and, if necessary, improving our interpersonal skills when dealing with trainees. A supervisor's intelligence, content mastery, or therapeutic charisma are, without excellent relationship skills, insufficient predictors of effective supervision.

Clear Thinking and the Capacity to Communicate a Coherent Model of Therapy

The supervisor must be able to conceptualize and articulate a workable therapeutic approach from the methods and content of training and supervision. While a "pure," narrowly defined model may be workable with some trainees, it will be inadequate with others who seek a broad working base. And an ill conceived, overly inclusive, and nonintegrative eclectic approach will also be untenable. This principle reminds us that supervision, like therapy, is far from a contentless or a mainly process-oriented activity: specific content presented in a systematic way is necessary for successful training outcomes.

Building and Using a Systemic Framework of Supervision

Therapists benefit conceptually and pragmatically from a systemic vision. Similarly, the supervisor needs a systemic approach to supervision. This provides the supervisor with a conception of the interrelationships and interconnections among the different spheres of the therapeutic and training systems. The principle of the isomorphic nature of training and therapy can be this kind of organizing and action-suggesting template.

The Supervisory Attitude

Respect, one of the basics of a useful supervisory attitude, is as essential to training as it is to therapy. Supervisors are not immune to the destructive therapeutic stance of *deficit detective*,[10] long known to be a problem for many therapists. It is sometimes difficult for supervisors to implement their "search for strengths" and "resource mobilization" principles with trainees, despite their success in this regard with their clinical families. Supporting and catalyzing trainee strengths is no less cardinal an activity in the training domain. This dimension transcends the technology of interventions, therapeutic or supervisory, and brings us into the basic human arena of empathy and caring. Respecting our trainees—their struggles, efforts, experiences, and opinions—and effectively communicating our respect, are preeminent aspects of supervision. *Acceptance* is another foundation of a helpful supervisory attitude. The capacity to challenge and not be unduly constrained by our values, biases, and stereotypes is essential to both therapy and training. Accepting our own and others' human frailties does not mean succumbing to them, nor does it mean abdicating our responsibility always to do our best with each trainee.

Supervisor Development

In teaching and supervision, giving is essential. Supervisors frequently feel depleted after a long week of many therapy, teaching, and supervision hours. What are the ways in which we monitor and take care of our own developmental and growth needs in this stressful work? What are the signs that indicate our need for professional renewal? As Whitaker might say, it is acceptable for supervisors to assert that they want to "get something for themselves" out of the supervisory and training experience. When supervision feels like an onerous task, something is obviously wrong. Interestingly, however, therapist, but not supervisor, burnout has been more thoroughly addressed in the literature (Maslach & Jackson, 1982). As research expands in family therapy training and supervision, the processes and effects of supervisor impairment will most surely demand more focus. Supervisors' sources of support, validation, and challenge cannot only be trainee change or therapeutic outcome. Professional organizations and networking affiliations, local colleagues, and work contexts flexibly organized to facilitate interprofessional growth are important sources of strength and regeneration.

Finally, like therapy itself, training therapists is serious business, but when we unwittingly check our perspective and sense of humor at the entrance to the observation room, we are suddenly in jeopardy of losing our humanness and, indeed, compassion itself—a pair of any supervisor's most powerful allies.

Acknowledgment

The author gratefully acknowledges George Saba and Gayle Dakof for their comments on an earlier version of this chapter. Work on this chapter was supported in part by a research grant to the author from the National Institute on Drug Abuse (Grant No. R01 DA 3714), "Structural–Strategic Family Therapy with Drug Abusing Adolescents."

Notes

1. For Levinson (1972), "Categories which appear widely unrelated in content will reflect the same patterning of form, will be, in a word, transformations or isomorphs of each other. It is important to realize that this is not idle analogizing. It is a literal belief that structure, or form, is constant in spite of changing content" (p. 36).

2. The focus here is multidimensional and interactional; no one factor is conceived as in and of itself the most or least important. Further, these factors should be considered in relation to and in interaction with each other. They are presented individually and sequentially for organizational and heuristic purposes.

3. Clinical skills are defined as the therapist's ability to intervene with a family during a session. These are distinguished from perceptual or conceptual skills, which form the basis for the intervention(s) but do not, in and of themselves, allow the therapist to implement the therapy approach.

4. These questions are posed as areas of exploration for the supervisor. The list is suggestive rather than exhaustive, and highlights some generic areas of inquiry for supervisors wanting to clarify their premises about supervision. Individual supervisors will add areas in need of specification, depending on the therapy model they teach, and a number of other variables, including personality and training setting factors.

5. The term "construction" is used to communicate the subjective and partial process of articulating "the predominant variables brought forth by supervisor and trainee in the training setting." Naming factors that might account for any phenomenon should not be seen as the identification of the "true" nature of that phenomenon. There will probably always be factors that cannot be identified, specified, or known about. Further, even if all variables could be "isolated," there remains the problem of understanding emergent qualities and interaction effects.

6. The expanding and contracting concentric circle imagery is one visual metaphor to assist in a certain way of thinking about complex, multilayered, and multifaceted systems and their interaction. Other visually oriented metaphors might be more useful to any given supervisor.

7. The creation of a strange contradiction, which itself might disorient the trainee, is quite possible here. Urging the trainee in the early stages not to become overly involved with the political machinations of an

agency might be seen as acontextual, the very antithesis of that viewpoint we are trying to teach. However, *understanding* the systemic difficulties in one's agency and trying to change them (e.g., lobbying for the "freedom" to see families) are distinctly different activities. Beginning trainees need to focus on skill acquisition; this is a full-time activity.

8. This is not to say that a supervisor's sharing of personal or professional matters is inappropriate at earlier stages of supervision. Rather, supervisor self-disclosure about himself or herself, as it relates to the supervisee's development and future, is most natural for many supervisors at later stages of the supervisory relationship.

9. Obviously, such supervisory freedom is given in a context of demonstrated therapist competence. Supervisors are reinforced to allow therapist autonomy through increased skill development on the therapist's part. The supervisor's ability to provide increasing latitude regarding therapist autonomy is thus conceived contextually; it is a function of and exists in interaction with therapist change, as well as with the change in the specific case the therapist is seeing.

10. Deficit detectives see pathology and dysfunction everywhere. For them, people are objects on which to practice their DSM-III proficiency; strengths and resources are impossible to locate in their clients and trainees.

References

Berger, M., & Dammann, C. (1982). Live supervision as context, treatment, and training. *Family Process, 21,* 337–344.

Breunlin, D. C. (Ed.). (1986). *Stages in family therapy.* Rockville, MD: Aspen Systems Corporation.

Breunlin, D. C., Karrer, B., McGuire, D., & Cimmarusti, R. Cybernetics of videotape supervision. Chapter 12, this volume.

Breunlin, D. C., Liddle, H. A., & Schwartz, R. C. Concurrent training of therapists and supervisors. Chapter 13, this volume.

Carter, B., & McGoldrick, M. (Eds.). (1981). *The family life cycle.* New York: Gardner.

Coppersmith, E. I. (Ed.). (1983). Special issue on the family and larger systems. *Journal of Strategic and Systemic Therapies,* 2(3), 1–86.

Draper, R. (1982). From trainee to trainer. In R. Whiffen & Byng-Hall (Eds.), *Family therapy supervision: Recent developments in practice.* New York: Grune & Stratton.

Duhl, B. (1983). *From the inside out and other metaphors: Creative and integrative approaches to training in systems thinking.* New York: Brunner/Mazel.

Everett, C. A., & Koerpel, B. J. (1986). Family therapy supervision: A review and critique of the literature. *Contemporary Family Therapy,* 8(1), 62–74.

Falicov, C. J. Learning to think culturally. Chapter 21, this volume.

Framo, J. L. (1976). Chronicle of a struggle to establish a family unit within a community mental health center. In P. Guerin (Ed.), *Family therapy: Theory and practice.* New York: Gardner Press.

Haley, J. (1973). *Uncommon therapy.* New York: W. W. Norton.

Haley, J. (1975). Why a mental health clinic should avoid doing family therapy. *Journal of Marriage and Family Counseling, 1,* 3–12.

Haley, J. (1976). *Problem-solving therapy.* San Francisco: Jossey-Bass.

Haley, J. (1980). *Leaving home: The therapy of disturbed young people.* New York: McGraw-Hill.

Hess, A. K. (Ed.). (1987). Special section: Advances in psychotherapy supervision. *Professional Psychology: Research and Practice,* 18(3), 187–259.

Holloway, E. L. (1987). Developmental models of supervision: Is it development? *Professional Psychology: Research and Practice,* 18(3), 209–216.

Kagan, J. (1984). *The nature of the child.* New York: Basic Books.

Kniskern, D. P., & Gurman, A. S. Research on family therapy training and supervision. Chapter 23, this volume.

Lebow, J. (1987). Training psychologists in family therapy in family institute settings. *Journal of Family Psychology,* 1(2), 219–231.

Levinson, E. (1972). *The fallacy of understanding.* New York: Basic Books.

Liddle, H. (1978). The emotional and political hazards of teaching and learning family therapy. *Family Therapy, 5,* 1–12.

Liddle, H. A. (1980). On teaching a contextual or systemic therapy: Training content, goals and methods. *American Journal of Family Therapy, 8,* 58-69.

Liddle, H. A. (1982a). Family therapy training and supervision: Current issues, future trends. *International Journal of Family Therapy, 4,* 81-97.

Liddle, H. A. (1982b). On the problems of eclecticism: A call for epistemologic clarification and human scale theories. *Family Process, 4,* 243-250.

Liddle, H. A. (Ed.). (1983). *Clinical implications of the family life cycle.* Rockville, MD: Aspen Systems Corporation.

Liddle, H. A. (1985a). Beyond family therapy: Challenging the boundaries, roles, and mission of a field. *Journal of Strategic and Systemic Therapies, 4*(2), 4-14.

Liddle, H. A. (1985b). Redefining the mission of family therapy training. *Journal of Psychotherapy and the Family, 1*(4), 109-124.

Liddle, H. A. (1988). Developmental thinking and the family life cycle: Implications for training family therapists. In C. Falicov (Ed.), *Family transitions: Continuity and change across the life cycle.* New York: Guilford Press.

Liddle, H. A. (in press). Family therapy training and supervision: A critical review and analysis. In A. Gurman & D. Kniskern (Eds.), *Handbook of family therapy* (2nd ed.). New York: Guilford Press.

Liddle, H. A. Breunlin, D. C., Schwartz, R. C., & Constantine, J. (1984). Training family therapy supervisors: Issues of content, form, and context. *Journal of Marital and Family Therapy, 10,* 139-150.

Liddle, H. A., Davidson, G., & Barett, M. J. Outcomes of live supervision: Trainee perspectives. Chapter 25, this volume.

Liddle, H. A., & Halpin, R. (1978). Family therapy training and supervision literature: A comparative review. *Journal of Marriage and Family Counseling, 4,* 77-98.

Liddle, H. A., & Saba, G. (1982). Teaching family therapy at the introductory level: A model emphasizing a pattern which connects training and therapy. *Journal of Marital and Family Therapy, 8,* 63-72.

Liddle, H. A., & Saba, G. (1983a). Clinical implications of the family life cycle: Some cautionary guidelines. In H. A. Liddle (Ed.), *Clinical implications of the family life cycle.* Rockville, MD: Aspen.

Liddle, H. A., & Saba, G. (1983b). On context replication: The isomorphic relationship of training and therapy. *Journal of Strategic and Systemic Therapies, 2,* 3-11.

Liddle, H. A., & Saba, G. (1984). The isomorphic nature of training and therapy: Epistemologic foundations for a structural–strategic family therapy. In J. Schwartzman (Ed.), *Families and other systems.* New York: Guilford Press.

Liddle, H., & Saba, G. (in press). *Supervising family therapists: Creating contexts of competence.* Philadelphia: Grune & Stratton.

Liddle, H. A., & Schwartz, R. C. (1983). Life supervision/consultation: Conceptual and pragmatic guidelines for family therapy training. *Family Process, 22,* 477-490.

Maslach, C., & Jackson, (1982). Burnout in health professions: A social psychological analysis. In G. Sanders & E. Suls (Eds.), *Social psychology of health and illness.* Hillsdale, NJ: Lawrence Erlbaum.

Matarazzo, R. G., & Patterson, D. R. (1986). Research on the teaching and learning of psychotherapeutic skills. In S. L. Garfield & A. E. Bergin (Eds.), *Handbook of psychotherapy and behavior change.* New York: Wiley.

Meyerstein, K. (1977). Family therapy training for paraprofessionals in a community mental health center. *Family Process, 10,* 477-494.

Minuchin, S. (1985). *Family kaleidoscope.* Cambridge, MA: Harvard University Press.

Montalvo, B. (1973). Aspects of live supervision. *Family Process, 12,* 343-359.

Morrison, J. (1979). Changing a mental health team's attitudes towards family therapy. *American Journal of Family Therapy, 7*(1), 57-60.

Ribordy, S. (1987, December). Training family therapists within an academic setting. *Journal of Family Psychology, 1*(2), 204-218.

Ryder, R. (1987). *The realistic therapist.* Newbury Park, CA: Sage Publications.

Saba, G., & Liddle, H. A. (1986). Perceptions of professional needs, practice patterns and critical issues facing family therapy trainers and supervisors. *American Journal of Family Therapy, 14,* 109-122.

Sluzki, C. E. (1974). On training to think interactionally. *Social Science and Medicine, 8,* 483-485.

Schwartz, R. The trainer-trainee relationship in family therapy training. Chapter 10, this volume.

Schwartz, R. C., Liddle, H. A., & Breunlin, D. C. Muddles of live supervision. Chapter 11, this volume.

Schwartzman, J. (Ed.). (1985). *Families and other systems*. New York: Guilford Press.

Tucker, B., Hart, G., & Liddle, H. (1976). Supervision in family therapy: A development perspective. *Journal of Marriage and Family Counseling, 2,* 269–276.

Tucker, B., & Liddle, H. A. (1978). Intra- and interpersonal process in the group supervision of beginning family therapists. *Family Therapy, 5*(1), 13–28.

Whiffen, R., & Byng-Hall, J. (Eds.). (1982). *Family therapy supervision: Recent developments in practice.* London: Academic Press; New York: Grune & Stratton.

Whitaker, C. A., & Keith, D. B. (1981). Symbolic–experiential family therapy. In A. Gurman & D. Kniskern (Eds.), *Handbook of family therapy.* New York: Brunner/Mazel.

Wright, L. M., & Coppersmith, E. I. (1983). Supervision of supervision: How to be "meta" to a metaposition. *Journal of Strategic and Systemic Therapies, 2*(2), 40–50.

10

The Trainer–Trainee Relationship in Family Therapy Training

RICHARD C. SCHWARTZ
Institute for Juvenile Research, Chicago

Imagine the following family therapy training scenario:

The trainer decides that Joe, the trainee, has been inducted into siding with the mother and calls in to the session. Buzz! Joe does not flinch, does not make any movement toward picking up the phone; the family members glance at the phone but keep talking, and seconds tick by while the trainer wonders what to do. The trainer buzzes again, still with no response, and finally gets up and knocks loudly on the door of the therapy room. After another long pause, Joe exits the room and preempts the trainer's complaints by saying angrily, "I was in the middle of something important and I resent being interrupted."

To say the least, the relationship between this trainer and trainee is not optimal. But how did it evolve to this point? Does the trainee not understand the etiquette of live supervision, that interruptions are frequent and to be welcomed? Or is he rejecting the authority or competence of a trainer who is too young, too inexperienced, or of a different therapeutic orientation? Perhaps the trainee is ambivalent about learning family therapy, or anxious because he is exposing his work, and so is indirectly telling the trainer to be careful with him.

On the other hand, it may be that the trainer has been extremely rigid with or critical of the trainee, resulting in an escalation that reached a climax in that scene. Perhaps the trainer felt insecure about his competence and was hypercritical or intrusive as a result. The trainer could be involved in similar escalations over competence with his supervisor or colleagues, or may feel disqualified in the training setting. In addition, the family may be so difficult that frustration and performance issues are played out between trainer and trainee.

These are but a few of the possible factors that could be a part of the context of the scenario above. In reality, most of these factors were operating years ago when the author was the young, inexperienced trainer in that scenario and was put in the position of supervising an older, veteran family therapist.

The point is that the degree to which the family therapy trainer and trainee define a mutually rewarding relationship is not only dependent on the delicate mix of their personal styles of relating. This type of relationship is embedded within a training context full of overt and covert stresses like those suggested above. The stresses are particularly influential where trainees and trainers are exposing their self-esteem to the pressures of live and video supervision.

The task facing the trainer of family therapy has become complex; in addition to dealing with the above complexities, it is no longer enough to teach some theory, demonstrate a few skills, and then react to the trainees' verbal reports of their cases. Now the modern family therapy trainer is a molder of trainee epistemology, as well as a master of new videotape and live supervisory technologies. A trainer cannot consider himself or herself successful until the trainee has leaped to new heights in conceptualization. Without the advantage of being a therapist to the trainee, the trainer is expected to reshape the trainee's view of the world, not to mention his or her interactions with clients and with people in general.

This change in expectations of family therapy training, from merely educating therapists to transforming them, and doing so in relatively short periods (one- or two-year training programs), has greatly increased the importance of and the strain on the relationship between the trainer and the trainee. The trainer–trainee relationship has become a major instrument for this transformation and, as such, needs careful preparation and monitoring. This chapter will discuss some factors and issues that family therapy trainers might consider in their attempts to create an atmosphere conducive to helping trainees shift their conceptual maps and levels of skill, and allowing for the growth of the trainer.

The isomorphic nature of the processes of training and therapy has been recognized and developed elsewhere (Liddle & Saba, 1983, 1985; Liddle & Schwartz, 1983). This isomorphism is particularly evident in the ways that the trainer–trainee relationship mirrors aspects of the trainee–family relationship. This mirroring is a recurrent theme throughout this chapter and is certainly relevant to the initial stages of building a relationship, whether it be with a trainee or with a family.

DIFFICULTIES IN THE TRAINER–TRAINEE RELATIONSHIP

Families enter therapy with a wide variety of motives for and understandings about their participation. These motives are often quite different from those of the therapist, and many initial sessions may be spent as the family and therapist co-evolve a mutually acceptable frame for their work together. From the therapist's perspective, the degree of distance between his or her frame and the family's frame will be an index of the amount of "resistance,"[1] or difficulty in joining the family, he or she can expect.

Frame for Training

In a similar way, the degree of fit between the expectations that the trainer and trainee have for the training experience will often determine the degree of initial difficulty in their relationship. For example, if the trainer subscribes to the ethic that successful family therapy training involves total transformation of epistemology, but the trainee simply wants to add some techniques to his or her treatment armamentarium, the potential for a resistant relationship is high. This situation is somewhat analogous to that of a family therapist who faces parents who are convinced that their son's problem resides totally in their child. In both situations, the degree to which the trainer or therapist believes it crucial to change the trainee's or family's frame immediately is often the degree to which he or she is resisted. As in the joining stages of therapy, the prudent trainer will use the trainee's language, and will show some degree of accommodation to and acceptance of the trainee's epistemology, while demonstrating family therapy's effectiveness and excitement through videotaped examples or through encouraging the trainee to try new skills. Like most products of high quality, family therapy sells itself. As has been observed before (Haley, 1973), the process of doing family therapy, by itself, transforms epistemology. In addition, the initial defensiveness of many trainees is based less in logical conceptual differences and more in the terror trainees feel in anticipation of an encounter with a wild family or of having their work observed. After surviving a few of these experiences, many trainees will show remarkable changes in their attitude toward learning if they have not been pushed into a corner through defensive exchanges with the trainer.

On the other hand, there are many contexts where it behooves the trainer to modify his or her frame for the training experience. Training psychiatric residents, for example, when 80% of their time is spent thinking psychoanalytic thoughts, or training family practice residents whose goals do not include becoming family therapists, are very different endeavors from training family therapy externs who want to "be family therapists," not just to be able to do some family therapy or to view problems in context. To avoid frustration, trainers in the former contexts learn to change their expectations for training (see Chapter 16 by Combrinck-Graham and Chapter 18 by Ransom, this volume).

Accepting the Trainer

Even after a better fit has evolved between the trainer's and trainee's frames for training, several factors remain that will influence the potential for difficulty in the trainer–trainee relationship. For example, the trainee may be motivated to become a family therapist, but have trouble accepting the trainer as a person capable of helping him or her to become one. There are several factors that influence this process. The closer the trainees are to the trainers in age, years of clinical experience, academic degree, or perceived family therapy competence, the more difficult it may be for them to define a comfortable, complementary teacher–student relationship. This will also be true where the trainee is interested in a different model of family therapy than the trainer's. In fact, a study of conflict in trainer–trainee relationships found that conflicts over differences in orientation were far more difficult to resolve satisfactorily than conflicts over the trainer's style of supervision (Moskowitz & Rupert, 1983).

Trainer Attitude

Such difficulties will be hard to avoid if the trainer is not generally secure in his or her abilities as a teacher/supervisor, and confident in his or her level of knowledge. The trainer needs to feel self-confidence, as well as confidence with the trainee. When this is not the case, the inevitable challenges to the trainer's conceptual model may turn into symmetrical escalations that can permeate all aspects of the training. In other words, the task of family therapy training is easiest and most rewarding for the trainer who is not out to prove himself or herself, or to elicit adoration, but instead enjoys and learns from the training process. Such a trainer recognizes that different people have different styles of learning and welcomes the challenger as much as the true believer for helping him or her learn how to train.

Thus, it is the trainer's attitude toward his or her job that will often determine (1) how rapidly an acceptable frame for the training is negotiated, (2) how many challenges escalate into "resistance," and (3) how much both trainer and trainee use their relationship to learn from each other. In other words, if the trainer's self-image is not wrapped up in (attached to) transforming the trainee, then the trainee will be free to transform. This is not to imply that the trainer is detached or does not care about the outcome of the training; rather, it means that he or she will not consider himself or herself a failure if a transformation does not occur, or if the trainee does not worship him or her, and knows that he or she will still learn from the process. Such an attitude is difficult to maintain if the trainer works in a context that is not supportive or does not take training seriously.

Despite the trainer's ability to maintain such an attitude, some trainer–trainee relationships will still be fraught with difficulty. There are some trainees the trainer simply may not like, no matter how hard the trainer tries to maintain a systemic view of that person's behavior; and, of course the trainee may not like the trainer. In other cases, contextual factors, sometimes unknown to the trainer, may be at work preventing the trainee from fully accepting the training. This is often a problem when the trainer is a consultant, because he or she will have less awareness of the operation of the system to which he or she is consulting. For example, the administration or high-level supervisors in an agency may strongly subscribe to traditional individual models.

Manifestations of Difficulties

Difficulties between the trainer and trainee can manifest themselves in myriad ways. The trainer may catch himself or herself being overly critical of the trainee's comments and actions, or, at the other extreme, being afraid to be critical and, consequently, being insincerely supportive. In addition, the trainer may slip frequently into defensive or rhetorical monologues or arguments that betray more family therapy chauvinism than he or she really feels. This can even reach the point where the trainer hopes the trainee will fail with a family so he or she will be vindicated.

While interacting with the trainee, the trainer needs to be able to distinguish problematic conflicts or escalations in their relationship from the learning style of certain trainees. For example, some trainees may strongly disagree with or challenge the trainer's suggestions. Yet, while in the presence of the family, the same trainee may follow the suggestions with enthusiasm. These trainees seem to learn best through dialectical exchanges and if the trainer does not overreact, both can benefit. Indeed, this trainer–trainee pattern is far less troublesome than the situation where the trainee's verbal response to a clear and simple suggestion is enthusiastically positive but the trainee's performance of the recommended intervention is halfhearted, or even self-sabotaged. Of the two patterns above, the former, if it does not persist indefinitely, is likely to be a function of learning style, while the latter may indicate the existence of unresolved trainer–trainee relationship issues.

The struggles, the overt and covert escalations, that characterize an ill-defined trainer–trainee relationship can disrupt the whole training system. In such cases, the trainer, trainee, and family all would be better off if the supervision did not occur. Along these lines, it has been observed that, during live supervision, transactions between trainer and trainee will be replicated or reflected in the trainee's interactions with the family (Liddle & Saba, 1983, 1985; Liddle & Schwartz, 1983). The experienced trainer will use an awareness of this phenomenon to benefit the training systems by engaging in transactions with the trainee that he or she wants to be replicated with the family. In highly resistant training situations, however, the trainer may not be aware of or able to shift out of the symmetrical escalations (for example) with the trainee, who subsequently enters such an escalation with a family member, which in turn triggers further challenge from the trainer, and so on (see Chapter 11 by Schwartz *et al.*, this volume, for more on these issues).

Urgency to Reduce Level of Difficulties

Difficulties in the trainer–trainee relationship are a large problem only if it is important for the trainee to change quickly. This is the case when the trainee has few skills for engaging or restructuring families—or, worse, believes he or she should immediately confront or interpret or "bring to a head" family interactions—and is currently working with families. In this situation, the trainer will feel some urgency to raise the trainee's level of competence in family therapy before the trainee loses or tortures many families. In other situations, for example where the trainee has low competence in family therapy but will not be seeing families for some time, or where the trainee has an adequate level of competence in family therapy, the element of urgency is absent, so the trainer has time to try any number of strategies to reduce the difficulty between them.

Table 10-1 categorizes difficult trainer–trainee relationships by the degree of urgency to change the trainee. While the level of difficulty may be high for the relationships in quadrants 1, 2, and 3, the trainer has many more options than for quadrant 4. The real challenge for trainers is with quadrant 4 relationships.

Reducing Difficulties

For difficulties placed in quadrants 1 and 2, the trainer can initially adopt a peer posture with the relatively competent trainee, by supporting his or her ideas and interventions until the difficulty has abated. For quadrant 3 difficulties, the trainer can introduce new ideas to the trainee in a suggestive manner, not forcing him or her to accept the ideas too quickly, in order to preempt the expected objections. The trainer can also frame family therapy ideas in the trainee's "language" and, in general, introduce an alternating restrain/encourage rhythm with the trainee as the trainee's enthusiasm waxes and wanes.

The strategies mentioned above may be all that is needed in some quadrant 4 situations, but in other cases the urgency felt by both trainer and trainee reduces the trainer's ability to remain in a supportive, restraining, suggestive, or peer posture for any extended period. Directives need to be given by the trainer and accepted by the trainee, or else families will be lost or tortured.

TABLE 10-1. Difficult Trainer–Trainee Relationships

		Trainee is currently or soon will be working with families	
		No	Yes
Family therapy competence	High	1	2
	Low	3	4

Since most trainers are also therapists, they have encountered many situations in therapy that are analogous to the quadrant 4 relationship, and they should have a variety of techniques for eliciting the cooperation of family members who are initially quite resistant. Unfortunately, it does not occur to many trainers that these are parallel situations; consequently, they deal with difficulties in the trainee relationship in less thoughtful or effective ways than in their roles as therapists. The point is that many quadrant 4 predicaments can be resolved quickly if the trainer puts as much systemic thought into those situations as he or she might put into dealing with similar patterns in therapy.

Thus, depending on the trainer's orientation toward therapy in quadrant 4 situations, he or she may want to "meta-communicate" with the trainee about their relationship, or attempt less direct strategies, such as giving an "illusion of alternatives" or making a suggestion and predicting that the trainee will not or should not carry it out. Whatever task the trainer selects, it is important to bear in mind that the difficulty he or she experiences is not necessarily indicative of a trainee trait but often is instead an artifact of trainer–trainee interactions and the training context. Consequently, the onus lies on the trainer to attempt to reduce, or otherwise use constructively, these difficulties.

AREAS OF FOCUS

During live or video supervision, trainees can focus on one of the following areas: (1) the trainer's or other observer's evaluation of their performance, that is, wondering what the observers think of what they are doing; (2) their own behaviors or feelings as they interact with the family, that is, watching their own posture, tone of voice, level of anxiety, and so on; (3) the family's interactions with each other and with them, as well as assessing and developing strategies to alter those interactions; or (4) formulating or following a general plan of treatment that transcends the current session.

Some difficulty in supervision is inevitable because of the evaluative nature of the training context, where the trainee's self-concept as a clinician is on the line. This is particularly true in live and video forms of supervision, where the trainee's mistakes cannot be hidden. Given this evaluative context, many trainees are likely to listen carefully for the relationship component (i.e., what the supervisor might be saying covertly about their relationship) of any messages they get from the supervisor, until they sense a comfortable definition of their relationship. Thus they are often preoccupied with focus 1 above.

As is true in many human endeavors, a preoccupation with how others are evaluating one's performance (focus 1 above) will interfere with learning and performance. In live supervision it is natural and relatively unavoidable for trainees to be worried initially about how they are appearing to the trainer or training group. The trainer's feedback to the trainee will play an important role in determining whether or not the trainee's evaluative preoccupation persists, and paralyzes the trainee. It is usually best for the trainer to free the trainee's attention from domination by this evaluative focus as quickly as possible.

REDUCING THE EVALUATIVE FOCUS

There are several ways that the trainer can help trainees become less anxious about their performance, or the trainer's opinion of it. The first way is for the trainer to provide more clarity of definition to their relationship by implying or stating overtly as soon as possible that he or she believes that the trainee is, or has the potential to be, a good therapist. This is usually the trainee's ultimate concern and, once this is resolved, any criticism becomes less threatening. Such a message need not be insincere if the trainer subscribes to a model of family therapy that believes that most people can become competent. Such a model orients one to search for and activate strengths rather than defects in trainees and in family members. If the trainer cannot give some form of this message relatively early in the training, then perhaps it is better not to proceed with the training. Once this message has been given and received, the training relationship may shift dramatically toward harmonious complementarity.

A second method of reducing this evaluative focus is for the trainer to develop and display an attitude regarding the trainee's performance that implies that while the trainer cares how the trainee does, the trainer's identity as a competent trainer does not depend on the trainee's performance or the family's outcome. With this attitude comes the implication that mistakes by the trainee are expected and not to be feared; indeed, at times, small errors might even be prescribed. With this attitude and a clear definition of the relationship, the trainer can make positive or negative comments about the trainee's performance, and the trainee will be able to focus on the content of the feedback without worrying about how that performance has affected the trainer's overall view of the trainee.

A third method is to negotiate a training contract with the trainee and periodically renegotiate it throughout the training. Such a contract can include (1) a discussion of the trainee's learning style and how the trainer can present himself or herself to best complement that style (e.g., authoritative versus suggestive); (2) a discussion of the meaning of the various elements of the supervisory process (e.g., "A phone call does not always mean you screwed up," or, "You have [or do not have] power to override my directives"); (3) a clear definition of the role of observing group members (e.g., "when the trainee comes behind the mirror you are [are not] free to comment"); and (4) an attempt to anticipate and discuss problems that the group will encounter or has encountered because of their idiosyncratic blending (e.g., "Some of you are more advanced and will feel impatient"). Negotiating such a contract at the outset of training is important and can help the group to an auspicious launching, but we have found that to do so at the outset alone is rarely enough. Scheduling periodic individual meetings with trainees to go over the contract again is worth the trouble, even if no problems are apparent.

A final method of reducing trainees' evaluative focus is to create a noncompetitive atmosphere within the training group. One way to do this is for the trainer to show fallibility, to be quick to point out his or her own mistakes rather than blaming trainees for poor performance, while at the same time maintaining a sense of leadership and confidence. Another way to remain noncompetitive is to monitor the distribution of praise and criticism given to group members such that drastic imbalances are avoided. Finally, a certain distance should be maintained in the "generational boundary" between trainer and each trainee so that "cross-generational coalitions" are avoided, and so that the trainer is free to push trainees beyond their comfortable ranges of therapy behavior. This "generational boundary" should gradually diminish as the trainees increase in competence.

INTERNAL FOCUS

If the trainer successfully employs some of the foregoing methods to create a noncompetitive, nonthreatening relationship with each trainee and atmosphere in the training group, the question remains of how to help trainees achieve the proper balance among the other three areas of focus. For example, it is important at times for the trainee to focus on the second area, that is, to be aware of and attempt to change his or her own behaviors, attitudes, and feelings while with the family. If, however, this internal focus dominates the trainer's attention throughout a session, it can be as much of an impediment to learning or to effective therapy as the first area of focus.

A good rule of thumb in training, therapy, or life in general, is to not prescribe changes that should happen spontaneously (Watzlawick et al., 1974). One sure way of getting a trainee to become obsessed with both the first and second (evaluative and internal) areas of focus is to tell him or her to relax, to be funny, to act confident, or the like. Not only will the trainee lose sight of what the family is doing, but often will not be able to comply with the directive, which will compound the trainee's internal, evaluative monitoring.

To avoid such predicaments during live supervision, the wise trainer keeps most of his or her suggestions at the behavioral or conceptual level and uses the relationship with the trainee to change the trainee's demeanor when such change is needed. If the trainer wants the trainee to be more intense, for example, the trainer can deliver a behavioral suggestion in an intense tone of voice, or enter into an intense exchange over some aspect of the session with the trainee, instead of directly instructing him or her to *be* more intense. If the trainee's style is to be commented on directly, it is often better to tell the trainee to *act as if* he or she was more intense, happy, relaxed, or the like, rather than to *be* that way.

In the process described above, the importance of the trainer–trainee relationship as an instrument for changing the ambience of the training system is evident. Just as the therapist must be able to "use himself or herself" in a variety of ways to push the family beyond their interaction thresholds, the trainer also uses himself or herself to broaden the trainee's range of behavior with the family. For example, the overly nice trainee may need to be challenged at some level by the trainer before he or she will be more challenging toward the family. In postsession discussions, after such a challenge, the trainer can discuss how the trainee might behave differently, and whether any adjustments in their relationship are needed because of the challenges.

The internal focus will dominate the trainee's attention to some degree at other times, in addition to the "be spontaneous" predicaments described above. This will be the case, for example, when a trainee tries a skill or technique for the first few times. During these times the trainer should be prepared for the trainee to display an increased degree of myopia or "tunnel vision." During live supervision the trainer can keep the trainee "covered" during these tryouts, that is, keep an eye on and make suggestions according to the family's interactions and reactions while the trainee is internally absorbed and less able to read the family's feedback. If the trainer can anticipate the ebb and flow of the trainee's external awareness as the trainee tries new skills, the trainer will not be frustrated with or disappointed in the trainee during these times, and can help the trainee be more patient with himself or herself.

INTERACTIVE FOCUS

The third area of focus, the in-session interactions among family members and between the family and the trainee, will also be heavily influenced by the trainer–trainee relationship. It is very tempting in all kinds of supervision for the trainer to "take the eyes" of the trainee, that is, to keep the trainee covered at all times by making observations and hypotheses for the trainee such that the trainee does not have to see. This temptation is greatest during live supervision, where issues of the trainer (1) wanting to show competence, or (2) feeling responsible to the family to make sure the session goes perfectly, or (3) being unable to trust the trainee's judgment, will foster an overprotectiveness and intrusiveness that tend to "robotize" the trainee.

Early in training, when every skill is a new one and the trainee has an underdeveloped conceptual map to guide his or her observations, some degree of robotization may be necessary or unavoidable. Trainees have various reactions to this stage of training, often depending on the clarity of expectations and level of comfort in the trainer–trainee relationship. If those issues are settled, most trainees, knowing that this is a temporary stage, appreciate the help during this period, but problems will result if it is not so temporary (see Chapter 11 by Schwartz et al. and Chapter 25 by Liddle et al., this volume). A training system that begins with a robotizing style develops a certain amount of inertia to remain in that style. It can become very comfortable for trainer, trainee, and family alike for the trainer to be very active. To overcome this inertia, "to give back the trainee's eyes," requires a good deal of energy and conscious restraint on the part of the trainer.

"BIG PICTURE" FOCUS

The ability of the trainee to pay attention during or between sessions to the fourth area of focus, the "big picture" of the evolution of treatment, will also largely depend on aspects of the trainer–trainee relationship. For example, the trainer may tend to "take the trainee's mind" in the same way that he or she was "taking the trainee's eyes." That is, if the trainer does most of the planning for each session, or the monitoring of events and feedback relative to a global treatment plan, then the trainee's conceptual talent will be underdeveloped (Schwartz, 1981).

Again, however, the early stage of training may call for some degree of this kind of robotization as well. While a trainee is worried about organizing the next session or mastering simple techniques, he or she will not be able to catch more than brief glimpses of the forest because these trees loom so large. Here again the trainer must find an adequate and changing balance between keeping the trainee covered conceptually, while increasingly pushing the trainee to construct his or her own strategies between sessions and to read feedback and make in-session adjustments to it. Finding this kind of balance is the art of family therapy training.

SYSTEMIC PERSPECTIVE

Thus far this chapter has discussed the influence and importance of the trainer–trainee relationship in the smooth functioning of the training–therapy system and in helping the trainee focus on the areas of the system that will facilitate learning. As mentioned in this chapter's introduction, successful family therapy training now also involves an epistemological shift from a linear to a systemic perspective of the human drama. The intellectual aspect of this shift can and should be conveyed through classes and readings. The practical translation of this conceptual shift into the behaviors and attitudes of the therapist, however, is conveyed through the trainer–trainee relationship (Colapinto, 1983).

The way the trainer talks about family members and their problems, about the trainee's performance and interactions with the family, about the trainer–trainee relationship or the trainee's work context, will have a potent impact on the trainee's acquisition of an attitude that sees all interactions or behavior in a larger context. This does not imply that the trainer must strive to be systemic at all times. Indeed, orgies of linearity are useful parts of systemic models (see Chapter 3 by Pirrotta & Cecchin, this volume). As long as trainer and trainee both recognize that such forbidden pleasures are steps on the path toward a more systemic understanding and that many effective interventions may be based on a less than fully systemic view, then they can allow each other the freedom to experiment with "partial realities," while acknowledging that they are partial. In other words, the trainer strives to maintain a systemic view and to model such a perspective for the trainee, but does not allow this view to become a straitjacket that stifles intuitive brainstorming, or a club with which to beat the trainee's linear epistemology into submission.

SUMMARY

The struggle to find a balance between a self-assertive tendency and an integrative tendency that characterizes all living systems (Koestler, 1978) is particularly difficult in training relationships. A thread running throughout this chapter is the trainer's dilemma of how much to allow the trainee to depend on him or her, and how much to allow the trainee to learn through his or her own mistakes, to find his or her own way. The trainee also struggles with his or her desire to feel autonomous and need for guidance and security. These ambivalences are compounded by the technology of family therapy training (live and video supervision) whereby the potential for robotization is increased, as is the pressure on both trainer and trainee to perform.

In recognition of these central training issues, this chapter outlined considerations and guidelines for the trainer to maintain an appropriate and evolving balance between these tendencies for self-assertiveness and integration, while attempting to minimize difficulties in the trainer–trainee relationship, to help the trainee focus on areas that will promote learning, and to convey a systemic perspective.

Note

1. The author acknowledges the problems inherent in the traditional use of the term "resistance" to mean a *thing* that is a trait of a person or family. For this reason, the term "difficulty" is used, which, though less specific, has fewer linear connotations.

References

Colapinto, J. (1983). Beyond technique: Teaching how to think structurally. *Journal of Strategic and Systemic Therapies*, 2, 12–21.

Haley, J. (1973). Beginning and experienced family therapists. In A. Ferber, M. Mendelson, & A. Napier (Eds.), *The book of family therapy*. Boston: Houghton Mifflin.

Koestler, A. (1978). *Janus: A summing up*. New York: Random House.

Liddle, H., & Saba, G. (1983). On context replication: The isomorphic relationship of training and therapy. *Journal of Strategic and Systemic Therapies*, 2, 3–11.

Liddle, H., & Saba, G. (1985). The isomorphic nature of training and therapy: Epistemologic foundation for a structural-strategic training model. In J. Schwartzman (Ed.), *Families and other systems*. New York: Guilford Press.

Liddle, H., & Schwartz, R. (1983). Live supervision/consultation: Conceptual and pragmatic guidelines for family therapy trainers. *Family Process*, 22, 477–490.

Moskowitz, S., & Rupert, P. (1983). Conflict resolution within the supervisory relationship. *Professional Psychology: Research and Practice*, pp. 632–641.

Schwartz, R. (1981). The conceptual development of family therapy trainees. *American Journal of Family Therapy*, 9, 89–90.

Watzlawick, P., Weakland, J., & Fisch, R. (1974). *Change*. New York: W. W. Norton.

11

Muddles in Live Supervision

RICHARD C. SCHWARTZ
Institute for Juvenile Research, Chicago

HOWARD A. LIDDLE
University of California, San Francisco

DOUGLAS C. BREUNLIN
Institute for Juvenile Research, Chicago

When family therapists began to watch each other's work from behind one-way mirrors, and, later, to interrupt sessions with comments or directives to the therapist, live supervision was born (Kempster & Savitsky, 1967; Montalvo, 1973). Used extensively, this procedure has become a highly valued and expected aspect of training for most family therapy approaches (Berger & Dammann, 1982; Birchler, 1975; McGoldrick, 1982; Rickert & Turner, 1978; Roberts, 1983). However, live supervision is an intricate undertaking that contains several possible muddles for the inexperienced or naive supervisor. Depending on whether or not these pitfalls are avoided, trainees recollect their live supervision experience as either one of the highlights or one of the low points of their training (see Chapter 25 by Liddle *et al.*, this volume).

In an effort to clarify the skills needed for live supervision, we outlined in another paper a stage-oriented set of conceptual and pragmatic guidelines for the practice of live supervision (Liddle & Schwartz, 1983). The present chapter extends this framework by providing examples of implementation dilemmas and possible solutions in difficult live supervision situations. Scenarios of the common muddles of live supervision are offered, and workable explanations and solutions for each situation are proposed. In addition to providing some problem-solving hints to the supervisor, this chapter is intended to help supervisors think contextually about the everyday problems they encounter in live supervision. We hope to promote the notion that supervisory impasses are not things or problems to be fixed but, rather, are interactional processes that always include the supervisor and have, for a variety of reasons, the possibility of occurring simultaneously in several subsystems of the training context.

TENDENCY TOWARD ROBOTIZATION

Before turning to the scenarios, we will discuss two tendencies that underlie most of the muddles depicted in them. The first is the tendency toward robotization of the trainee. In this process, the trainee becomes little more than an automaton, mechanically carrying out the supervisor's every command, and exhibiting little initiative or creativity. In combination with ineffectual implementation or inadequate conceptualization on the part of the trainee, the structure and process of live supervision often contribute to robotization.

One common artifact of live supervision, the so-called MEGO ("Mine Eyes Glaze Over") syndrome, often attacks trainees during their first live supervision experiences. Such assaults are frequent because to expose oneself to the critical eye of an authority and newly acquainted peers can be intimidating for any trainee, no matter what steps are taken to minimize the evaluative nature of the experience. Preoccupied with evaluation of their performance, many trainees become tentative, insecure, and anxious when working with a family. Their work in this context is less competent than it might be in their practice. The supervisor who is observing the trainee's discomfort and the consequent ineffective therapy may try to help the trainee by making many detailed phone calls or consultations, or even entering the room to take over the session. This behavior is likely to be welcomed by the struggling trainee in the throes of MEGO. However, such an interactional sequence often initiates the robotization process. This process can be rigidly maintained if either the trainer, the trainee, or both assume, on the basis of the trainee's inauspicious beginning, that the trainee is not competent and requires significant guidance.

In addition to the beginning trainee's expectable stage fright and consequent MEGO reaction, there are other frequently occurring obstacles to optimal trainee functioning at the onset of live supervision. Often trainees must struggle to understand and adopt a model of therapy that is foreign to their previous training. During this time, the trainee may appear to lack direction and to be unclear about the direction of each intervention the trainer requests (and, further, may not communicate this lack of clearness or understanding), and consequently may lack confidence. Until the trainee has found a way to function with the new model of therapy in live supervision, he or she has little choice but to rely on the supervisor.

Additionally, the supervisor may be requesting behaviors of the trainee that are quite dissimilar from his or her previous training, personal style, or beliefs. Until the struggles that these requests provoke are successfully addressed, the trainee may seem tentative and lacking conviction.

Supervisors, too, may create robotization. For example, beginning supervisors, or those who feel insecure in their role, may inappropriately take over the session in an attempt to impress the training group. Moreover, robotization may occur as a result of supervisory mistakes. Although supervisors might not like to face their mistakes, it nevertheless remains a possibility that the supervisor has offered a misguided or mistimed intervention, or has misjudged the therapist's ability to implement it. In any of these cases, the trainee may accurately read the feedback that things are not going well in the session. The supervisor, being more removed from the feedback by virtue of the one-way mirror, and perhaps also reluctant to admit a mistake, may call for the trainee to persist along the original path, initiating sequences of trainee tentativeness and supervisor overactivity.

Some degree of robotization is inevitable in live supervision, and, if it is a temporary process, there are times when it may be helpful and necessary, such as during early stages of training. But robotization is harmful when it is prolonged to the point at which it erodes trainees' confidence in their ability to generate and deliver competent interventions, or to develop an effective treatment plan. It can also be harmful to the trainee when it is motivated by the supervisor's insecurity or need to be central or idolized.

In addition, the supervisor's learning is also hampered by this process because he or she functions as a therapist-once-removed rather than as a supervisor focused on learning how to teach the trainee.

ISOMORPHIC SEQUENCES

The second tendency that is commonly involved in the muddles of live supervision has to do with the isomorphic nature of the live supervision context: patterns of interaction at one level of the training/therapy system that tend to mirror or replicate patterns at other levels. Thus, interactions between supervisor and trainee may resemble interactions between trainee and family members, or those among the family members themselves (Liddle & Saba, 1983, 1985; Liddle & Schwartz, 1983; Liddle, Chapter 9, this volume).

Supervisors who are unaware of this tendency toward isomorphism can find themselves amid escalating and unproductive more-of-the-same sequences. For example, in a session with a family characterized by hostile, challenging exchanges, a family member may overtly challenge the supervisor's competence. Frustrated, the trainee may, in turn, challenge the supervisor's directives more overtly. If, in turn, the supervisor defensively criticizes the trainee, then the isomorphic sequences remain intact and the replicating hostile exchanges within the training/therapy system are likely to continue to escalate; the family and/or the therapist will show more "resistance."

If, however, the supervisor is aware of this isomorphic process, he or she will be able quickly to identify and then to change such escalations, and also to use this tendency toward isomorphism to the advantage of the training/therapy system; a supervisor can alter his or her relationship with a trainee not only to break isomorphic escalations but also to create a more productive series of sequences in the system.

SCENARIOS OF LIVE SUPERVISION

In this section we will examine how these two tendencies (robotization and the isomorphic replication of sequences) are commonly manifested in impasses of live supervision, and we offer some suggestions for resolving or avoiding them. To do this, we will present a series of scenarios, each of which is followed by several hypotheses about its origins and several suggestions for altering the scenario.

First Scenario

The supervisor is making many calls during a session because the trainee carries out the instruction of each call, but then seems aimless or tentative and perplexed as to what to do next, and waits until the phone rings before making the next intervention. The supervisor continues to phone frequently.

This is a common occurrence in live supervision and, as will be discussed below, it may or may not indicate a problem, depending on several factors, including the stage of training, the stage of therapy, the trainer–trainee relationship, and the broader context in which the supervision occurs.

STAGE OF TRAINING

If this scenario is taking place early in the training process, it may not be a problem. For reasons mentioned earlier—initial stage fright, difficulties in learning a new model of therapy, and awkwardness in performing new behaviors—beginning trainees will often seem tentative and overly dependent on their supervisor. This natural reluctance or lack of initiative will not generate destructive sequences between the supervisor and trainee if both can keep the episode in perspective.

There are many steps a supervisor can take to maintain perspective, however, and thereby reduce the duration and negative consequences of this initial dependence. First, the supervisor can assess and discuss with the trainee (prior to the beginning of live supervision, or when necessary before each session) the likelihood of such a scenario developing. They might discuss the degree to which the trainee has been influenced by and has adopted other models of therapy, the degree to which the other approaches are not syntonic with the supervisor's model, and the trainee's degree of familiarity with the supervisor's model. In addition, the supervisor should routinely inquire about, acknowledge, and normalize trainee fears and anxiety. Further issues for this supervisory discussion might include how much initiative the supervisor expects the trainee to take at any particular stage of training, and how comfortable the trainee feels about having to depend on the supervisor's input.

Indirect strategies can also be used to deal with extreme expressions of trainee nervousness or expressions of undue dependence on the supervisor (see Chapter 6 by Mazza, this volume). Statements such as, "For a while you may not be able to do much more than repeat the words that I say over the phone," or, "You'll make any number of blunders from which I may have to rescue you," can both reduce trainee anxiety and decrease the likelihood of these behaviors.

Second, during this early stage of training, the supervisor should strive to be as clear as possible in the presession discussion about the overall goals and plan for the session. Although at this stage the trainee often does not have an understanding of the model and goals of therapy, a clearly articulated session plan can allow the trainee to reach certain destinations on his or her own. A focused and crisp preparatory discussion as close to the beginning of the session as possible can obviate the need for many corrective calls during the interview.

When the robotization process is related to a clash of models between what the trainee has previously learned and the model the supervisor is trying to teach, the supervisor and the trainee are well advised to spend time outside of the live supervision context talking about the conflicts (interpersonal and paradigmatic) that are emerging as a result of the clash of models. If these conflicts can be acknowledged, anticipated, and openly discussed, they become far less debilitating. In cases where discrepancies between models are great, it may be necessary for the trainer to "walk the trainee through" some sessions until the trainee gains more confidence in the unfamiliar model and, also, sees that the supervisor's approach can be beneficial.

The supervisor's understanding and framing of the robotization process is instrumental in its management. Just as a robotization scenario does not necessarily indicate a problem if it occurs early in the training, the same is true if it occurs temporarily during a later stage of training. Each time a trainee encounters a new set of skills or a new family, he or she may lose confidence, become tentative, and begin another dependent cycle with the supervisor. This may also occur periodically throughout the training as trainees go through the conceptual crises that often occur in attempting to understand a systemic paradigm. During such crises it is common for trainees to question not only their previous conceptual models and modes of therapy, but also their conceptual and therapeutic abilities.

Such periods of robotization occurring later in training will remain temporary and will not lead to difficulties if the supervisor and trainee deal with them in much the same way as we suggest the early periods are handled. If these later robotization periods are anticipated and are openly discussed when they arise, they will not disrupt the rhythm of training.

SUPERVISOR TEMPTATION AND URGENCY

If this scenario persists, however, it may reflect a problem. The supervisor and trainee may be co-evolving a complementary relationship in which the supervisor is doing the therapy and simply using the trainee as a channel for his or her interventions. As discussed earlier, such an arrangement is seductive: the insecure supervisor may want to impress the training group, or may want to feel assured that the family is receiving competent treatment; the trainee is relieved of the burden of generating interventions and yet can feel a part of successful treatment; and the family may be eager to hear from the "experts" behind the mirror. As the process of robotization continues, it can become increasingly difficult to reverse—the trainee will feel and act more and more incompetent, thus perpetuating the supervisor's belief that he or she must take over.

For this reason, among others, the trainer should intervene only when necessary. The immediacy of trainer intervention, which is the strength of live supervision, can also lead to one of its weaknesses. Prudent supervisors constantly question the need for their interventions; impatience or an inclination to show off one's cleverness are unacceptable reasons for supervisory intervention. We offer the following considerations for supervisors to keep in mind when trying to decide whether to intervene.

There will be many occasions when the supervisor notices certain trainee behaviors that need to be altered, yet the performance of the different behavior is not crucial to the outcome of the session taking palce. If trainee robotization is a particular concern, it may be best to practice restraint on those occasions, discuss the matter during the postsession meeting, and intervene only at points where the outcome of the session appears to be at stake. The degree of urgency of a particular intervention will vary, of course, depending on the model of therapy being taught, the time left in the session or overall treatment plan (that is, whether the intervention could be made later), and the possible consequences to the therapy or the trainee if the supervisor does not intervene.

A related issue is the supervisor's judgment of the probability of the trainee implementing the intervention on his or her own, without supervisory guidance. As the trainee and supervisor synchronize their models, it is common for a trainee to begin, without a supervisory prompt, the exact intervention the supervisor was formulating minutes before. It is always preferable for the trainee rather than the supervisor to initiate an intervention. Thus the supervisor must weigh the urgency of the intervention against the likelihood of it being initiated at a slightly later point by the trainee. In addition, when the supervisor believes the need for an intervention is urgent, it is also important to judge whether the trainee is capable of carrying out the intervention. Asking trainees to perform an intervention for which they are unprepared can produce trainee failures and possibly numerous consequent supervisor calls that disrupt and frustrate the entire training/therapy system. On the other hand, it is important not to underestimate or unduly protect trainees. Thus a realistic assessment of the trainee's intervention repertoire or stage of development is crucial.

Since the same intervention can be carried out effectively in any number of ways, the supervisor should also consider whether the modification about to be requested does not merely represent a difference in style between supervisor and trainee. It is often difficult to let trainees find their own therapeutically appropriate style of intervention when their personal style is different from and perhaps antithetical to the supervisor's style. Of course, if alteration of trainee style is something that is a supervisory target, and part of the learning contract, interventions that are related to style are appropriate.

SUPERVISOR MISTAKES

As mentioned previously, one of the more difficult explanations of robotization for a supervisor to entertain is simply that the supervisory suggestions are questionable in terms of content, timing, or overall direction. Thus, the trainee's reluctance in the first scenario to go beyond the instructions in each call may be a demonstration of sensitivity to the family's appropriate lack of responsiveness or cooperation.

During live supervision, the supervisor is simultaneously confronted with several sets of needs. For example, the family's presenting difficulties and interactional patterns must be considered along with the trainee's overall and session-specific training objectives. The supervisor can become so preoccupied with the trainee's stylistic or implementation difficulties that previously clear thinking about the family becomes at least temporarily confused. This mistake can be compounded or maintained by the emotional distance between the supervisor and the family prompted by the one-way mirror (Berger & Dammann, 1982). Particularly in cases where trainees have previously shown competence, robotization may be a warning to the supervisor to reassess the therapeutic direction being promoted.

Under these circumstances, we recommend bringing the trainee behind the mirror for a consultation with the supervisor and the training group. In addition to assessing the trainee's understanding of the direction of therapy, the group can discuss the appropriateness of the direction, or particular interventions. Including the group in a consultation about a possible mistake or change is not always easy for supervisors to do, especially if they feel insecure about their own competence. But such an effort, particularly if the reassessment proves successful, can have several beneficial effects on the training group. Trainees are likely to feel less pressure to be perfect if the supervisor can acknowledge some imperfections. They will feel less like passive observers and more like integral, contributing members of the training system, and they are likely to respect and model the supervisor's flexibility.

Second Scenario

In an early stage of training, the trainee is not direct with the family. The direction for the session has been made clear during the presession meeting, yet during the interview the trainee is verbose and ambiguous. The supervisor calls in to request a more succinct and clear delivery. The call fails to alter the trainee's pattern, however, and the session proceeds amid vague and cautious therapist–family member exchanges.

FEAR, IGNORANCE, OR ISOMORPHISM

Many of the explanations given for the first scenario, particularly those relating to performance anxiety, might also apply here. Additionally, these problems might be the result of vague supervisory suggestions. The supervisor may have suggested a broad intervention, such as "create an enactment," rather than one that includes specific steps: "Ask them to face each other, then . . . ."

There are several reasons that the supervisor frequently needs to be concrete. First, the trainee may be unfamiliar with the intervention requested, and selection of the most effective wording or tone of voice will be indicated by this knowledge deficit. Second, the trainee's lack of directness may be related to a fear of offending, challenging, or hurting one or more family members. Third, the training system may be engaged in isomorphic sequences of vagueness in which abstract or indirect interactions at all levels of the system are mirroring, influencing, and compounding each other. In the scenario presented here, perhaps the supervisor was too abstract in his or her directives to the trainee, who in turn acted confused and tentative with the family members, who then remained indirect and indefinite with each other. At some point the supervisor may recognize that the therapy is muddled and offer additional unclear directives, which will merely maintain the sequence.

A change in the supervisor's style can influence this scenario. If the supervisor's instructions became more concrete, the trainee would most likely follow suit and change his or her style. Instead of saying, "I want you to unbalance with the father," or, "Be more concise," the trainer could say, "I want you to move your chair next to the father, look directly at him and say . . . ."[1] If the trainee's vagueness has been due primarily to a lack of understanding of the model or intervention, concrete delivery of the suggestion by the supervisor can often be sufficient to allow the therapist to change. If trainee vagueness is related primarily to fear of the family and/or situation, then, since he or she can no longer avoid what is feared through vagueness, the trainee will have to come behind the mirror to discuss the fears openly with the supervisor or perform the intervention despite trepidations. Finally, if the trainee's vagueness seems related to isomorphic sequences, then greater concreteness at one level of the training system can alter the unclear sequences and initiate more clarity at other levels.

Supervisors, of course, also may lack clarity, often because of a lack of familiarity or comfort with the attempted interventions. Incompetent or novice supervisors can hide incomprehension of details in abstract requests of the trainee and then blame trainees, overtly or to themselves, for the resulting inept performance.

The optimal duration of a concrete style of supervision depends on several factors. For example, if the trainee is new to family therapy, then it is appropriate to "walk the therapist through" many early session interventions in a concrete fashion. If, on the other hand, a more advanced trainee has run into a new, difficult, or complex intervention, then the supervisor should shift temporarily to a concrete style. Again, the supervisor must be sensitive enough to balance tendencies toward trainee robotization with promoting therapist independence.

Third Scenario

An advanced trainee is challenging parents to be more consistent and firm with their rebellious adolescent son. The trainee's message to the parents is clear, direct, and concrete, but his demeanor is light, amiable, and playful. As instructed, the parents directly and concretely communicate their expectations to their son, but their tone does not match their words. Watching, one wonders whether the son will believe that they mean business. Acting on this possibility, the supervisor phones in to challenge the therapist to be more serious with the parents. The supervisor's tone, however, also lacks intensity. Not unexpectedly, the sequence recurs.

Again, an isomorphic sequence is involved, this time centering on the use of the light, polite manner within the training/therapy system. One common reason for the transmission and continuation of this sequence is a reticence about disturbing relationships at one or more levels of the system. The parents of this scenario may be afraid of their teenager's reaction to their increase in believable limit setting, and the therapist may have similar worries about how the parents might react to a change in the intensity of his or her interactions with them. Finally, the supervisor may also be apprehensive about a possibly intense exchange with the trainee.

In this case the supervisor can use the principle of isomorphism to change interaction throughout the training/therapy system. By shifting to a more intense demeanor with the trainee, the supervisor may increase the intensity of the exchanges between the trainee and the parents, and between the parents and their son. Of course, the supervisor may need to use varying degrees of increased intensity at different times. On one occasion it may suffice for the supervisor to state the same words ("I want you to sound more serious"), but with more gravity in his or her voice. At another time, the supervisor may have to challenge the trainee more directly in both word and tone. For example, "What is keeping you from asking these parents if they believe this issue is important?" when asked in a serious tone, will probably allow a message of seriousness and urgency to be transmitted.[2] In this way the supervisor can generally maintain a certain extent of control over the emotional climate of a session by varying the tenor of the supervisor-therapist relationship. As discused in Chapter 9 by Liddle, this volume, this is often a more effective way to modify intensity than to tell the trainee to be more intense, humorous, solemn, or so forth, because such a directive to "be spontaneous" can focus trainees in a paralyzing way on their performance.

Supervisors should be reminded that these shifts in intensity in the supervisory relationship can be misinterpreted by anxious trainees, eager to achieve the approval of their supervisor. This relationship, which can be a fragile one, especially at the early stages, is essential to trainee change and a positive therapeutic outcome. Time spent in attending to and checking on the status of the supervisor–supervisee relationship is generally a good investment in the various intended outcomes in the training and therapy system.

Fourth Scenario

The supervisor phones the trainee and gives a directive to create an enactment. The therapist attempts the intervention halfheartedly and fails. The supervisor phones again and, with greater intensity, explains the directive in a step-by-step fashion. The trainee attempts the intervention once again, this time with even less enthusiasm, and once again fails. The supervisor asks the trainee to come behind the mirror, and confronts the therapist about the lackluster attempts. The trainee responds by questioning the supervisor's judgment regarding the timing of the intervention. These symmetrical exchanges between supervisor and trainee continue to escalate throughout the session. The interview loses focus, and family does not return.

There are a number of ways to view such difficulties. Here we will focus on one explanation that again relates to the style of the supervisor.

Let us assume that the trainee in this scenario has not accepted the learner role, or the supervisor as a teacher. Many of the possible reasons for his or her dissatisfaction with this complementarity have been discussed in Schwartz's chapter on the trainer–trainee relationship (Chapter 10). For example, it may be that the supervisor and trainee are too close in age, experience level, or perceived family therapy competence for the trainee to feel comfortable taking a subordinate position. If this is the case, then each time the trainer uses a *directive* style that defines him as the authority ("I want you to do this now"), the trainee may react with less than enthusiastic compliance, no matter how appropriate the directive. Such sequences can quickly escalate, as they did in the scenario, to the point at which the supervisory direction becomes the battleground for a covert struggle over relationship definition.

Frequently, if the supervisor recognizes this struggle in these terms and begins to shift toward a less hierarchical style, the trainee will begin to express fewer concerns about the supervisor's judgments. This change includes moving from a directive to a *suggestive* style when giving the trainee input. For example, instead of saying, "I want you to do this now," the supervisor might say, "What would you think about doing this?" or, "This is what I would do here; how does that feel to you?" In addition, the supervisor might make extra attempts to solicit and incorporate more of the therapist's ideas.

Certainly there are occasions in live supervision when the supervisor needs to be unabashedly directive, particularly when therapeutic situations warrant immediate action (Liddle & Schwartz, 1983). In such cases, however, it is possible to minimize the hierarchy during the pre- or postsession meetings. When such a shift in supervisory style does not effectively diminish the escalating struggle in their relationship, the supervisor may have to address suspected relationship issues more directly in frank discussion with the trainee.[3]

A final note on this scenario: it is important not to overreact to minor escalations or challenges in live supervision, as they are an expected part of this often intense training and therapy context. As shown in earlier scenarios, this last situation does not necessarily represent a problem if such escalations are not chronically disruptive to the training/therapy system. Indeed, some trainees learn effectively through lively, polemical exchanges, and these interactions can help supervisors clarify their positions as well. It is a mistake to interpret and react to all challenges as indicative of supervisor–trainee relationship problems.

These four scenarios are examples of some of the more common impasses we have experienced in doing live supervision. There are many others, of course, but if supervisors can be mindful of the tendency toward robotization, as well as the isomorphic replication of sequences across system levels, a perspective can be gained that helps to avoid or preempt many problems and, when problems are unavoidable, to generate creative solutions.

DEUTERO-LEARNING

A final muddle in live supervision is not easily illustrated by a specific scenario. We are concerned with the deutero-learning of family therapy trainees within and outside of live supervision. We use Bateson's (1972) term "deutero-learning" to denote the way that trainees learn to learn about families, therapy, or themselves. In highly directive forms of training, trainees learn to look to their trainers rather than to their own observations or intuition for conceptual and technical solutions or innovations. This tendency, especially if it fails to shift over time, is a major concern of both proponents and critics of live supervision. Trainees are often told how to think and behave as family therapists, rather than having to discover these things for themselves. They learn to rely on their wise supervisor—beyond the point at which it is developmentally appropriate—rather than on themselves for creative ideas or interventions. Many alumni of intensive training programs, especially programs that emphasize live supervision, report that, even years after graduation, when they get stuck with a family they think of what their original supervisors would say, then respond in that way. The creativity and flexibility of these trainees is often limited by their perceptions of their supervisor's creativity and range of interventions.

Certainly live supervision per se does not *create* this dependent style of deutero-learning. It is possible for trainees to learn to look to themselves even while their work is observed and critiqued by more experienced supervisors. But the development of an autonomous deutero-learning style in trainees requires more sensitivity and conscious restraint on the part of the supervisors in programs using live supervision than in programs in which live supervision is not used. In addition to the previously discussed robotization factor, which plays an obvious role in deutero-learning, many trainees will naturally tend to marvel at their trainer's ability to assess and plan so clearly, and will believe themselves incapable of such work. What most trainees do not know is that in at least one specific way live supervision is easier than therapy; the supervisor has more time and distance, two factors that can facilitate greater clarity and precision of thought. In the therapy room, obviously, the therapist feels the immediacy of the family's presence and feedback all the more.

Thus, the art of training consists in helping trainees learn theory and technique, while also learning to monitor, trust, and use their own abilities. Supervisors must be able to motivate but not dominate; to restrain "savior" leanings while competent trainees struggle to accomplish and learn about therapy in their own ways; to cast aside prideful motivations and give ample credit for changes in others; to solicit, listen to, and validate the trainees' ideas; and to be courageous enough to admit their own fallibility. Supervisors can use live supervision to create a safe context for mutual discovery and stimulation.

Notes

1. The practice of feeding trainees lines has distinct disadvantages and advantages. Depending on such factors as the stage of training and the degree to which the trainee can understand an intervention, offering concrete examples of how interventions might or should be delivered can be a very helpful supervisory method, and not necessarily one that fosters dependency and stifles creativity.

2. Challenges of this sort must be carefully done by the supervisor. Factors such as the stage of training and of the supervisory relationship and individual style variables affect a supervisor's decision to challenge trainees in this way.

3. A primary point throughout is that it is the supervisor's responsibility to initiate such things as discussions about the supervisory relationship. "Waiting until the trainee is ready to discuss it" (as evidenced by the trainee's taking the initiative in bringing up relationship struggles with the supervisor) can be a convenient but irresponsible excuse that keeps supervision ineffective.

References

Bateson, G. (1972). *Steps to an ecology of mind.* New York: Ballantine.

Berger, M., & Dammann, C. (1982). Live supervision as context, treatment, and training. *Family Process, 21,* 337–344.

Birchler, G. (1975). Live supervision and instant feedback in marriage and family therapy. *Journal of Marriage and Family Counseling, 1,* 331–342.

Kempster, S. W., & Savitsky, E. (1967). Training family therapists through live supervision. In N. Ackerman, F. Beatman, & J. Sherman (Eds.), *Expanding theory and practice in family therapy.* New York: Family Service Association of America.

Liddle, H., & Saba, G. (1983). On context replication: The isomorphic relationship of training and therapy. *Journal of Strategic and Systemic Therapies, 2,* 3–11.

Liddle, H., & Saba, G. (1985). The isomorphic nature of training and therapy. In J. Schwartzman (Ed.), *Families and other systems.* New York: Guilford Press.

Liddle, H., & Schwartz, R. (1983). Live supervision/consultation: Conceptual and pragmatic guidelines for family therapy training. *Family Process, 22,* 477–490.

McGoldrick, M. (1982). Through the looking glass. In R. Whitten & J. Byng-Hall (Eds.), *Family therapy supervision: Recent developments in practice.* New York: Grune & Stratton.

Montalvo, B. (1973). Aspects of live supervision. *Family Process, 12,* 343–359.

Rickert, V., & Turner, J. (1978). Through the looking glass: Supervision in family therapy. *Social Casework, 59,* 131–137.

Roberts, J. (1983). Two models of live supervision: Collaboration team and supervisor guided. *The Journal of Strategic and Systemic Therapies, 2*(2), 68–83.

12

Cybernetics of Videotape Supervision

DOUGLAS C. BREUNLIN
BETTY M. KARRER
Institute for Juvenile Research, Chicago

DENNIS E. McGUIRE
Carthage College, Kenosha, Wisconsin

ROCCO A. CIMMARUSTI
Center for Family Development, Chicago

During the past two decades, both the conceptual and the technical bases of family therapy have grown exponentially. These advances are due, in part, to the widespread use of direct observation of family therapy via methods such as live supervision and videotape playback. Surprisingly, until recently, neither the potential hazards nor the articulation of skills required for effective use of these methods was given much attention. Although there is a growing literature on live supervision, and even guidelines for its effective and benevolent use (Berger & Dammann, 1982; Liddle & Schwartz, 1983), far less has been written about videotape supervision (VTS) (Bodin, 1969, 1972; Kramer & Reitz, 1980, Whiffen, 1982).

In this chapter we present a model that enables the competent supervisor to make effective and benevolent use of VTS. We first describe the complexity of VTS, then discuss our choice of second-order cybernetics as an organizing theory for understanding and using VTS. Finally, we offer a set of guidelines, and discuss pragmatic considerations for undertaking VTS.

THE COMPLEXITY OF VTS

Videotape supervision is a far more complex process than has been heretofore recognized in the literature. This complexity becomes apparent if one examines the total process of VTS. A therapist, functioning in a subordinate role as a supervisee, conducts and simultaneously records a therapy session with the intention of reviewing the tape with a supervisor at some later time. The recording captures the actions of therapist and family members, but not the mental and affective internal processes that guided and/or affected the therapist's decision making during the session. Afterwards, the therapist is left with memories and some degree of satisfaction about the session, which form an impression that may be quite different from the session itself. Later the therapist may review the tape alone in preparation for VTS, and form yet more impressions about the session.

Finally, the therapist and supervisor convene to view the tape, sometimes with other therapists watching. The experience has the potential to make the therapist very anxious.

Some preliminary remarks are made, and then segments of the tape are played. The therapist observes the segment and offers comments that are influenced by many variables: assumptions about therapy, memories and satisfaction of the session, impressions from an earlier viewing, the immediate reaction to seeing the segment, the amount of felt anxiety, and the nature of the supervisor–therapist relationship. The supervisor's task is to respond to the therapist's comments in a manner that will foster the therapist's clinical development. Given that the segment represents only a fraction of the session, and that the supervisor may have no way of knowing how much each of the variables mentioned above has biased the therapist's comments, responding appropriately is very difficult. Finally, from this discussion, the therapist is expected to derive a plan for improving subsequent performance.

VTS, therefore, is an experience wherein neither past nor future performance can be accessed directly. Rather, past and future must be mediated in the present through VTS. The supervisor's efforts to be helpful can easily backfire, producing defensiveness, anxiety, and little learning.

To avoid these potential hazards and to use VTS effectively, supervisors need a framework to understand and organize the highly complex process of VTS. The framework must connect the therapist's internal process (cognitive and affective) with the interactions during the session. The connection between internal and interactive process is then related to three contexts: (1) the session itself, (2) the memories of the session, and (3) during the VTS. These processes are further elaborated later in this chapter in the section on "Guidelines for VTS."

VTS: A Neglected Art

Given the complexity and potential hazards of VTS, it is surprising that the articulation of guidelines for its use has been neglected. This neglect derives, in part, from the use of one of two theoretical frameworks for VTS that enabled its complexity to be simplified and its hazards downplayed. The first framework, psychodynamic theory, simplified VTS by emphasizing the therapist's internal process while minimizing the interactive process. The second framework, first-order cybernetics, emphasized the interactive process and minimized the therapist's internal process. While both theories offered useful ways to understand VTS, neither fully addressed the total process, and both have the potential to create many pitfalls for the supervisor.

We prefer another theoretical framework, that of second-order cybernetics, because it connects internal and interactive processes. Before turning to this framework, however, we consider briefly the relative merits and problems derived from the use of psychodynamic theory to focus primarily on internal process, and the use of first-order cybernetics to focus on interactive process.

Psychodynamic Theory and Internal Process

Early writings on VTS were based on psychodynamic theory (Berger, 1970), and emphasized that effectiveness in family therapy correlates with the therapist's ability to understand, control, and communicate his or her own internal process (Ackerman, 1966). With this theory, the family was viewed as a stimulus, triggering the therapist's internal process and creating a family countertransference. Supervision was geared primarily toward understanding this internal process, with the intent of increasing therapist self-awareness, flexibility, and congruence (Kramer & Reitz, 1980). In VTS, segments of tape were used to examine how internal process organized the therapist's behavior. Internal process was accessed through a videotape playback by focusing on incongruities between channels of communication. The tape could reveal a leakage or betrayal of feelings, affects, and attitudes through facial expressions, body movements, and tone of voice that were incongruous with the therapist's verbal communication. For example, a therapist may cross his legs and turn away while at the same time speaking to a mother in an apparently supportive manner. This incongruity, then, became a pathway to the therapist's internal process. For instance, the supervisor may ask, "What were you feeling when you turned away from the mother as you spoke?" The psychodynamic approach to VTS purports that as a therapist becomes increasingly aware of his or her internal process, verbal and nonverbal communication becomes more congruent, and the therapist becomes more effective.

This approach to VTS poses several problems. First, research has documented that the experience of confronting one's body image and incongruities through tape review creates in the observer a state of psychophysical arousal that activates defenses (Geertsman & Reivich, 1965; Holzman, 1969). If excessive, this arousal can negatively affect learning. The very process of VTS, therefore, affects the therapist's internal process in a manner quite independent of the internal process that existed at the time of the actual session. Other variables, such as anxiety about overall performance, dissatisfaction with the session, and concerns about the supervision–therapist relationship, can also increase arousal and further interfere with the therapist's ability to recall the internal process of the therapist during the session. For VTS to access internal process accurately, therefore, excessive arousal must be avoided (Kramer & Reitz, 1980).

Second, the emphasis on the psychodynamics of internal process means that less attention can be paid to the cognitive process, which enables the therapist to think consciously about and decide how to interact with the family. Finally, psychodynamic theory's emphasis on internal process can limit the attention given to interactive process, or make it appear that one can choose between internal and interactive process as a focus (Whiffen, 1982), when, in fact, the two processes are inseparable.

First-Order Cybernetics and Interactive Process

Any difficulty accessing internal process disappears if one adopts a theory that minimizes its importance. This is the case with first-order cybernetics (Fishman, 1982; Keeney, 1983, Sluzki, 1985), where both family and therapist are defined as "black boxes." The internal working of the boxes is not considered; only their respective inputs and outputs bear relevance. This theory defines the therapist as an objective observer separate from the family. From this position, the therapist defines the family as a system, and assesses the family's interactive process as system output. With this assessment, the therapist devises interventions that function as inputs into the family system designed to alter interactive process.

First-order cybernetics produced a shift in supervision from a focus on internal process and the personal growth of the therapist to the family's interactive process and the development of therapist skills required to change it. Therapists were taught observational and conceptual skills to assess a family's interactive process, and therapeutic skills to devise and implement effective interventions (Cleghorn & Levine, 1973; Falicov, Constantine, & Breunlin, 1981; Tomm & Wright, 1979). Live supervision, with its immediate impact, emerged as the preferred supervisory modality for teaching therapeutic skills (Birchler, 1975; Hare-Mustin, 1976; Montalvo, 1973), and, presumably because it was less immediate, VTS was reserved for the refinement of observational and conceptual skills (Falicov et al., 1981).

Despite the widespread use of first-order cybernetics as a theory to understand both therapy and supervision, little has been written about its application to VTS, perhaps because there seemed little to be said about a straightforward process whereby a supervisor and therapist reviewed a tape with the goal of analyzing the interactive process and discussing possible interventions to change it.

First-order cybernetics, by neglecting the therapist's internal process, creates another set of problems in VTS. First, the therapist can never be an objective observer completely separate from the family. The very act of observing helps to create the interactive process the therapist seeks to observe. Thus, the internal process that guides the therapist's observations plays an important role in creating the interactive process displayed by the family. The videotape of a session, therefore, does not portray "raw data" of a family's interactive process, equally acessible to both supervisor and therapist. Rather, the tape portrays only the actions of an observing system that can only be understood by including the internal process that guided the therapist's observations.

Second, during VTS the internal process of the therapist continues to work. Even when VTS does not focus on the therapist, it still involves self-confrontation that can create excessive arousal. By approaching a videotape as raw data of interactive process, the supervisor ignores the fact that the therapist's performance is frozen on tape for all to see. Arousal may, therefore, become excessive even when the therapist has only been asked to describe and discuss the family's interactive process. If arousal becomes excessive, it will alter the therapist's internal process and negatively affect the therapist's ability to concentrate, stay on task, and learn.

Finally, using VTS to analyze an intervention simply as a therapist output ignores the internal process involved in the design and implementation of the intervention. Moreover, that internal process is uniquely defined by the context of the session; consequently, a therapist's choice of intervention cannot be understood without consideration of the internal process that went into its making.

Organizing the Complexity of VTS: Second-Order Cybernetics

To organize and manage the complexity of VTS, a theory that considers both internal and interactive process, and a framework to apply the theory to VTS, are needed. The "cybernetics of cybernetics," or second-order cybernetics, constitutes such a theory. Keeney (1983) noted that second-order cybernetics "attempts to move to a perspective in which the two separate boxes (therapist and family) can be opened and seen as a whole recursive system" (p. 77). Second-order cybernetics defines the therapist/observer as part of the observed system. No longer does the therapist analyze interactive process as the raw data of a family system's output. Rather, the therapist/observer, using an internal process, makes and shares observations with a family that elicit an interactive process from them that in turn influences subsequent behavior and observation. This recursive cycle defines a therapist–family system, which becomes the focus of VTS, and can only be understood through consideration of both internal and interactive process.

Making and sharing observations are but two levels of a larger internal process by which a therapist draws distinctions about, and participates in, the creation of an interactive process exhibited by the family (Keeney, 1983). We have identified six levels of distinction that form the essentials of the therapist's internal process. First, the therapist selects a class of information from which to make observations. Examples of classes are the family's history, their behaviors outside the session, their affective communication, or their behavior inside the session. Second, the therapist mentally organizes this information into some meaningful pattern. Third, the therapist decides how the pattern should change. Fourth, the therapist decides how to offer the proposed change to the family in the form of an intervention. Fifth, the therapist reads the family's feedback to determine the response to the intervention. Sixth, the therapist decides whether to continue the intervention or begin again with new information. Once therapy is underway, all these levels operate simultaneously, making the therapist's internal process highly complex.

We believe the internal process of drawing distinctions can be viewed as largely cognitive, but the therapist's cognition is always influenced to some degree by affective process, either triggered by the family or arising independently of it. When we access internal process, therefore, we are less concerned with the psychodynamic properties of self-awareness and congruence, and more concerned with therapists having a clearly articulated cognitive map that organizes the six levels of distinction. Supervisors who combine psychodynamic and cybernetic theory may still wish to include the affective component in their consideration of internal process.

During VTS, then, the therapist's comments about a tape segment are considered an attempt to understand the recursive cycle between internal and interactive processes that existed during the session. Just as the therapist's distinctions about a family create a partial reality of that family, so also the therapist's distinctions about his or her performance in a session are just a partial reality of that performance. The supervisor's responses during VTS become meta-distinctions about this reality, the intention of which is to create another reality about the performance that will foster the therapist's clinical development.

A framework that applies second-order cybernetics to VTS, and organizes and manages its complexity, must satisfy four criteria. First, it must delimit the enormous amount of tape stimulus potentially available to the supervisor. Second, it must relate internal and interactive process. Third, it must distinguish and connect different information available from the session itself, from memories of the session, and also from the review of a videotape of the session. Fourth, it must control for the stressful effects of VTS, and provide a way to maintain arousal at a useful level.

To develop a framework for VTS that satisfies these criteria, we have formulated six guidelines. The guidelines suggest a format for VTS; however, some variation is always necessary to accommodate the pragmatics of the context in which VTS occurs. We will, therefore, present the guidelines and then discuss some pragmatic considerations that affect format.

GUIDELINES FOR VTS

Guideline 1: Focus VTS by Setting Goals

A common pitfall of VTS is the failure to focus the discussion (Whiffen, 1982). A supervisor may attempt to review the entire tape (implying that everything can be covered), randomly sample segments of the tape, or discuss one aspect of a segment while the therapist discusses another. Any of these approaches fails to provide a clear focus, reducing the learning potential of VTS, and dramatically increasing the potential for arousal.

The infinite stimuli of a videotape can be delimited with goals that are established prior to the videotaped session, and agreed on by both therapist and supervisor. By goals we mean those related to the therapist's clinical development, not case goals. Goals should be precise, limited in scope, and operationalized. They should be set at the cutting edge of the therapist's ability, and achievable in an approximate way while allowing for refinement. To arrive at a goal, therapist and supervisor must first agree to focus on one or more levels of distinction. For example, if the supervisor and the therapist are just beginning to work together, it is important that they agree on the class of information (level one) from which the therapist will make observations. If the class of information of interest to the therapist is history, while that of the supervisor is in-session behavior, it would be counterproductive for the supervisor to focus on the therapist's ability to read feedback. The supervisor assures that the goals are moderately difficult by encouraging the therapist to select a level of distinction within his or her ability. For example, therapists must be able to see isomorphic sequences before they can organize these sequences into a pattern (level two) and before they can make distinctions about ways that pattern can change (level three) or what interventions might change the pattern (level four).

Once the level of distinction has been set, the supervisor and therapist can select a specific therapeutic task that becomes the objective of the session. The therapeutic task often derives from one of the models of family therapy. For example, using the MRI model (Fisch, Weakland, & Segal, 1982; Watzlawich, Weakland, & Fisch, 1974), the task may be to organize the family's description of events into a pattern that defines an attempted solution to a problem (level two).

Specifying goals gives the therapist a clear training task for the session, and a clear expectation of the focus of VTS. The therapist, then, approaches VTS with less anxiety because all of his or her work is not subject to scrutiny. Also avoided is the common pitfall whereby at the outset of VTS the supervisor asks for the therapist's goals for the session and receives a vague reply, or a response the therapist believes *ought* to have been the goals. In either case, VTS will be less connected to the actual session, making it difficult to maintain a focus. Goals also circumscribe the tape by delimiting the segments that can be productively reviewed, because a segment is only reviewed if it portrays the therapist attempting the goals in some approximate way. With goals established, then, the past performance of a session and future performances are connected in the present experience of VTS.

Guideline 2: Relate Internal Process across Contexts

A videotape captures and freezes a session's interactive process, but not the internal process. During VTS, therefore, the therapist relies on recollection to connect the two processes. These recollections are also influenced by the therapist's memories of the session and by immediate reactions to seeing the session on tape. The validity of any connection between internal and interactive process, then, is related to the supervisor's ability to separate the internal processes arising from three contexts: (1) the session itself, (2) memories of the session, and (3) the videotape playback of the session. This effort is most successful when the supervisor asks the therapist to define each internal process shortly after or during the time frame of its occurrence.

By focusing on a particular level of distinction during a session, goals help to define internal process. Although all levels are required to conduct the session, the therapist remains most aware of, and can remember best, the level preselected by the goals. During VTS, then, the supervisor refers to these goals when asking the therapist to connect internal and interactive processes. For example, if the therapist's goal was to create an enactment, the supervisor may show a segment where an enactment is taking place and ask the therapist to describe the internal process that led to any number of decisions such as the therapist's frame to motivate the family for the enactment, the therapist's punctuations to sustain the enactment, or the therapist's termination of the enactment.

Therapists recall only part of a session. Therapists-in-training more often remember problematic parts, missed opportunities, and less-than-perfect interventions. Hence, their memory of sessions is usually low in satisfaction. In an evaluative context like supervision, low satisfaction may cause the therapist to dread VTS. Dread generates anxiety, making it more difficult for the therapist to accurately recollect the session during VTS. Instead, the therapist offers excuses for the decisions made in therapy. For example, the statement, "I was afraid mom would not come back, so I let the enactment die," probably does not reflect the actual internal process that led to a decision not to stick with an enactment in the session.

The danger that memory and low satisfaction will contaminate recollection of internal process is reduced if therapist and supervisor discuss the session soon after its completion. The supervisor begins this discussion by allowing the therapist to ventilate feelings about the session in general, and then asks the therapist to relate his or her experience of the session to the agreed-on goals. If goals were established at the right degree of difficulty, the therapist's experience should be that the goals were approximated. Consequently, the therapist should be moderately satisfied. Moderate satisfaction minimizes dread and the anxiety that distorts internal process, and also motivates the therapist to want to review the tape.

At the beginning of VTS, first the goals, then satisfaction in relation to goals, are again reviewed. Only then is a tape segment played. When a segment is played, the therapist's internal process will still be affected by the experience of self-confrontation. The level of arousal created by this experience should be moderate. Below we offer a separate guideline pertaining to arousal.

Finally, it is important that the therapist comment on the segment before the supervisor, otherwise the supervisor's comments serve as yet another variable influencing the therapist's internal process. For example, if the supervisor comments first, the therapist may respond with a comment that he or she thinks the supervisor wants to hear, rather than attempting to recollect internal process as it actually occurred in the session.

Guideline 3: Select Tape Segments That Focus on Remedial Performance

By remedial, we mean those aspects of a therapist's work that he or she is capable of changing. Three aspects are essentially nonremedial and should, therefore, be avoided. First, some aspects of a therapist's style are so much a part of his or her basic presentation of self that they are not readily amenable to change. For example, a therapist's slow and deliberate speaking pattern may prove nonremedial, and may even put a therapist in a "be spontaneous" bind if attempts are made to change it. Second, some aspects of performance may represent a level of skill not currently attainable by the therapist. For example, a therapist may be unable to read feedback because he or she has not yet learned to organize behavior into a pattern. Third, even when the skill level is appropriate, it can become functionally nonremedial if the tape segments selected portray the therapist failing. For example, if the goal was for a therapist to be less central, any segment that shows the therapist talking too much would be functionally nonremedial.

If the supervisor establishes goals with an appropriate degree of difficulty, and selects segments wherein the therapist is portrayed approximating the goals, then the focus will be remedial, and there will be ample opportunity for a critical discussion and goal refinement. To avoid a nonremedial focus, segments should be selected before VTS, either by the supervisor who assumes this responsibility, or by the therapist (who must be able to do so without having the unmediated review unduly contaminate internal process) (Whiffen, 1982). This issue is discussed further under pragmatic considerations.

Guideline 4: Use Supervisor Comments to Create a Moderate Evaluation of Performance

The therapist's comments on a tape segment connect internal and interactive process by comparing observations of the segment with the established goals. This comparison represents an evaluation defined by the discrepancy between goals and observation of performance. In effect the therapist is saying, "I see myself coming this close to achieving my goals in this segment." If the discrepancy is small—that is, the performance nearly matches the goals—the evaluation will be favorable. As the discrepancy increases, the evaluation will become more negative.

Fuller and Manning (1973), reviewing the literature on videotape playback, found that *moderate* discrepancies between goals and observations of performance are optimum for learning. If there is no discrepancy, then there is no challenge for learning. Large discrepancies lead to unfavorable self-evaluations, which in turn produce intense therapist discomfort and increase arousal. Moderate discrepancies indicate an approximation of goals, and challenge the therapist to improve.

The supervisor's response shifts the therapist's evaluation to a moderate level by increasing or decreasing the discrepancy between goals and observations of performance. In effect, the supervisor's comments are observations that serve as meta-distinctions to those of the therapist, and expand the connection between internal and interactive process.

If the therapist's discrepancy is too large, the supervisor has several options to reduce it. First, the supervisor can make observations about performance overlooked by the therapist. This option is particularly helpful for therapists who tend only to view their work negatively. Second, the supervisor can expand the connection between internal and interactive process. For example, a therapist commenting on a goal to use the family's language may observe a segment and conclude that, instead, she allowed the family to talk about history. The supervisor may respond by noting that the family's history is, in fact, part of their language. Consequently, without knowing it, the therapist was using the family's language. The initially large discrepancy would then become more moderate. If the discrepancy cannot be reduced, then the goals were too difficult. This should be acknowledged, and goals refined to a more appropriate level.

If the discrepancy is small, the supervisor must first decide whether the therapist is not observing something that would result in a larger discrepancy, or whether the goals have truly been achieved. In the former case, the therapist may, for any number of reasons, have difficulty critically evaluating his or her performance, or may simply be unaware that the goal allowed for a more sophisticated performance than was given. The supervisor's task is to define a moderate discrepancy by noting that, while the goals were approximated, the segment suggests areas where performance could be refined. For example, if the goal was to sustain an enactment, the therapist may observe the segment and conclude that the enactment was sustained very well. The supervisor, on the other hand, may see many ways that the enactment could have been productively sustained even further. The supervisor may first ask the therapist to comment on the internal process that led to a decision to end the enactment, and then ask the therapist to reconsider how to use the interactive process to sustain an enactment for longer periods of time. If the supervisor agrees that the discrepancy is indeed small, then the therapist is complimented and told that it is time to refine the goals to a higher level.

Guideline 5: Refine Goals Moderately

When goals are refined, the supervisor must decide whether to refine the current level of distinction, or to shift levels. The supervisor should recall that what seems easy in discussion of a tape may prove far more difficult in practice. For example, if VTS involves a discussion about the many in-session behaviors of the family (level one), it does not necessarily follow that in the next session the therapist could actually organize those behaviors into a pattern. To refine a goal that would have this expectation may set the therapist up for failure by targeting a nonremedial behavior. The rule of thumb for goal refinement is similar to that for other aspects of VTS: make the refinement moderate. VTS then becomes part of the recursive cycle of setting goals, practicing, reviewing in VTS, refining goals, and so on. For example, a moderate refinement of goals would be for the therapist to link the enactment with a between-session task in order to enhance the therapist's repertoire.

Guideline 6: Maintain a Moderate Level of Arousal

We define "arousal" as a state of tension, activation, or readiness, related to a number of psychological and physiological factors (such as worrying, off-task behavior, heart rate, perspiring, and adrenalin flow). Arousal has been viewed as a negative phenomenon by most psychodynamic supervisors, or disregarded by supervisors using the "black box" view of the therapist. We prefer to consider arousal as existing on a continuum: too much arousal negatively affects learning; too little arousal contributes to a state of placidness and a lack of interest in learning; while a moderate level of arousal creates an optimal state of readiness, engagement, and vigor conducive to learning and the acquisition of new skills. In VTS, moderate arousal increases a desire for self-evaluation and a willingness to learn by exploring the supervisor's meta-distinctions. When this occurs, a positive cycle develops wherein moderate arousal facilitates on-task behavior which in turn facilitates openness and learning that further moderates arousal, and so on.

Excessive arousal interacts with cognitive activity to produce worry rather than on-task behavior (Deffenbacher, 1978). Worry, in turn, produces rumination, self-doubt, and asociated discomfiting physiological responses, like increased heart rate and perspiration, which further increase arousal. This escalating negative cycle produces a tendency toward flight and an avoidance of learning.

Too little arousal is most often the result of allowing the tape to play uninterrupted, creating the hypnotic effect of watching television, and concomitant boredom for both therapist and supervisor. Little learning then takes place.

Arousal cannot be quantified during VTS. Instead, the supervisor reads cues emitted by the therapist to approximate the level of arousal. If the therapist looks forward to VTS, responds to it as a challenge, remains actively engaged in the discussions, and follows through with refined goals, then arousal is more than likely moderate. If, on the other hand, the therapist creates excuses for not having a tape, grows defensive in the discussion, appears to be upset, and fails to follow through with refined goals, then arousal is more than likely escalating.

All of the guidelines discussed above are designed to facilitate a moderate level of arousal. First, by establishing clear and realistic goals, the supervisor limits the focus of VTS. Second, by connecting internal process across contexts, the supervisor takes into account the effects of satisfaction and self-confrontation. Third, the segments selected and the discussion of them focus on remedial behaviors. Fourth, the supervisor mediates evaluation by adjusting the discrepancy between goals and observation of performance to a moderate level. And finally, the goals are refined moderately. When these guidelines are followed and arousal is moderate, the therapist approaches VTS eager to make observations that critically assess performance. The message the supervisor listens for is, "That's adequate, but I see how I can improve." This message fixes the therapist at the cutting edge of his or her ability, and conveys motivation for improvement.

PRAGMATIC CONSIDERATIONS

The guidelines above suggest a format for VTS. Therapist and supervisor meet sometime before a session and establish goals. The therapist then conducts and videotapes the session. Soon after the session the therapist and supervisor meet and discuss the experience, including the level of satisfaction. At some point before VTS, relevant segments are selected. When therapist and supervisor convene for VTS, goals and satisfaction are reviewed first. Then tape segments are played. The therapist makes comments that relate observations to goals, and the supervisor responds with meta-distinctions that create a moderate evaluation. As a result of this discussion, goals are refined, and the process is repeated.

Unfortunately, this format takes time, and in the real world of supervision, adequate time frequently is not available. Instead, therapist and supervisor schedule VTS haphazardly, use old tapes for review, and proceed without adequate preparation. The immediate access to tape stimuli makes this "shoot from the hip" approach appear plausible. However, the complexity of the total process of VTS is such that more harm than good is the likely outcome (Whiffen, 1982).

If an agency or training program has a commitment to VTS, and time is a constraint, then a limited use is preferable to a more frequent but random approach. Brief sessions (10 to 15 minutes) between supervisor and therapist can be used to establish goals and review the session for satisfaction. If segments are preselected, usually 45 minutes of VTS is sufficient to review several segments and refine goals. With about one hour and fifteen minutes a week, supervisor and therapist can productively utilize VTS.

The selection of tape segments for subsequent review merits further discussion. Ideally, this is the task of the supervisor, but few supervisors have the luxury to review tapes regularly. The task can be assigned to the therapist, but this creates unmediated viewing, and introduces another context and an associated internal process into the supervisorial system. We have found that, at the outset of a training program or the beginning of a therapist–supervisor relationship, unmediated tape reviews lower satisfaction, increase arousal, and hinder rather than facilitate VTS. Once a positive cycle of learning has been established, the therapist can be counted on to critically review a tape and select appropriate segments without adverse effects.

A third option exists if the session is also supervised live. In this instance, the conscientious supervisor records relevant counter numbers from the video cassette recorder during the session (Cornwell & Pearson, 1981). Then only a spot review is needed to arrive at a final selection of segments. Of course, live supervision introduces yet another level of complexity to the total process, with associated advantages and disadvantages (Hodas, 1985). The advantage is that the supervisor actually sees the session and can be helpful during it. The disadvantage is that the supervisor will participate in the creation of the therapist–family system and in the functioning of the therapist's internal process. Separating these effects during VTS can be very difficult.

We have described a framework for using VTS to advance therapist goals. VTS is also used by many supervisors for case management (Whiffen, 1982). While a small amount of tape is helpful to orient a supervisor to a family, too great a focus on videotape for case management poses several problems. First, it is time-consuming and inefficient. Second, it is very easy to drift from case management goals to therapeutic goals in an unfocused and arousal-generating manner. We believe case management goals are advanced most productively through a judicious and limited use of videotape review, and ample discussion.

SUMMARY

We believe VTS merits the same rigorous attention afforded to live supervision. This chapter is an attempt to use the theory of second-order cybernetics to define the total process of VTS, and to present a set of guidelines that begins to organize that process. We believe that the careless use of VTS can actually impair therapist learning and development. Our guidelines are intended to make VTS a benevolent and efficient form of supervision that will motivate therapists to advance their clinical skills.

References

Ackerman, N. W. (1966). *Treating the troubled family*. New York: Basic Books.

Berger, M. M. (Ed.). (1970). *Videotape techniques in psychiatric training and treatment*. New York: Brunner/Mazel.

Berger, M., & Dammann, C. (1982). Live supervision as context, treatment and training. *Family Process, 21,* 337–344.

Birchler, G. R. (1975). Live supervision and instant feedback in marriage and family therapy. *Journal of Marriage and Family Counseling, 1,* 331–342.

Bodin, A. (1969). Video-tape applications in training family therapists. *Journal of Nervous and Mental Disease, 143,* 251–261.

Bodin, A. (1972). The use of video-tapes. In A. Ferber, M. Mendelsohn, & A. Napier (Eds.), *The book of family therapy*. Boston: Houghton Mifflin.

Cleghorn, J., & Levin, S. (1973). Training family therapists by setting learning objectives. *American Journal of Psychiatry, 43,* 439–446.

Cornwell, M., & Pearson, R. (1981). Cotherapy teams and one-way screens in family therapy practice and training. *Family Process, 20,* 199–209.

Deffenbacher, J. L. (1978). Worry, emotionality and task generated interference in test anxiety. An empirical test of attentional theory. *Journal of Educational Psychology, 70,* 248–254.

Falicov, C., Constantine, J., & Breunlin, D. C. (1981). Teaching family therapy: A program based on learning. *Journal of Marital and Family Therapy, 7,* 497–506.

Fisch, R., Weakland, J., & Segal, L. (1982). *The tactics of change: Doing therapy briefly*. San Francisco: Jossey-Bass.

Fishman, H. C. (1982). Assessment in structural family therapy. In H. A. Liddle (Ed.), *Diagnosis and assessment in family therapy*. Rockville, MD: Aspen.

Fuller, F. F., & Manning, B. A. (1973). Self-confrontation reviewed: A Conceptualization for video playback in teacher education. *Review of Educational Research, 43,* 469–528.

Geertsma, R. H., & Reivich, R. S. (1965). Repetitive self-observation by videotape playback. *Journal of Nervous and Mental Disease, 141*(1), 29–41.

Hare-Mustin, R. T. (1976). Supervision in psychotherapy. *Voices, 12,* 21–24.

Hodas, G. R. (1985). A systems perspective in family therapy supervision. In R. L. Ziffer (Ed.), *Adjunctive techniques in family therapy*. Orlando, FL: Grune & Stratton.

Holzman, P. S. (1969). On hearing and seeing oneself. *Journal of Nervous and Mental Disease, 148*(3), 198–209.

Keeney, B. P. (1983). *Aesthetics of change.* New York: Guilford Press.

Kramer, T., & Reitz, M. (1980). Using video playback to train family therapists. *Family Process, 19*(2), 145–150.

Liddle, H. A., & Schwartz, R. C. (1983). Live supervision/consultation: Conceptual and pragmatic guidelines for family therapy trainers. *Family Process, 22,* 477–490.

Montalvo, B. (1973). Aspects of live supervision. *Family Process, 12,* 343–359.

Sluzki, C. E. (1985). A minimal map of cybernetics. *The Family Therapy Networker, 9*(3), 26.

Tomm, K., & Wright, L. (1979). Training in family therapy: Perceptual, conceptual and executive skills. *Family Process, 28,* 227–250.

Watzlawick, P., Weakland, J., & Fisch, R. (1974). *Change, principles of problem formation and resolution.* New York: W. W. Norton.

Whiffen, R. (1982). The use of videotape in supervision. In R. Whiffen & J. Byng-Hall (Eds.), *Family therapy supervision: Recent developments in practice.* New York: Academic Press.

13

Concurrent Training of Supervisors and Therapists

DOUGLAS C. BREUNLIN
Institute for Juvenile Resarch, Chicago

HOWARD A. LIDDLE
University of California, San Francisco

RICHARD C. SCHWARTZ
Institute for Juvenile Research, Chicago

> *Real education is not learning something, but becoming something.*
> —Edward Fischer

This book addresses the ways in which supervisors help therapists become competent in the practice of family therapy. Rather than view this process as leading to a clearly demarcated end point signifying a complete therapist, we prefer to view training along developmental lines. From this perspective, we define "becoming a therapist" as an activity in which one will always be engaged; like development, it is never-ending. Supervisors have an interesting and curious role in relation to this process. They initiate and facilitate the process of becoming a family therapist, but they never complete it.

Our rationale for this view has four components. First, there are, theoretically at least, no clear limits to therapeutic competence. As in karate, there are many "belts," and even the black belt, signifying master, has degrees. Second, as therapists mature and advance in their profession, they are given greater responsibilities that require new knowledge, more skills, and greater competence. Third, because the field of family therapy is itself evolving, therapists rarely have the luxury to consider themselves completely trained. Finally, therapists change and experience families differently as they mature through their own life cycle (Nichols, 1986; Schwartz, 1982).

At some point in this process, depending on factors such as the individual, training opportunities, and work setting, therapists become motivated and/or coerced to achieve sufficient competence to become supervisors. At one level, becoming a supervisor provides another perspective from which to learn about therapy and, hence, to continue the process of becoming a family therapist. Practicing supervision enhances the quality of one's therapy. In addition, becoming a supervisor gives the therapist a new set of skills and another professional identity, one that places the therapist in a position of greater prestige and responsibility in the family therapy field. The perspective about therapy obtained through supervision enables a gifted supervisor to draw distinctions about family therapy that have the potential to advance our field. In time and with favorable circumstances (e.g., supportive work context, individual motivation, and some reinforcing success) talented supervisors communicate these ideas in the family therapy literature. Most of the leaders in the field of family therapy have been or continue to be supervisors.

The training of supervisors, therefore, plays an integral and vitally important role in the evolution of the family therapy field. Surprisingly, very little attention has been devoted to this task. Accumulated experience and/or informal apprenticeships were once the only pathways available to becoming a supervisor. Recently, a few programs have been designed to train supervisors (Constantine, Piercy, & Sprenkle, 1984; Liddle, Breunlin, Schwartz, & Constantine, 1984; Wright & Coppersmith, 1983). Taught by experienced supervisors, these programs convene several therapists and supervisors, and essentially train them concurrently. Such concurrent training is desirable because, just as family therapy is best learned by actually seeing families, so also supervision is best learned by closely monitoring and guiding that supervisor/trainee's supervision. Supervisors learn their craft by supervising actual trainees under real-life circumstances, and, in the present view, this training should occur in a context in which there can be live supervision of supervision.

Concurrent training programs can be exciting and are always a challenge, but they involve enormous complexities that can yield considerable difficulty if ignored. This chapter extends our earlier work (Liddle *et al.*, 1984) and subsequent experience with simultaneous training of supervisors and therapists. We will develop conceptual and pragmatic considerations that have aided our management of the complexity of such programs and produced successful training outcomes for supervisors and therapists. The primary emphasis will be on the position and training of the supervisor in the context of a concurrent training experience.

COMPONENTS OF A SUPERVISOR/THERAPIST TRAINING PROGRAM

Supervisor/therapist training programs bring together three groups of professionals at different points along the continuum of becoming a family therapist. The first group, the *therapists*, are attempting to learn family therapy. The second group, the *supervisor/ trainees*, are experienced therapists who are learning supervision. The third group, *supervisor/trainers*, possess high-level therapy and supervision skills, have a commitment to continued professional development, and see participation in a supervisor–therapist training program as a viable way to actualize this commitment.

As learning occurs, the more experienced group members are expected to learn, in part, by helping members of the less experienced groups. At one level, therapists pursue a process of becoming family therapists by seeing families and receiving assistance from the supervisor/trainees. At a second level, supervisor/trainees help the therapists and simultaneously pursue the process of becoming supervisors by receiving assistance from supervisor/trainers. At the third level, the supervisor/trainers oversee the work of both supervisor/trainees and therapists, and use this experience to continue professional stimulation and development. Since the program also provides clinical services to families, competent therapy and supervision must be provided while the therapists and supervisor/trainees simultaneously learn and change.

To organize a program of this nature, careful attention must be paid to its inherent complexity (Constantine et al., 1984; Liddle et al., 1984; Wright & Coppersmith, 1983). The program must have appropriate training formats, procedures, and well articulated content areas, preferably in the form of training objectives which are complementary: the teaching and learning of one group cannot occur at the expense of another.[1]

Throughout the duration of the training program, the formats call for the groups sometimes to meet separately, and at other times, when different goals are being pursued, together. Ongoing therapy seminars are given for the therapists, and a separate seminar is taught for the supervisors. In these formats, focus can be maintained on the distinct training objectives of supervisors or therapists, respectively. The primary format for joint meetings of both groups is a training system where a supervisor/trainer, supervisor/trainee, and therapist work together so that live supervision of supervision can be conducted. In this format, the training objectives of all three groups overlap; when the system is well conceived, organized, and monitored, this can be achieved in a complementary fashion. Other joint formats are a regularly scheduled meeting between a supervisor/trainer and supervisor/trainee where supervision in the training system is discussed, and regularly scheduled meetings between a supervisor/trainee and therapist where therapy conducted in the training system is discussed. An example of a supervisor-therapist program structure as described above is shown in Figure 13-1.

In each of these formats, the training objectives of each person must be clearly defined, first, so that participants know what they are attempting to learn, and second, to anticipate the interactive effects of the training objectives when the supervisor/trainee and therapist are working together on a case. All trainees in this setting must be clear about the structure of the training system, which includes knowledge of lines of communication, responsibility, and authority about a case.

TRAINING OBJECTIVES

Supervisor/trainers, supervisor/trainees, and therapists pursue common generic training objectives that cluster into three categories: *systemic thinking, technical skill,* and *professional identity.* Although some objectives are shared by the three groups, they always exist at different levels of sophistication. For example, all three groups pursue systemic thinking, but differ enormously in how refined their systemic thought is, and the purposes to which they put it. Objectives also differ in many other ways. The technical skills of supervision and therapy are distinct, and the professional identity of a supervisor clearly differs from that of a therapist.

Systemic Thinking

To think systemically, one must learn theoretical concepts and mental processes to perceive, organize, and describe interaction and recursiveness in human systems. Most therapists enter family therapy training with little or no previous exposure to systemic

Composition: 4   Supervisor/Trainers
4   Supervisor/Trainees
16   Therapist/Trainees

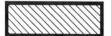 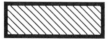 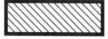 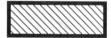

4 Supervision of Supervision Groups (Training System)

Each group is composed of :   1 Supervisor/Trainer
1 Supervisor/Trainee
4 Therapist/Trainees

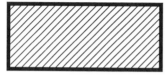   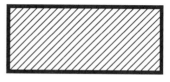

Supervision Seminar   **Didactic Therapy**

Composition: 4 Supervisor/Trainers   Composition: 16 Therapist/Trainees
4 Supervisor/Trainees   1 Instructor (Supervisor/Trainer
or Supervisor/Trainee)

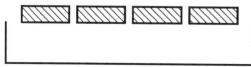   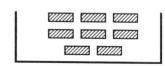

4 Supervisor/Trainer-Supervisor/Trainee dyads

Supervisor/Trainer-Therapist dyads

(Number depends on how many therapists are being
supervised by each supervisor/trainee)

FIGURE 13-1. A model of formats for a concurrent supervisor/therapist training program. From the Supervisor Externship and Clinical Externship Program of the Family Systems Program, Institute for Juvenile Research, Chicago.

thinking. Supervisor/trainees, having been trained as family therapists, might think systemically, but frequently cannot articulate the systemic view in a teachable way or have not expanded their systemic thinking to include the supervision system.

For supervisor/trainee and therapist to collaborate on the conceptualization of a case together, they both must think systemically, but the supervisor/trainee must recognize that they operate at different points along a continuum of systemic thinking. While this difference exists in all supervisor–therapist relationships, it is particularly problematic when the participants are in training because both formulate training objectives to advance along the continuum of systemic thinking, and both naturally want to use every training opportunity to progress. For example, a beginning therapist may first master a content area of systemic thinking (e.g., boundary regulation or double binds), and have as an objective the perception of this content area in observed interaction. The supervisor/trainee, on the other hand, may have as a training objective the task of seeing the same interaction in a more complex manner. In this example, the training objectives of the therapist and supervisor/trainee are not necessarily synchronized. If the supervisor/trainee tries to teach the more refined systemic thinking to the therapist, the therapist will be lost. The supervisor/trainer must decide how to orchestrate the two sets of training objectives so that both supervisor/trainee and therapist can learn, and the family can receive adequate service. In the above example, the supervisor/trainer must help the supervisor/trainee assess the therapist's ability to think systematically, and to accept the need to help the therapist at that level. The supervisor/trainer also finds another training format, or a more experienced therapist, to allow the supervisor/trainee to work on his or her objectives of refining systemic thinking.

The supervisor/trainer recognizes that the development of systemic thinking involves an oscillation between periods where new information is introduced and competes with the old—creating confusion—and periods of clarity and consolidation where the new and old are integrated and/or the previous notions abandoned. New information for a therapist is likely to come from increments in and refinements of existing knowledge in the field. For the supervisor/trainee, new information often comes through attempts to incorporate advances and cutting-edge issues in systemic thinking entering the field of family therapy.[2]

Since the supervisor/trainee is assigned the task of helping the therapist to think clearly, he or she cannot afford to operate in a period of confusion while offering supervision. This situation is not easily avoided, because the supervisor/trainee's systemic thinking is challenged throughout the training program. Supervisor/trainees must learn to not overreach in the conceptual realm with their supervisees; that is, they need to utilize only those aspects of their thinking in which they can be clear.

It is the responsibility of the supervisor/trainer to orchestrate the progress of supervisor/trainee and therapist so their efforts to learn systemic thinking and the corresponding skills complement each other. Of course, supervisor/trainers also have periods of confusion. These occur because supervisor/trainers are committed to remaining current with developments in the field, and because most are attempting to articulate new ideas through writing or research.

Technical Skills

A supervision/therapy training program imparts both supervision and therapy skills. While therapists master the latter, supervisor/trainees must learn both. Supervisor/trainees must know therapy skills to assess the strengths of therapists, and to establish objectives for therapists to develop those skills. The isomorphic nature of therapy and supervision (Liddle *et al.*, 1984; Liddle & Saba, 1983a, 1983b, 1984) also provides a schema that allows for the translation of therapy skills into the domain of training and supervision. For example, structural–strategic therapy skills, such as searching for strengths, supporting and challenging, creating workable realities, building intensity, and enactment, have an equivalent in supervision (Liddle *et al.*, 1984). Supervisor/trainees learn when and how to use these skills to help therapists. For instance, a supervisor/trainee may possess the skills to create workable realities with families, but struggle to use these same skills to help a therapist review a difficult session.

Supervision skills fall into two categories: those required to understand and structure complex supervisory processes such as live, videotape, and group supervision, and those required to do supervision. The first category enables a supervisor to orchestrate supervision by effectively using assessment of context, timing, and sequencing. Examples of such skills are getting live supervision started, deciding whether to increase or decrease the amount of live or videotape supervision, assessing the supervisor–therapist relationship (see Chapter 10, this volume), or gauging the impact peers may have on a therapist's behavior in a supervision group. The second category provides the behavioral repertoire essential to practice supervision. Examples of such skills are the behaviors associated with effective phone-ins (Liddle & Schwartz, 1983; Wright & Coppersmith, 1983; Chapter 11, this volume), selecting and focusing on an appropriate segment of videotape (Chapter 12), and formulating a training contract (Chapter 9).

When supervisor/trainees have difficulty with the technical skills of supervision, they are naturally tempted to fall back on therapy skills. This is most evident when the supervisor/trainee attempts to do the therapy—using the therapist as a mere extension of his or her therapeutic style. Alert for this tendency, the supervisor/trainer, in a position to supervise the supervision, helps the supervisor/trainee refocus on the technical skills of supervision. This can take the form of a reminder of one of supervision's basics: supervisors supervise—they do not conduct indirect therapy on the case being seen (Chapter 9).

Professional Identity

The development of a professional identity as a therapist or supervisor is an integral part of the process of becoming (Friedman & Kaslow, 1986; Hess, 1986). A training program initiates and fosters professional identity, but never fully completes its work. Experience, association with colleagues and superiors, and continuing education opportunities nurture professional identity throughout one's career.

A key component essential to developing professional identity during a training experience is professional self-confidence. With self-confidence, trainees can realize their potential under stressful training conditions. Without it, they often make mistakes, appear incompetent, and jeopardize their fragile professional identity.

We believe that training programs contribute to the development of professional identity by paying careful attention to training objectives that facilitate professional self-confidence. In the case of concurrent training, the objectives must allow for experiences where both supervisee/trainees and therapists work on their self-confidence.

Becoming a family therapist is difficult, often demoralizing work. Therapists-in-training must think and behave in new ways while encountering bewildering and sometimes frightening families. Professional self-confidence is not automatic merely because one has completed a family therapy training program, and many therapists at some point question their judgment for considering or continuing in such a demanding and difficult line of work.

Successful treatment outcome is a potent elixir for therapists worrying about their professional competence. When a therapist is a beginner, the supervisor is often largely responsible for a positive treatment outcome, but the supervisor must give the trainee realistic credit for his or her contributions to the outcome. Crediting therapists with as much success as possible, while not necessarily focusing on their own perceived contributions to outcome, can be difficult for supervisors-in-training, because they also struggle with concerns about professional competence. These supervisor/trainees experience doubts about their ability to help the therapists; when clinical success comes, the supervisor/trainee often feels the urge to claim it as much as the therapist, sometimes in an understandable attempt to gain approval from the supervisor/trainer. Although this behavior on the supervisor/trainee's part is understandable as an artifact of this complex, multitiered training context, it should also be seen as a problematic process requiring the supervisor/trainer's attention.

The supervisor/trainer needs to possess a clear identity, and carry primary responsibility to model for the supervisor/trainee an appropriate attitude and demeanor toward successful outcome. This stance is one in which it is not necessary to elicit statements of credit from one's trainees. Rather, the supervisor/trainer and supervisor/trainee's role is congratulating, supporting, and enumerating resources in their trainees—giving them appropriate credit and reward for change.

After the therapy session, when the supervisor/trainer and supervisor/trainee meet separately, the supervisor/trainer can support and credit the supervisor/trainee for areas of strength, thus establishing a context in which the supervisor/trainee's competence is supported, accomplishments enumerated, and doubts addressed apart from the therapist.

The supervisor/trainee's posture toward therapy and the therapist are crucial to the emerging identity of the therapist. Therapists in training, appropriately, borrow from and are inspired by the convictions of their supervisor, helping them to survive periods of doubt. Supervisor/trainers are also responsible for conveying to all the trainees the realization that therapy is not magic. Supervisor/trainers convey curiosity about effective methods, and a commitment to excel, but they do not attribute overall feelings of professional competence and identity or lack thereof to specific clinical outcomes (Schwartz, 1985). Throughout the training program the supervisor/trainer works to develop the supervisor/trainee's professional identity and increased self-confidence, emphasizing that experience is the ultimate facilitator of these attributes.

Although some models of family therapy emphasize one category of training objectives over another, we believe that competence in all categories is ultimately essential to become a family therapist and a supervisor.[3] Focusing on all three categories simultaneously is difficult, and sometimes it is problematical to try. It is often preferable to work on one particular skill cluster at a time. By identifying and focusing on a particular training objective, confusion is avoided, the probability of positive outcome increases, and all parties are better able to evaluate their own and others' performances.

If therapists and supervisor/trainees entered a training program with the same potential to learn, and progressed uniformly in all categories of training objectives, programs could be standardized. But therapists as a group and supervisor/trainees as a group mature at different rates on the categories of skills. Some develop systemic thinking without undue struggle and confusion, while others quickly excel in learning technical skills, often relying on superior interpersonal skills to do so. Programs, therefore, must acknowledge differences among trainees, and allow categories to be pursued in idiosyncratic ways.

ORGANIZATION OF THE TRAINING CONTEXT: TRAINING FORMATS

To impart training objectives successfully, a concurrent training program must be well organized and make flexible and creative use of training formats. The primary format is a training system composed of a supervisor/trainer, supervisor/trainee, and several therapists-in-training, in which therapy and supervision are practiced under the guidance of an experienced supervisor/trainer (see Figure 13-2). Other formats support and augment this training system. For supervisor/trainees there is an ongoing supervision seminar attended by all supervisor/trainers and supervisor/trainees, and individual meetings between the supervisor/trainer and supervisor/trainee who work together in a particular supervision group. For therapists, there are didactic therapy seminars and individual meetings with their supervisor/trainees (see Figure 13-1).

The various training formats make synergistic contributions to the training process. Each format has its own goals and, when combined in a complementary fashion with other formats, can produce the desired result. Careful sequencing and sound judgment regarding the timing of training objectives in various formats are essential for successful training (Liddle *et al.*, 1984).

The Supervision Seminar

This format relieves supervisor/trainees of the intensity of live supervision, and enables them to pursue all categories of training objectives without immediate performance demands. By combining supervisor/trainers and supervisor/trainees, the very formation of the seminar defines the participants as members of the supervisory subsystem. In this subsystem, supervisor/trainees can learn from, identify with, and model themselves after experienced supervisors; a context is created in which supervisor/trainees can, with support and focus, continue the process of consolidating their professional identity.

Supervisor/trainees begin their work on systemic thinking in the seminar by preparing and delivering an epistemological declaration (Liddle, 1982; Liddle *et al.*, 1984). Geared to the supervisor/trainee's level, the epistemological declaration tends to empha-

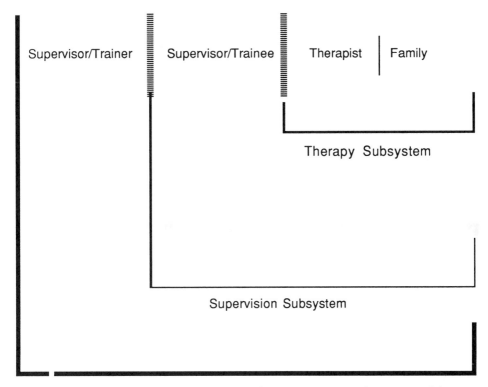

FIGURE 13-2. Supervision of supervision training system for concurrent training of supervisors and therapists.

size a particular model of family therapy. Reliance on a family therapy model allows the supervisor to refer to the model's literature and to approximate its theoretical clarity. The models, however, are viewed as partial realities of the field of family therapy, and, as the training program progresses, supervisor/trainees are encouraged to expand their systemic thinking through careful integration of compatible models. Such integrative attempts should not be confused with undisciplined eclecticism, which can do more to confuse than to clarify systemic thinking (Liddle, 1982). Supervisor/trainees question the commonalities and differences among models, and extract supervisory decisions. For example, questions regarding the use of direct versus indirect strategies, or when to shift from one approach to another, challenge the supervisor/trainee to think in a more complex fashion about a case. The development of an integrated model prepares the supervisor to think critically, question the literature, and remain open to new ideas (Lebow, 1987). Having learned to learn, supervisors continue to expand their thinking beyond their tenure in the training program, and thus remain current with our rapidly evolving field.

Another activity has proved useful in the supervision seminar. After the first wave of epistemological declarations have been made (these are seen as constantly evolving statements of theories-in-use), midway through the training year, tapes of live supervised therapy sessions with audio overdubs of supervisor communication are played. These tapes enable supervisor/trainees to receive example-grounded and situation-specific feedback on systemic thinking and technical skills away from the performance demands of live supervision of supervision. Here supervisor/trainees are prompted and helped to develop clear guidelines about how supervisory decisions are made.

Discussion of tapes is also devoted to the advantages and implementation difficulties of constructing a personalized, integrated therapeutic framework (Lebow, 1987; Liddle, 1982). The critique of tapes not only focuses on supervisory issues, but also allows theoretical matters to be debated, most frequently the complex territory of integration. In this seminar we are constantly reminded of the inseparability of supervisory and clinical issues. Therapeutic matters must be considered with the question in mind: "How will my trainees be able to understand and/or put into practice this concept or method?"

Supervisor/Trainer–Supervisor/Trainee Conferences

Each supervisor/trainer and supervisor/trainee pair assigned to a training group meet weekly. The supervisor/trainer can give the supervisor/trainee feedback without adversely affecting either supervisor/trainee and therapist relationships or the supervisor/trainee's credibility in the training system. Specific training objectives receive attention (e.g., providing more specific positive feedback and support of the therapists), and plans are made to practice them when the training system next convenes. Finally, and importantly, the meeting monitors and provides a means to develop further the complex relationship between supervisor/trainer and supervisor/trainee.

The conferences are a time of teaching, learning, and sharing. The supervisor/trainer supports those areas of competence achieved by the supervisor/trainee, and brings into focus areas in need of improvement. In a basic sense, the meetings allow the supervisor/trainee to be with a respected teacher in a setting in which he or she can be a learner. The pressures of becoming and being a supervisor are impressive, and the opportunity to be in a trainee position (which does not necessarily infer passivity, low status, or an extremely disparate hierarchy) is necessary for supervisor/trainees.

Meeting of Supervisor/Trainee and Therapist

Each supervisor/trainee meets weekly with the therapists he or she supervises to review progress on the therapists' training objectives, to discuss theoretical and clinical issues that have arisen in the weekly supervision or the therapists' readings, and to develop further and monitor the supervisory relationship. These conferences draw a boundary around the sometimes fragile supervisor/trainee and therapist subsystem, and represent a time when supervisor/trainees can feel more free to experiment with their still evolving role as supervisors. An analogy could be drawn to training clinicians. Live supervision is important, yet performance demands always exist, even after the therapist becomes accustomed to it. Trainees, therefore, are expected also to see cases away from the watchful and intense live supervision eye, thus giving them time to practice the style and skills being forged in the more emotionally intense and closely monitored live supervision and seminar time. The supervisor/trainee and therapist meetings serve some of the same function. They allow the participants time and a setting in which each can, in the context of seeing cases and doing supervision, formulate, practice, and recalibrate their developing roles as supervisors and therapists. When these meetings are productive, they strengthen the hierarchy of the training system (i.e., clarify the organizational structure and roles), and enable both supervisor/trainee and therapist to deal more effectively with the stress of training.

Didactic Therapy Seminar

The didactic therapy seminar exposes therapists to systemic concepts and technical skills in an atmosphere where discussion and critical thinking are encouraged. The supervisor/trainees make presentations on clinical topics in the seminar, which provide them with teaching experience and give the therapists an opportunity to see their supervisor/trainees as competent teachers. The seminar also provides experiential labs—simulations where therapists can practice recently learned technical skills away from actual clinical situations with families.

The Training System

The training system uses live supervision. The supervisor/trainee and therapist conduct their supervision and therapy, respectively, while simultaneously pursuing all three categories of training objectives. As this process unfolds, the supervisor/trainee and therapist are both expected to deliver increasingly competent supervision and therapy, while the emphasis on the service (to families and therapist/trainees) and professional aspects of the training context is never lost.

Live supervision provides immediate help during actual practice, creating the potential for rapid, experientially anchored learning, and better service for the family, therapist, and supervisor/trainee. But live supervision is predicated on an assumption that the participants can be helped to function competently while learning new behaviors and ideas. This assumption is not easily realized in practice because the demands of live supervision can yield a variety of difficulties (e.g., dependency and/or anxiety) resulting in a (temporary, one hopes) impairment of performance and service delivered to the trainee or family (see Chapter 11, this volume). In this complex setting, there is a simultaneous evaluation of the performance (i.e., service provided) of both supervisor/trainee and therapist. Sometimes when a session goes poorly, one of these participants blames the other. This situation is exacerbated by the demands of live supervision. The supervisor/trainer is ethically bound to deliver the best possible service for all involved: family, therapist, and supervisor/trainee. If the family does not receive adequate therapy, or the therapist adequate supervision, the supervisor/trainer has the responsibility to devise a plan to correct the situation.

These common implementation difficulties of live supervision can be mitigated by paying careful attention to the gradual attainment of a workable hierarchy among the supervisor/trainer, supervisor/trainee, and therapist (Fine & Fenell, 1985; Liddle et al., 1984). For this hierarchy to work in an organizational sense requires the person lower to view the person higher as helpful in the sense of having more expertise and being able to teach it. It also calls for the person higher to view the person lower as competent in the sense of believing the lower person can, with guidance, perform adequately (see Chapter 25, this volume). Hence, from the bottom up, the family perceives the therapist as helpful, the therapist perceives the supervisor/trainee as helpful, and the supervisor/trainee perceives the supervisor/trainer as helpful. From the top down, the supervisor/trainer perceives the supervisor/trainee as competent, the supervisor/trainee perceives the therapist as competent, and the therapist perceives the family as competent.

Establishing and maintaining this hierarchy is the primary task of the supervisor/trainer. When the hierarchy works well, supervisor/trainee and therapist pursue their training objectives effectively and everyone experiences competence, even while they are practicing and learning unfamiliar skills. The complexity of the training system, however, renders it vulnerable to two common difficulties: failure to deliver good service in the form of therapy or supervision, and interpersonal conflict among its members. When these difficulties emerge, the supervisor/trainer is challenged to formulate a systemic assessment about the difficulty. Thinking and perceiving in terms of isomorphism (see Chapter 9, this volume) can be helpful in this regard. Failure to conceptualize the training system's difficulties contextually can result in the supervisor/trainer focusing on the supervisor/trainee, therapist, or himself or herself alone, and drawing the conclusion that one or another participant is incompetent.

Such acontextual focusing in training can easily create an escalating cycle where that trainee feels under increasingly negative scrutiny, experiences overpowering anxiety, acts less and less competent, and loses professional self-confidence. When difficulties arise in the training system, therefore, the supervisor/trainer first analyzes the training process in hopes of discovering a solution. This does not suggest that a supervisor/trainer should ignore the way a particular therapist or supervisor/trainee is handling a training objective; rather, it cautions against simplistic, reductionistic assessments and interventions.

Three processes in particular consistently demonstrate their potential to disrupt the concurrent training of supervisors and therapists: inadequate communication among members of the training system, boundary problems between levels of the system, and problems relating to insufficient experience differentials between members of the system.

INADEQUATE COMMUNICATION

The supervisor/trainer must be aware that professionals do not always communicate clearly with each other. Since the potential for breakdowns in the flow of communication increases with complexity, the multileveled nature of the training system makes it more prone to such process difficulties.

Inadequate communication can occur for several reasons: theoretical differences among participants alters meaning (the message sent does not equal the message received); the message sent may be unclear, too complex, or contain too many components; or the facility may render hearing and speaking difficult (there is no substitute for a well soundproofed observation room). Inadequate communication creates an effect like the parlor game of "secrets," where a message is passed around the room until the final meaning of the message differs significantly from the original. A suggestion given by the supervisor/trainer to the supervisor/trainee may ultimately be implemented by the therapist in a manner quite different from that intended. Such ambiguity increases the potential for conflict, and for someone to appear incompetent. When this occurs, service delivery is impaired, and someone may be unjustly blamed.

BOUNDARY PROBLEMS

These problems occur when participants violate the hierarchy by consistently seeking or giving help to someone who is not at the next hierarchical level in the training system. Such violations most often occur when a person believes their colleague at the adjacent hierarchical level, that person with whom they are supposed to interact, to be unhelpful or incompetent. The supervisor/trainee seems most prone to boundary violations, not surprisingly perhaps, because of the delicate position between the supervisor/trainer and the therapist.

In a typical problem situation, the therapist questions the supervisor/trainee's helpfulness and, acting on this doubt, mistrust, or lack of attraction, seeks supervisory help directly from the supervisor/trainer, the person perceived as more expert.

Such processes may be subtle or blatant. For example, the therapist may ask the supervisor/trainer what he or she thought of the supervisor/trainee's suggestion. Such boundary violations can appear to be innocuous, and infrequent ones probably are. But a consistent pattern of incidents that, not coincidentally, appear in times of stress in the training system can be destructive to the formation of a functional organization and positive tone, and can surely undermine the supervisor/trainee's confidence and evolving professional identity.

To guard against boundary violations, communication should follow levels of the training system: the supervisor/trainer communicating with the supervisor/trainee, the supervisor/trainee with the therapist, and the therapist with the family. This is particularly important during the early stages of the training program when everyone is eager to demonstrate his or her competence. Once the hierarchical organization has been established, communication (i.e., assistance or input) can bypass levels without creating difficulties; a therapist can ask the supervisor/trainer a question without threatening the supervisor/trainee. At this phase, too, the supervisor/trainer is free to provide observations and ideas about a therapist's case without undue concern about undermining the supervisor/trainee's authority or stature. Such open communication is ideal, and in training groups that meet weekly for at least nine months this process is not uncommon to see. At this advanced stage in the development of the training system, therapists can learn from both supervisors.

INSUFFICIENT EXPERIENCE DIFFERENTIALS

Process difficulties can also arise when supervisor and/or therapist perceives an insufficient disparity in their personal or professional experience levels. For instance, a mature therapist with children and considerable experience in another form of therapy may find it difficult to see a young unmarried supervisor/trainee as credible, even if the supervisor/trainee has had more family therapy training.

The best way to deal with this process difficulty is to ensure an experience differential by accepting only those applicants with considerable clinical expertise and experience. Clearly established and realistic selection criteria, advertising for the supervisor training program, and selection procedures help to assure that competent applicants are accepted. Selection mistakes create a situation in which the supervisor/trainer quickly realizes that he or she is really training at the level of therapy rather than of supervision skills. This is not to say that a supervisor training program does not teach supervisor/trainees about therapy. But when the supervisor/trainee's developmental level indicates a paucity of clinical knowledge or skill, his or her capacity to be an effective supervisor is severely compromised.

Guidelines for Avoiding Process Difficulties

From our experience with concurrent supervisor/therapist training programs we have induced five guidelines that can help supervisor/trainers minimize the occurrence and disruption of process difficulties.

First, convene the training system well prepared. The supervisor/trainer and supervisor/trainee should plan supervision during their individual meetings prior to live supervision of supervision. Preparation gives the supervisor/trainee, as well as the supervisor/trainer, direction and confidence (albeit in a different way, of course), and eliminates many instances where the supervisor/trainer has to overrule or take over for the supervisor/trainee because the latter is on the wrong track. Well prepared supervisor/trainees feel more comfortable in the supervisory role, making it more likely that they will be accepted by the therapist. When these processes are set in motion, the professional identity and competence of the supervisor/trainee is enhanced.

Second, clearly differentiate what is possible in teaching contexts versus practice contexts. Teaching is an essential part of a training program but is most effective in formats such as seminars where students can discuss and question what is being taught; this is the time for deliberation and dialogue, if not debate. The practice demands of live supervision do not permit these kinds of activities, at least not in the ways in which they occur in teaching formats. Teaching in traditional ways during live supervision introduces new information that can confuse and/or disrupt the plan for the session. Input should mainly be geared to help the supervisor/trainee implement an agreed-on aspect of therapy. The supervisor/trainer is then better able to observe the supervisor/trainee, therapist, and family interaction, to review and, if necessary, set new priorities for training objectives.

Third, for any supervision session, have workable, realistic objectives. For example, it is difficult to emphasize systemic thinking and technical skills simultaneously. If a supervisor/trainee is attempting to articulate an unfamiliar strategic concept through a phone-in, he or she should not be expected also to worry about the precise wording of the phone-in. Often, the supervisor/trainee or therapist becomes confused when either tries to think through, formulate, or assimilate a new idea while also trying to change behavior at the same time.

Fourth, set moderately difficult objectives for practice in a session. The supervisor/trainee and therapist should be challenged by objectives that extend their range of skills, but should not be asked to attempt something clearly beyond their current abilities. Obviously, the supervisor/trainer's judgment is critical in this regard. Just as unreasonable challenges can have debilitating effects, weak challenges fail to stretch the trainee.

Fifth, mediation and middle-stage outcomes are important foci in a training context. Small steps toward change should also be emphasized. Exclusive focus on the final outcome of a case can cause problems. Overattachment to the outcome of any particular session or case can lead to undue and overgeneralized conclusions about one's competence. The expectation of brilliant performances or spectacular outcomes should be left to the theatrical and sporting arenas, respectively. The supervisor/trainer's responsibility is to ensure adequate, competent training or service to the supervisor/trainee, therapist, and family. The achievement of this expectation may be demonstrated by the gradual, but noticeable, changes at all three levels of the training/treatment system.

Trouble-Shooting the Training System

Even when careful attention is paid to the formation of a workable training system, and one's personally derived guidelines are followed, difficulties can still emerge. The supervisor/trainer focuses on the performance of the supervisor/trainee or therapist and, depending on preference and style, can intervene more or less indirectly to institute a change in the training system process. Changes with the supervisor/trainer, at the top of the hierarchy, often have repercussions that affect the other levels. Sometimes a supervisor/trainer's construction that a supervisory decision, which ultimately led to an unsatisfactory clinical action, originated with him or her can free the training system from an increasing cycle of demoralization and blame. The supervisor/trainer can also take a subordinate position, and express fallibility, for example, by admitting a lack of surety regarding what to do in a difficult situation.

In a more direct fashion, the supervisor/trainer can, for example, increase the amount of positive feedback given in the group, or discuss the functioning of the training system with the training group. Sometimes a three-way meeting—including the supervisor/trainer, supervisor/trainee, and a particular therapist—that simply airs accumulated tensions can clarify and repair relationship difficulties that had produced conflict and impaired the training system's functioning. In addition to improving their level of functioning, these interventions often allow the supervisor/trainee and therapist to feel less pressure and to relax and enjoy the training process more.

Focusing Directly on Training Objectives

Direct focus on how the supervisor/trainee and/or therapist are performing with respect to their training objectives is crucial to successful training. Such emphasis makes the complex training experience less overwhelming and more manageable for trainees, allowing clear benchmarks for progress made and progress still to be made within and beyond training. With this focus, the supervisor/trainee or therapist is less likely to feel incompetent, which provides an atmosphere in which one's quest for professional identity can successfully occur.

As an example of focusing directly on training objectives, consider a supervisor/trainee who has difficulty communicating supervisory suggestions clearly. This situation can produce inadequate supervision, thus hindering the therapist's training and jeopardizing service to the family. Although the supervisor/trainer must intervene to assure adequate service, such intervention must be done with care and, as Haley termed his phone-in philosophy, with some reluctance as well. Just as supervisors hesitate to take over the therapy, supervisor/trainers hesitate to take over the supervision of their trainees' trainees. In most situations, the supervisor/trainer and supervisor/trainee can meet and formulate plans to target additional resources to practice the training objective. Additional reading, tape review, and simulations are common options in this regard.

There are two situations, however, where this wait-and-see approach is likely not to work. The first involves the presence of a complicated training issue with a therapist that requires immediate high-level supervisory skills that the supervisor/trainee does not yet have and, further, will be unlikely to master in a reasonable (or the needed) period of time. If the issue is not addressed, service to the family will suffer, as will the supervisory relationship between the supervisor/trainee and therapist. In this situation the two supervisors can agree that the supervisor/trainer will show the supervisor/trainee how to handle the complex training issue. If the supervisor/trainer's direct involvement with the therapist is limited to this issue, the professional identity of the supervisor/trainee will not be damaged during the process of providing necessary care for the case.

The second situation occurs when the supervisor/trainee simply does not change or learn quickly enough to deliver effective supervision. The supervisor/trainer must then become directly involved in conducting some of the supervision, but this does not necessarily include assuming complete supervisory responsibility for the duration of the case. The supervisor/trainer can target the objective needing support, define clear limits for his or her involvement, and frame the involvement as a temporary measure designed to bolster the service dimension of the training system. For instance, if a supervisor/ trainee has difficulty with conceptualization and formulation of treatment objectives in planning sessions, the supervisor/trainer may participate in the presession discussion and communicate directly with the therapist, but not be involved in the live supervision.

When all these solutions fail, sometimes it is preferable to discontinue the supervisor/trainee's involvement temporarily, rather than plodding ahead with the likelihood that the training system will become conflictual and paralyzed. Freed from the pressure to perform, the supervisor/trainee can observe the supervisor/trainer, then discuss the supervision in the seminar and individual meetings. When sufficient progress has been made the supervisor/trainee can again begin supervision.

CONCLUSIONS

This chapter proposes that becoming a family therapist is a never-ending process. Programs that undertake concurrent training of supervisors and therapists provide a rich context where three groups at different points in this process of becoming can interact in mutually beneficial ways. The complexity of this endeavor, however, is formidable, and many difficulties will be encountered if careful attention is not given to the structure and process of the program. We have described how the use of training objectives and the use of planned training formats can enable such a program to achieve its ambitious goals of simultaneously advancing all three groups along the continuum of competence.

Training in family therapy and in supervision accelerates but never completes the process of becoming a family therapist or supervisor. When supervisors have been well trained, they feel and accept the responsibility to continue their development. As supervisors gain experience, they gain confidence in their ability, and begin to contribute to the field by presenting papers at conferences and writing for publication. If our field is to remain dynamic, the goal of training must enable the therapists of today to be the leaders of the field tomorrow. When training of supervisors is clearly conceptualized—especially in terms of the delicate training and service balance—well organized, and closely monitored, and when it emphasizes a process of becoming, that goal can be realized.

Notes

1. It is beyond the scope of this chapter to present training objectives in detail. For further information, see Cleghorn and Levine (1973), Falicov, Constantine, and Breunlin (1981), and Tomm and Wright (1979).

2. For example, consider the confusion many therapists and supervisors are experiencing by their efforts to shift from a first- to a second-order cybernetic perspective.

3. See, for instance, Chapters 3 and 4, where systemic thinking is emphasized, and compare to Chapters 5 and 6, where technical skills are emphasized.

References

Cleghorn, J., & Levine, S. (1973). Training family therapists by setting learning objectives. *American Journal of Orthopsychiatry, 43*, 439–446.

Constantine, J., Piercy, F., & Sprenkle, D. (1984). Live supervision-of-supervision in family therapy. *Journal of Marital and Family Therapy, 10*, 95–98.

Falicov, C., Constantine, J., & Breunlin, D. C. (1981). Teaching family therapy: A program based on training objectives. *Journal of Marital and Family Therapy, 7*, 497–505.

Fine, J., & Fenell, D. (1985). Supervising the supervisor-of-supervision: A supervision-of-supervision technique or a hierarchical blurring? *Journal of Stategic and Systemic Therapies, 4*, 55–59.

Friedman, D., & Kaslow, N. J. (1986). The development of professional identity of psychotherapists: Six stages in the supervision process. In F. Kaslow (Ed.), *Supervision and training: Models, dilemmas and challenges.* New York: Haworth Press.

Hess, A. K. (1986). Growth in supervision: Stages of supervisee and supervisor development. In F. Kaslow (Ed.), *Supervision and training: Models, dilemmas and challenges.* New York: Haworth Press.

Lebow, J. L. (1987). Developing a personal integration in family therapy: Principles for model construction and practice. *Journal of Marital and Family Therapy, 13*(1), 1–14.

Liddle, H. A. (1982). On the problems of eclecticism: A call for epistemologic clarification and human-scale theories. *Family Process, 21*, 243–250.

Liddle, H. A., Breunlin, D. C., Schwartz, R. C., & Constantine, J. (1984). Training family therapy supervisors: Issues of content, form, and context. *Journal of Marital and Family Therapy, 10*, 139–150.

Liddle, H. A., & Saba, G. (1983a, September). On context replication: An isomorph of training and therapy. *Family Therapy News.*

Liddle, H. A., & Saba, G. (1983b). On context replication: The isomorphic nature of training and therapy. *Journal of Strategic and Systemic Therapies, 2*(3), 3–11.

Liddle, H. A., & Saba, G. (1984). The isomorphic nature of training and therapy: Epistemologic foundation for a Structural–Strategic training paradigm. In J. Schwartzman (Ed.), *Families and other systems.* New York: Guilford Press.

Liddle, H. A., & Schwartz, R. C. (1983). Live supervision/consultation: Conceptual and pragmatic guidelines for family therapy training. *Family Process, 22*, 477–490.

Nichols, M. (1986). *Turning forty in the eighties.* New York: Basic Books.

Schwartz, R. C. (1982). On becoming a familied therapist. *Family Therapy Networker, 6*, 44–46.

Schwartz, R. C. (1985). Has family therapy reached the stage where it can appreciate the concept of stages? In D. C. Breunlin (Ed.), *Stages: Patterns of change over time*. Rockville, MD: Aspen.

Tomm, K., & Wright, L. (1979). Training in family therapy: Perceptual, conceptual and executive skills. *Family Process, 18*, 227–250.

Wright, L., & Coppersmith, E. I. (1983). Supervision of supervision: How to be "meta" to a metaposition. *Journal of Strategic and Systemic Therapies, 2*, 40–50.

SECTION FOUR

CONTEXTS FOR TRAINING

Introduction

Family therapy training now occurs within a variety of settings, which differ widely in the nature, scope, and desired outcome of the training they offer. The scope of family training in a given setting can be inferred in part from that setting's definition of family therapy. The three basic kinds of settings each have a different definition. The degree-granting programs in marriage and family therapy accept the definitions of family therapy as a profession, orientation, and field, and therefore offer the most in-depth training. The free-standing institutes, by defining family therapy as a field and an orientation, also provide intensive family therapy training; compared to degree-granting programs, however, institute training is less comprehensive because it is offered on a part-time basis and extends over a shorter period of time. The disciplines of psychology, psychiatry, and social work are not inclined to define family therapy as a profession or an orientation, preferring instead to define family therapy as a modality or as a field with a body of knowledge and set of skills from which to borrow ideas. Family therapy training in these settings is necessarily less intense and more often secondary to a broader training mission. We can begin to appreciate the diversity, and compare and contrast the family therapy training offered by the seven settings represented in this section, by examining four definitions of family therapy. This analysis reveals that the settings are producing a heterogeneous pool of professionals who define and practice family therapy in a multitude of ways.

FOUR DEFINITIONS OF FAMILY THERAPY AND THEIR IMPACT ON TRAINING

At various times in its history family therapy has been given a variety of meanings. The present discussion concerns four of these definitions: family therapy as (1) a profession, (2) an orientation to human problems, (3) a treatment method, and (4) a field of study with a body of knowledge about families and how to treat them. Because of the interconnection of any field's clinical and training domains, and the fluid nature of the still maturing field of family therapy, we will examine these definitions in the context of their implications for training.

Family Therapy as a Profession

When asked what they do for living, many mental health professionals reply, "I'm a family therapist." Clinicians refer to themselves as family therapists for many reasons, two primary ones being that they believe they belong to a profession bearing that name, and that the term best describes the duties of their work. In the former case, credentials are required to assure that one belongs to the profession of family therapy. In the latter case, the task defines one's identity. For example, social workers who enjoy working with families and see 20 families a week may well conclude that "family therapist" rather than "social worker" is the more appropriate description of their identity.

Whether or not family therapy is or ever will be recognized as a distinct profession is still an unanswered and hotly contested question. Many feel that family therapy would be best served if it emerged as a distinct profession, while others argue that family therapy exists in the public domain, is a body of knowledge, set of skills, and an orientation to human problems, and should never be subjected to the constraints that recognition as a profession would impose.

The degree-granting programs in marriage and family therapy in various universities clearly define family therapy as a profession. Sprenkle (Chapter 14) notes that the emergence of a professional organization (the American Association for Marriage and Family Therapy, or AAMFT), a body of literature, and a code of ethics, coupled with the growth of graduate programs in family therapy, are clear evidence of an emerging profession of family therapy. By offering a degree in marriage and family therapy with curricula heavily focused on family therapy, these programs socialize and constrain their graduates to view themselves as part of a distinct profession—the profession of family therapy.

Free-standing institutes only sometimes define family therapy as a profession. Most institutes offer a certificate, which is a sort of credential. More important, the exclusiveness, enthusiasm, and prestige associated with family therapy at these institutes proselytize many trainees, who complete the program well trained and eager to specialize in family therapy, and who identify themselves as family therapists.

Because many universities prepare students for traditionally recognized disciplines only, graduates from these programs do not consider themselves to be family therapists. We find, for example, social workers or psychologists who might have a family therapy orientation and practice family therapy, but do not necessarily consider or call themselves family therapists. Nevertheless, many graduates from these disciplines go on to obtain postdegree training in family therapy and develop such a strong affiliation with family therapy that they either abandon their affiliations with their original profession or adopt two identities.

Family Therapy as an Orientation to Human Problems

When family therapy is defined as an orientation, it becomes synonymous with the systemic view. In fact, defined as an orientation, the term "family therapy" is something of a misnomer, because one can apply the systemic view not just to the family, but also to any unit, including the individual and larger systems.

For family therapy to be defined and taught as an orientation, the setting must be able to give preeminence to the systemic view. Sprenkle (Chapter 14) notes that degree-granting programs in family therapy, housed as they are in departments of family studies, home economics, and sociology, can emphasize the systemic view because it does not compete with other clinical or theoretical traditions. Likewise, most free-standing institutes were established precisely to achieve the freedom to pursue specialization and focus on a systemic view.

In the discipline-related settings such as departments of psychology, psychiatry, and social work, systemic thinking, as a newcomer, must compete with the discipline's established theoretical traditions (Liddle, 1987b). Berger (Chapter 19), for instance, notes that the long-standing traditions of individual psychology may clash with the systemic view; consequently, systemic thinking, when taught, is often presented as one of several theories. Likewise in psychiatry (Chapter 16), the systemic view and the medical model may be viewed as incompatible.

Family therapy, defined as an orientation, also encounters resistance in settings where other therapies have traditionally formed the basis of clinical training. The clinical emphasis sometimes associated with family therapy as orientation is rejected outright in these settings, with the result that sometimes family therapy is not taught at all, or taught only as another modality of treatment.

In such settings, teachers interested in the systemic view can initially separate it from family therapy by first introducing systemic thinking on its own. For example, Combrinck-Graham (Chapter 16) introduces systemic thinking at all levels of the bio-psychosocial continuum, from the biology of cells to the functioning of an inpatient ward; only in their third year do psychiatry residents encounter family therapy as a form of psychotherapy. By then they have grown accustomed to systemic thinking. In Chapter 20, Bardill and Saunders suggest that the systemic view could serve as an umbrella theory uniting social work's two divisive camps, the people changers and the social changers. In fact, one of the editors of this volume (D.B.) graduated from such a social work program. Having approached social welfare and public policy from a systemic perspective, it seemed to him quite reasonable to think systemically about therapy. In this way, novice therapists can evolve to a view of family therapy as orientation.

Family Therapy as a Modality

Family therapy can also be viewed as a modality of psychotherapy. As such, it can be catalogued and compared with other psychotherapies, and criteria can be used to decide when family therapy is the treatment of choice. As a modality, family therapy may or may not be grounded in systems theory. The therapy may also be based on traditional theories such as psychodynamic theory, object relations theory, social learning theory, gestalt theory, or small-group therapy. More recently these theories have been combined with systems theory to create integrated models of family therapy. Examples are Nichols's integrative psychodynamic and systems approach (Chapter 7), and Functional Family Therapy, which combines systems and social learning theories (Chapter 8).

Defined as a modality, family therapy is less threatening in settings where many theories and types of therapy are taught, particularly in the mental health disciplines of psychology, psychiatry, and social work. In these settings, students take courses on family therapy just as they do for individual and group therapy.

The modality definition also fits well in settings where the overall training mission is broader than therapy, as is the case in all of the discipline-related settings. Family therapy is approached as but one task to be learned among others such as research skills, psychological assessment, taking social histories, or prescribing medicine.

Family Therapy as a Field

As a field consisting of a body of knowledge, family therapy exists in the public domain and is accessible to all of the settings according to their needs. The degree-granting programs in marriage and family therapy adopt this body of knowledge as the core of their curricula, and the free-standing institutes use large parts of it, often emphasizing the literature of a particular model of family therapy.

In the discipline-related settings, family therapy's body of knowledge is used in two ways. First, as described above, it can be used to teach family therapy as a modality. Second, some settings, particularly nursing and social work, possess their own language and body of knowledge about families; consequently, ideas drawn from family therapy's body of knowledge are assimilated into the preferred curricula of the discipline. For example, Wright and Leahey (Chapter 17) note that nursing has a wide variety of family assessment models that have incorporated family therapy concepts along with many concepts from nursing and sociology. Bardill and Saunders (Chapter 20) note that family therapy concepts and techniques might be covered in a course entitled "Social Work on Behalf of Children and Adolescents." This pattern of assimilation is probably preferred for several reasons, traditions within the disciplines are preserved, ambivalence about family therapy is minimized, and departments do not require faculty qualified to articulate the concepts of family therapy. Students exposed to family therapy in this manner may not recognize it as a profession, an orientation, or even a modality.

In some settings, particularly bachelor's-level nursing and family medicine, practicing therapy of any sort is not automatically sanctioned. Instead, since they recognize that nurses and family practice physicians must interact with families, these settings draw upon concepts and skills from family therapy that can be applied in a wide variety of interpersonal situations. For instance, Wright and Leahey note that nurses benefit from knowing how to take a "one-down" position with a difficult patient or family, and Ransom notes that family physicians, accustomed to having a "bag of tricks," are able to draw on many family therapy skills. These professionals are not initially trained to practice family therapy, but a talented nurse or family practice physician interviewing a family often appears to be doing just that. Additionally, some pursue specialist training in family therapy per se.

The various disciplines argue that, as a field, family therapy should have a more open dialogue with them because each has much to offer the other. Some family therapists who train in other disciplines agree. For instance, Ransom (Chapter 18) believes that family therapy has for too long lacked a serious dialogue with another discipline, and proposes that family practice can offer such an exchange.

Berger (Chapter 19) notes that psychology's strong research tradition has contributed much to family therapy. He also argues that psychology's theories of child development have for too long been neglected by family therapy. Likewise, social work's understanding of macrosystems and social policy, psychiatry's grasp of neuroanatomy, nursing's experience with the impact of illness on families, and family medicine's biopsychosocial treatment of illness all have much to offer family therapy. The *Journal of Family Systems Medicine,* edited by Don Bloch, and the new publication of the Division of Family Psychology of the American Psychological Association, *Journal of*

Family Psychology edited by Howard Liddle, are two examples where dialogues between family therapy and another discipline are now vigorously pursued (Liddle, 1987a). Like all new endeavors, family therapy first established itself by closing its boundaries and adopting extreme positions with respect to other disciplines (Schwartz, 1985). As family therapy matures and gains more widespread acceptance, however, it appears to be increasingly receptive to interaction with other disciplines.

Not surprisingly, then, the settings for training have produced a group of professionals who define and practice family therapy in a variety of ways. For all these professionals, however, a key question is how much training is necessary to ensure clinical competence.

Training for Clinical Competence

We begin this discussion by noting that there are many pathways to clinical competence in family therapy. Indeed, the pioneers of family therapy, who are widely recognized as master clinicians, never received formal training in family therapy. They honed their skills through trial and error afforded by experience. But a generation later family therapy has evolved to become a far more complex and sophisticated endeavor. This factor, coupled with the availability of a multitude of training opportunities, has created a context where the vast majority of clinicians seek training before attempting to practice family therapy.

Although the settings vary enormously in their training missions, when the goal is to train clinicians all agree that training should include three experiences: (1) didactic presentations (in the form of course work or seminars) where students learn about and discuss family therapy's body of knowledge; (2) clinical work with families; and (3) regular supervision with an experienced family therapy supervisor. The settings, however, vary greatly on the desired amount and mixture of the three experiences. Unfortunately, to date no research has documented how to combine these training experiences to produce clinical competence. One existing benchmark is provided by the AAMFT, which has established criteria for its clinical membership that include the following: course work in marital and family therapy from or equivalent to a master's degree in marriage and family therapy (approximately 33 semester hours), 1,000 hours of clinical work with families, and 200 hours of supervision from a qualified family therapy supervisor. Although the numbers designated by this criterion may be questioned, the spirit is sound because it recognizes that competence in family therapy requires thorough training. Another requirement of AAMFT clinical membership is 2 years of practice experience and supervision following completion of a qualifying degree. Thus, requirements for clinical membership cannot be achieved through a single training experience.

Students committed to developing clinical competence in family therapy can choose from several pathways. One involves obtaining a graduate degree in marriage and family therapy, followed by clinical supervisory experience in family therapy. This pathway involves an accelerated and concentrated experience in family therapy with ample course work, clinical experience, and supervision. Another pathway involves pursuit of a graduate degree from a discipline, followed by clinical and supervisory experience and postgraduate training at a free-standing institute (see Sutton, 1985, for a comparison of a degree-granting and institute training programs). Students who pursue a degree in a discipline and know of their interest in family therapy from the outset can accelerate their family therapy training by selecting settings where family therapy is emphasized. Key questions to ask in selecting a graduate program are the number and caliber of faculty available to teach family therapy courses, and the availability of clinical sites (for internships and field placements) offering clinical work with families and supervision. Programs with family therapists on faculty actively cultivate such sites and direct committed students to them (for example, see Solomon, Ott, & Roach, 1986, for a listing of family therapy internships in psychology).

Another trend in discipline-related programs is toward a specialization in family therapy. For example, Bardill and Saunders (Chapter 20) propose a master's degree in social work that also meets AAMFT accreditation requirements, and Berger (Chapter 19) and Wright and Leahey (Chapter 17) describe programs in academic psychology and graduate nursing, respectively, that offer a family therapy specialization. Combrinck-Graham (Chapter 16) notes that a systemically oriented residency in psychiatry, in part because of its length (4 years) affords many training opportunities to residents, including 300 hours of family therapy supervision.

One important message about the relationship between clinical competence and training repeated throughout this book is that ultimately becoming competent is a never-ending process that extends well beyond any period of formal training (see Chapters 7 and 13, in particular). Thus, key training objectives in all settings are teaching students to remain curious about family therapy and to learn to learn. To some extent the settings can function as a set of building blocks toward increasing competence further, where master's level, doctoral, and postgraduate training facilitate this process.

References

Liddle, H. A. (1987a). Editor's Introduction I: Family psychology: The journal, the field. *Journal of Family Psychology*, 1(1), 5–22.

Liddle, H. A. (1987b). Editor's Introduction II: Family psychology: Tasks of an emerging (and emerged) discipline. *Journal of Family Psychology*, 1(2).

Schwartz, R. C. (1985). Has family therapy reached the stage where it can appreciate the concept of stages? In D. C. Breunlin (Ed.), *Stages: Patterns of change over time*. Rockville, MD: Aspen.

Solomon, J., Ott, J., & Roach, A. (1986). A survey of training opportunities for predoctoral psychology interns in marriage and family therapy. *Journal of Marital and Family Therapy*, 12(3), 269–280.

Sutton, P. M. (1985). An insider's comparison of a major family therapy doctoral program and a leading nondegree family therapy training center. *Journal of Psychotherapy and the Family*, 1(4), 41–52.

14

Training and Supervision in Degree-Granting Graduate Programs in Family Therapy

DOUGLAS H. SPRENKLE
Purdue University, West Lafayette, Indiana

This chapter describes family therapy training and supervision in one of the most promising, yet still relatively undeveloped contexts—degree-granting graduate programs. First, I will discuss the problem of defining what such programs are, and give a history of their development. Reasons for their slow start, but recent rapid growth in number and quality, will be explored. Next, the major training issues facing these programs will be explored. Attention will be given to their goals, the advantages and disadvantages of this training context, and the methods and materials employed in training, supervision, and the supervision of supervision. Finally, I will reflect on the current and future contributions of these programs.

DELIMITING THE FIELD

Deciding what to include as a degree program in family therapy is not easy. Even among the 28 (as of December 1987) programs accredited by the Commission on Accreditation for Marriage and Family Therapy Education, only 3 offer master's degrees or doctorates in marriage and/or family therapy per se. The rest offer degrees in a broad field of study (e.g., child development and family studies, sociology, home economics, counseling and guidance) with a *specialization* in family therapy. Nonetheless, the quantity and quality of course offerings and supervised practice in the AAMFT programs are well monitored to assure that these are far more than programs in name only. Unfortunately, the same cannot be said for some nonaccredited "programs," which (despite impressive brochures) are little more than a few course offerings by overextended, if well meaning, faculty.

Although the Commission on Accreditation standards cannot ensure excellence, they go a long way to eliminating gross programmatic incompetence. They require that a graduate program have a history—not only of graduates but also of moral and financial support by the program's department, school, and university. The basic institution in which program resides must be regionally accredited. The vitae of all faculty are scrutinized, as are all course syllabi. After completing a detailed self-study, an outside review team from the organization's Commission on Accreditation makes a site visit to examine facilities; to interview students, faculty, and administrators; to attend classes and practica; and to write a report for the Commission delineating strengths and concerns about the program.

The Commission requires that the program have an integrated curriculum that meets certain educational objectives. While course offerings are not rigidly prescribed, the Commission on Accreditation has published a model two-year curriculum that serves as a guide to identifying substantive content areas (AAMFT, 1981). The 1981 model was the same for the MS and the PhD. It did not specify additional requirements for the latter degree, although there was an implicit recognition that universities expect additional course work, further training in research, and a dissertation for a doctorate. As of this writing, the Commission is in the process of writing a revised model that will probably contain master's–doctoral distinctions. Readers should contact the Commission in care of the American Association for Marriage and Family Therapy (AAMFT) Office in Washington, DC, for the latest Accreditation Manual. The major impression one gets from studying these documents is that the Commission clearly believes the field has a substantive body of theory, content, research, and professional issues that should be a part of training, and that this knowledge cannot simply be handed on to the student through apprenticeship training from a master clinician or as a by-product of clinically oriented endeavors (Nichols, 1979b).

This is not to suggest that supervised clinical practice is slighted in these programs. Rather, supervision is embedded in a much broader context of training. The Commission on Accreditation required in its 1981 standards that all students must document the completion of a minimum of 500 direct face-to-face clinical contact hours prior to graduation. Furthermore, it was expected that the ratio of supervision hours to treatment hours should never be less than 1 to 5 (AAMFT, 1981).

Nonaccredited academic "programs" vary considerably in the extent to which they approximate these requirements. Since they have not subjected themselves to outside review, little can be said about them with certainty. In a survey completed in 1980, Bloch and Weiss (1981) reported on the existence of 55 degree programs (of which about 40 are *not* on the current list of accredited programs). This report noted 9 programs offering an MSW, 23 offering the MS, 1 granting an MS with an advanced certificate in marriage and family therapy, 5 combination MA and PhD programs, and 15 programs offering a PhD, PsyD, or DSW. One MA and one PhD in pastoral counseling were also included. Unfortunately, however, clear operational definitions of what constitutes a program were not given, and self-selection appears to be the major criterion. In another directory of marriage and family therapy graduate programs and training centers (Joanning & Castle, 1983), about 20 graduate degree programs are described, in addition to those that are now accredited. Since the descriptions of these programs are brief and were provided by the schools in a mail survey, it is difficult to evaluate them objectively.

To summarize, there are 28 AAMFT-accredited programs. Seventeen universities offer the master's only, seven grant the doctorate only, and two give both degrees. Hence, the 28 programs are housed in 26 universities. There have been as many as 40 other degree-granting programs identified in surveys taken in the early 1980s, and there are undoubtedly other programs not yet identified. Until they are willing to pursue the accreditation process, it is extremely difficult to ascertain their quality. For this reason, most of the remaining commentary on degree programs will refer to the accredited programs.

HISTORY OF DEGREE PROGRAMS IN FAMILY THERAPY

Although the number of accredited programs is still not large, the recent rate of growth can be considered explosive. The 28 accredited programs December 1987 represent almost a 400% increase since only 1979, when there were just 7 accredited programs. This rapid growth rate, however, must be seen in light of the previous three decades, in which expansion could best be described as slow.

Although AAMFT (originally the American Association of Marriage Counselors, or AAMC) was founded in 1942, it did not publish standards on "graduate education in marriage counseling" until 1959. In its early years the organization was more concerned with establishing standards for marriage counselors (1949) and with centers for marriage counseling (1953). It also assumed that marriage counseling was a professional activity that persons entered with a previous, recognized graduate degree in another discipline. Marriage counseling was learned as a postgraduate intern (Nichols, 1979b). This made sense in that early practitioners considered marriage counseling as supplemental to their primary occupations as psychologists, psychiatrists, social workers, ministers, and so forth (Broderick & Schrader, 1981).

The 1959 standards on graduate education in marriage counseling recognized the pioneering work of certain universities that had begun to develop graduate programs in marriage counseling, and suggested that it could be recognized as a separate area of graduate education and a professional field in its own right (Nichols, 1979a). It is interesting that these early standards called for a 4-year minimum doctoral program with internship. It was assumed that as the field developed, training would cease to be primarily at the postdoctoral level and would be shifted to doctoral programs in the discipline itself. During the 1950s, somewhat loosely defined doctoral programs could be found at Columbia University Teachers College, the University of Southern California, Florida State University, and Purdue University (Nichols, 1979a).

Ironically, however, the growth that has subsequently occurred in the 1960s, 1970s, and 1980s has been mostly at the master's level. AAMFT's 1971 standards concerning training centers in the marriage and family counseling clearly gave credence to the master's degree as the entry level to the field. By 1974, standards for graduate degree programs in marriage and family counseling were applicable to both master's and doctoral programs (a condition that remained in the 1981 standards).

Several factors may be responsible for the emergence of the master's degree as the basic degree in the discipline:

1. Frankly, there were simply too many entry points to the field, and not enough control by AAMFT, to mandate a doctoral standard.
2. For persons with a previous doctorate, it was simply too much to expect that they would complete the rigors of a second one, particularly when there were post-degree training centers available (Nichols, 1979a). In truth, the imposition of a specialized doctorate flew in the face of the reality that most early practitioners envisaged their family work as supplemental to their primary occupations.
3. The first licensing law (in California in 1962) was passed at the master's level, and most other states have followed this standard (Nichols, 1979a).

4. In most states family therapy continues to be an unregulated profession, and acceptable standards for the field are determined by what the public will tolerate. Apparently the public will accept training at the master's level, either because there is a great demand for services and master's-level clinicians are available, and/or because the public is not as impressed by the doctorate as some professionals are.

Nontraditional Context

An important feature of the history of the early programs is the context in which they developed—a context that continues to have considerable influence today. The early doctoral programs developed in nonclinically oriented departments where there was an *existing* emphasis on marriage and the family. A clinical component was then added to this emphasis. The two primary academic disciplines were sociology and home economics, which encompassed home and family life, child development, and family relations departments. Departmental locations were more influenced by the interests and clinical commitments of certain key individuals than by widespread consensus that marriage counseling belonged within a given discipline, such as sociology (Nichols, 1979a). It is significant that these programs did not develop within traditional clinical disciplines, such as clinical psychology. Being born in family-oriented departments rooted the young discipline in the broader context of family theory and research, and made it less likely to be considered merely "one counseling technique" that can be used to intervene in human problems. The early ties to sociology also forced the program leaders to think interactionally and to give considerable emphasis to the social context of behavior. While only one of the accredited programs today remains housed in sociology (at the University of Southern California), the sociological emphasis is still strongly felt in the other programs that are, with very few exceptions, housed in multidisciplinary departments.

Family Studies and Clinical Training in the Same Department

Another legacy of the early programs, strongly evident today, was the placing of clinical training, and training in family studies and human development, in the same department (Nichols, 1979a). Not "farming out" the clinical component to other departments (e.g., psychology) has a distinct political advantage; it is much less likely that such programs will consume energy fighting epistemological battles over the contextual view of problem formation and change. Supervisors typically need not worry that their interactionally oriented work will be undermined by an intrapsychically oriented colleague. Persons attempting to teach family therapy within the context of clinical or counseling psychology departments are much more likely to face these struggles (Liddle, 1978).

CURRENT STATUS

Program Growth

It is interesting to speculate why there has been rapid graduate program growth, particularly at the master's level, in the past five years.

First, the growth of AAMFT, both in size and in prestige, has provided a significant impetus. People increasingly value the AAMFT credential and want to be sure that their training will facilitate membership. While a degree from an accredited program is not yet a membership requirement, AAMFT is becoming increasingly insistent that applicants have the equivalent of a strong master's program. The current membership application calls for 11 courses, in addition to clinical practice—a course of study that closely parallels the recommendations for graduate programs from the Commission on Accreditation. Programs, in turn, want the best students, and believe AAMFT recognition is an important factor in recruitment. The prestige of AAMFT endorsement of programs was greatly enhanced when, in 1978, the Commission on Accreditation gained official recognition as an accrediting agency for graduate degree and clinical training programs in marriage and family therapy by the United States Office of Education, Department of Health, Education and Welfare.

A second impetus for graduate degree programs has been the development of family therapy as a unique profession. As late as 1968, 75% of the members of the (then) AAMC did not see themselves as belonging to a new or unique profession (Peterson, 1968). In a recent study of 22 family therapy programs (representing university, free-standing, accredited, and nonaccredited types), family therapy was overwhelmingly (by 86.4% of the 297 students and faculty respondents) considered to be a unique clinical profession (Henry, 1983). Clearly, the proportions have shifted markedly in the past two decades.

I believe there is a positive feedback cycle operating between professional identity and graduate degree training in family therapy. The more the discipline is recognized as unique, the more legitimate and necessary a degree in the discipline becomes. The more degrees are actually granted in family therapy, the greater the professional identity of the field.

If family therapy follows the model of other disciplines, there will probably be growing pressure to limit access to the field by persons who have not received degrees in the discipline (as in the fields of medicine and law). Such pressure will be much more likely if licensure becomes widespread and degree programs become the avenue to licensure (as is the case in psychology). In her sociological analysis of professionalization, Larson (1977) has argued that professions represent a special class of labor organization in a capitalist society. In order to achieve market control, professions strive to control the production of practitioners and their knowledge, which necessarily entails the standardization of training, as well as the development of mechanisms to control the practice, such as licensure (Henry, 1983). Viewed less cynically, the growth of graduate programs can be seen as one of the requisites for an activity becoming a profession, the other components being a professional organization, a code of ethics, and a body of literature and related journals (Hall, 1968).

In my opinion, the field has reached "critical mass," and the movement in the direction of degree programs is inexorable. I agree wholeheartedly with Nichols (1979b) that ". . . there is adequate reason to assume that present trends will continue and that larger proportions of those entering the field in the future will do so directly by securing their basic education in marriage and family therapy at the graduate level" (p. 21). Another fascinating finding of the Henry (1983) study, which supports this conclusion, is that even the majority of students and faculty in free-standing (nondegree) programs regard the degree-granting option as the ideal MFT program.

Theoretical Diversity

A hallmark of the accredited programs is not only their theoretical diversity, but also their pride in such diversity. In a survey I completed of the 17 programs accredited in 1984, the number of (self-reported) theoretical approaches taught ranged from 2 to 6, with a median of 4. Ten of the 17 programs listed "systems" either as a general heading or as a type of approach. Among the specific approaches mentioned, the strategic (9 listings), structural (7), and structural–strategic (3) were among the most popular. Yet, perhaps surprisingly, 11 different programs listed either or both psychodynamic (5) and psychoanalytic (7) among the approaches taught. Other theoretical orientations receiving 4 or more listings included behavioral or learning (9), experiential (5), and Bowen (4). The implicit assumption that students are expected to do some integration of these diverse approaches was made explicit in the report of one program: "Students are to become familiar with at least three different approaches and synthesize them to a process that works for them." (Joanning & Castle, 1983, p. 28). This approach stands in contrast to the argument advanced by Liddle (1982) that it is premature to integrate theories and that such attempts result in a smorgasbord eclecticism that will not advance the field.

Most program directors believe that since there is so little empirical evidence supporting any one theoretical approach, intellectual integrity mandates the presentation of a broad spectrum of theories. It appears to me, however, that theoretical diversity is more evident in classroom instruction than in practica. At Purdue, for example, although all major approaches are taught in theory courses, the practica emphasize brief, problem-centered interactional approaches.

Program Goals

Training in family therapy should emphasize the synergistic interplay among the domains of theory, research, and practice (Sprenkle, 1976). The *sine qua non* of graduate degree-granting programs in family therapy is that they offer more than simply clinical supervision. Graduates should be what Olson (1976) calls champions of the "triple threat" of science. Practitioners are better practitioners because their work is guided by a theory of change (rather than by technique faddism) and is evaluated empirically. Practice, in turn, helps shape both theory and research. As a result of the capacity to function well in all three areas, students should be in a position to make original contributions to the field, as opposed to simply carrying forth a clinical tradition. The research–evaluative component is especially emphasized in doctoral programs.

Programs should be concerned with professional as well as scholarly development. Although attention to scholarship is rigorous and intense, professional education has some unique demands. Nichols (1979b) puts it well:

> Preparation of marriage and family therapists as a form of professional development differs from graduate education in an essentially cognitive discipline in which professional identification is at best a minor part of the educational experience. The basic commitment in the study of history and related academic disciplines, for example, is to the pursuit of truth and to the discipline or body of knowledge itself. The orientation of the professional is not only to truth but also to the ethical code of his profession and to the needs and interest of his/her

clientele. The peculiarities of professional development throw upon the faculty the responsibility for planning and guiding the shaping of professional persons in more focused ways than is necessary in most graduate education. Faculty need to make certain in so far as possible that comprehension of the ethical issues and the needs of clientele are gained as the student moves toward forming a self-identity as a member of the profession. This concern must go along with the screening of applicants for the program in terms of cognitive, ethical, and maturational readiness. There is an important professional culture that cannot be passed on through books and library materials. (pp. 24-25)

Everett (1979) also notes that the concern for professional socialization sets these programs apart from traditional graduate training in the social sciences and liberal arts. The freedom of the typical graduate student to select a variety of courses according to individual preference is inappropriate in professional education until a basic core of knowledge is mastered.

A developing goal of these programs is to promote training in supervision, and the supervision of supervision. Almost all of the doctoral programs offer specialized training in supervision. Doctoral graduates especially will frequently be in settings where they must supervise and evaluate clinical practice, as well as do it.

Obstacles to Program Development

Although these programs have proliferated rapidly in recent years, there have been several factors that have impeded, or may impede, growth in quality as well as quantity.

First, these programs rarely constitute a separate department. Therefore, family therapy programs share, and compete for, resources with the other programs (typically nonclinical) in the departments in which they are housed. Clearly this is a different educational model than in many professions, which have their own schools (medicine, law, social work, nursing, etc.). Not infrequently, nonclinical faculty in these departments do not appreciate the needs of family therapy programs, which are typically very expensive—requiring quality equipment, small classes, released time for supervision, and so forth. Nonclinically oriented administrators have the same misperceptions and frequently require clinical faculty to "donate" the time necessary for supervision. It is clearly the exception for faculty members to be given 100% of their teaching time for courses in marriage and family therapy, and even more rare to be fully compensated for supervision. Professional jealousies may also arise because family therapy courses are typically popular and out-draw other courses. It is not unusual for the large majority of the total applications to a given department to be for family therapy. As a result, the programs have the luxury of a higher degree of admissions selectivity; this may lead to concerns about elitism. Clinical faculty can also supplement their income through part-time private practice, which may compound feelings of separateness.

A second potential obstacle is university funding limitations and retrenchment. Even though graduate programs may themselves be successful, they cannot be guaranteed adequate financial support. Particularly in state-supported universities, departmental allocations are based, in considerable measure, on undergraduate enrollments or other factors beyond the control of MFT programs. There is very little money available today for new programs if they imply the creation of truly "new" faculty positions. Many so-called "new" programs are being created when existing faculty put new labels on what they are already doing, or assume voluntary overloads. Although these restrictions do not necessarily apply to private institutions, the very nature of family therapy education requires that these programs be very expensive. Probably none of the accredited programs are fully supported by student fees.

A third potential obstacle relates to the vagaries of state licensure laws and norms pertaining to third-party payments. If it remains true (as in most states) that (1) licensed psychologists have a monopoly on nonmedical third-party payments, and (2) graduates of family therapy programs have an increasingly difficult time becoming licensed as psychologists, the growth of family therapy programs could be limited. The future of (specific) marriage and family therapy state licensure, the education requirements for it, and the future of third-party payments connected with it are additional factors that will potentially abet or limit program growth.

METHODS AND MATERIALS

In this section the author will describe methods and materials utilized by 17 accredited programs based on a telephone survey of the training directors completed in the spring of 1984. In addition, specific details will be presented concerning the doctoral program in family therapy at Purdue University, which is an example of the more highly developed programs.

Academic Classroom Components

As previously noted, academic training in theory and research is the *raison d'être* of degree-granting programs. While the terms "supervision" and "training" are sometimes used synonymously in the literature, academic family therapy educators insist that supervision is a subset of training, and that the latter requires mastery of a body of academic knowledge that requires years of intensive study.

The Commission on Accreditation ensures a relative degree of uniformity in curriculum across programs. Students are expected to be versed in such important aspects of human development as personality theory, human sexuality, and psychopathology and behavior pathology. The academic study of the family includes such topics as family development, the interaction among important family subsystems, and the sociocultural context in which the family is embedded. All programs expose the students to major marital and family therapy treatment approaches. Students must also be trained in research design, methodology, and statistics. Important professional issues, such as ethics and legal questions, are covered. Since these programs are typically in multidisciplinary departments, they offer the student the capacity to interface marriage and family therapy with other related disciplines, such as child development.

Beyond these general guidelines, however, there are only a few resources that training directors can draw on to give direction to or improve classroom instruction. Winkle, Piercy, and Hovestadt (1981) have offered a model curriculum for graduate-level marriage and family therapy education based on a consensus of a national panel of approved supervisors and training directors. While there were more similarities than differences between this model and the AAMFT model, the panelists seem less concerned than was the AAMFT with course content areas derived from more traditional theories (such as individual psychotherapy theory). There was also more emphasis on the study of group dynamics and group psychotherapy. The panel would also require more semester hours than AAMFT.

Other resources include Liddle and Saba's (1982) description of an introductory family therapy course, which demonstrates parallel processes, such as joining, restructuring, and consolidation, used in both teaching and therapy. Nichols (1979a) has written a general article on doctoral degree programs in family therapy, and Everett (1979) has prepared a similar statement about master's programs. There are also a few articles describing the curricula of particular programs (e.g., Garfield, 1979; L'Abate, Berger, Wright, & O'Shea, 1979). More recently, Fred Piercy and I have published papers describing the content and teaching methods of courses in ethics, legal and professional issues in family therapy (Piercy & Sprenkle, 1983), and family therapy outcome research (Sprenkle & Piercy, 1984). These authors have also prepared a general article on the process of family therapy classroom education that delineates basic educational assumptions and a variety of techniques applicable to a wide variety of courses (Piercy & Sprenkle, 1984). These contributions notwithstanding, the literature on case supervision is much more extensive than that on the broader context of training.

AN ILLUSTRATION

The Purdue program has taken several steps to ensure more-than-basic training in theory and research, as well as to foster the aforementioned integration of theory, research, and practice:

1. Theoretical training includes a generic course in theory construction and theory evaluation, which facilitates the processes of the student developing his or her own theory of family therapy, and critically analyzing other theories. The substantive theories of marriage and family therapy are covered in a four-course sequence, in which the major thinkers are read in the original sources (as opposed to textbooks). The first course, called "Foundations of Marriage and Family Therapy," analyzes the original documents in cybernetics, epistemology, and systems theory on which the field is based. The works of such scholars as VonBertallanfy, Weiner, and Bateson are analyzed. The second course covers structural and strategic theories. The third focuses on communicational, behavioral, and experiential approaches. The final course covers neoanalytic and transgenerational models.

2. Training and research are rigorous and thorough. There are typical courses in research methodology (beginning and advanced), statistics (two advanced courses), and computer science. But a course specifically on family therapy research has also been created; it entails a critical review of all of the outcome research in the discipline, critically evaluates research designs and methods appropriate for family therapy, and points to major directions for future research. (A complete description of this course is found in Sprenkle & Piercy, 1984.) A separate course has also been developed on tools (instrumentation) and techniques for the assessment of family therapy. All students also participate in the ongoing program of outcome research at the Purdue Marriage and Family Therapy Center, where they receive the bulk of their clinical training. The client

families are given a battery of pretherapy, posttherapy, and follow-up measures, which the students gather, partially analyze, and utilize for feedback to clients.

3. Activities that encourage the integration of theory, research, and practice occur as part of this research program. Students fill out a modified Goal Attainment Scale (Kiresuk & Sherman, 1968) for each family. On an original form that I designed, students must (1) delineate mediating and ultimate goals for each family; (2) operationalize how the family would look at the end of therapy if things were "the same," "better," or "worse"; and (3) relate each of these goals, in turn, to a particular theory of family therapy. Therefore, the student is challenged to guide his or her practice with specific theoretical assumptions and to operationalize outcome in ways that can be checked against client and/or observer data (Piercy & Sprenkle, 1984).

4. Another integrative task is the preliminary examination that each student must complete toward the end of his or her program. The student prepares a scholarly referenced 20- to 30-page paper on his or her personal theory of family therapy and its relationship with the existing body of family therapy theory. This paper is then defended before the family therapy faculty and students. Application of the theory is demonstrated by presenting at least five videotaped therapy segments illustrating the precepts described in the paper. In addition, the student must also present research data indicating his or her effectiveness with at least one of the client families shown on videotape. Through these activities, once again, the domains of theory, practice, and research are linked in a meaningful way.

Clinical Practica

Perhaps not surprisingly, the 1984 survey of accredited programs revealed that client contact and supervision hours approximate AAMFT guidelines. Weekly direct client contact hours ranged from 2 to 15 hours, with a median of 8 to 10. Total client contact hours for the program depend on whether it offers the master's or the doctorate. The median for master's programs was 500 client contact hours (range, 250–800) and the median for doctoral programs was 950 hours (range, 480–1000).

The median number of individual supervision hours per week was 1.5. In addition, programs offered a weekly median of 2.5 hours of group supervision. Again, the total number of supervisory hours received would depend on the student's length of stay in the program. Based on the medians just reported, a typical student receives about 96 hours of individual supervision over two academic years (the time it typically takes to earn a master's degree), and 160 hours of group supervision during this same period. AAMFT regulations specify that supervision groups may not be larger than six students.

Table 14-1 notes the first, second, and third most commonly used supervision modalities in the 17 accredited programs. If one makes the assumption that the therapist's interaction with the family constitutes the "data" of supervision, and that the better modalities provide the supervisor with objective access to these data, then these results are encouraging. The two most subjective methods, review of case notes and case presentations, are used sparingly. Only two institutions reported case notes as the primary modality, and only 16% of the total votes cast for first, second, or third choices was shared by these two methods.

TABLE 14-1. Methods of Supervision in 17 AAMFT Accredited MFT Program

Method	First choice	Second choice	Third choice	Total votes
Review of case notes	2	1	1	4
Case presentations	0	2	2	4
Audiotape review	1	1	4	6
Videotape review	7	3	4	14
Live, feedback during session	7	4	1	12
Live, feedback after session	0	6	5	11
Total	17	17	17	51

Note: This table is based on a telephone survey of all accredited programs as of the spring of 1984. The reader should write for an up-to-date list of accredited programs from the Commission on Accreditation. The American Association for Marital and Family Therapy, 1717 K Street N.W., Washington, DC 20006.

Of the two mechanical means for gaining access to therapist–family interaction (audio and video recording) clearly the latter is more prevalent. In fact, the review of videotapes is tied with "live" supervision as the most popular first choice method, with 41% (7 of 17) of the programs reporting it as their first choice. This finding corroborates the Henry (1983) study in which university faculty also reported videotape review as the primary mode of supervision. In the 1984 study this method also gathered the largest number of first-, second-, and third-place total votes among the six methods.

Live supervision with feedback during the session was as popular as videotape review as a first-choice option. Taken together, the two forms of live supervision (totaling first, second, and third choices) are endorsed more than the mechanical or subjective methods. Forty-five percent (23 of 51) of the total vote was shared by the "live" methods. Of the two live modalities, it is also interesting that delayed feedback is a secondary choice to instant feedback; these data suggest that the intrusiveness of instant feedback has become quite acceptable. No program mentioned cotherapy or any additional modality among the top choices.

It is not the case that the type of supervision was dictated primarily by available facilities and equipment, since virtually all of the training programs have therapy rooms with observation windows, two-way phone connections between therapists and observers, and audio- and videotape equipment. However, the use of non-live methods was enhanced by the impracticality of observing all sessions. The majority of schools reported that they had an in-house family therapy clinic and that, in addition, students worked in community agency placements. In these contexts, live supervision was less likely. At the Purdue Family Therapy Center, for example, where live supervision is the norm, students videotape those sessions that are not observed.

As previously mentioned, the theoretical inclusiveness of these programs narrows somewhat at the clinical level. What actually occurs in practica is strongly influenced by the orientation of the particular supervisor. Even though these same persons may teach classroom theory courses, and cover orientations as divergent as psychodynamic and brief-strategic, it is rare that they employ these methods equally in their clinical work. On the other hand, I did not find a single accredited program in which only a single clinical orientation was practiced (as is the case with numerous free-standing institutes).

Training in Supervision

As previously mentioned almost all of the doctoral programs offer training in supervision.

The Purdue supervision seminar and practicum is among the more highly developed supervision sequences. It is predicated on the assumption that PhDs in family therapy will seldom function simply as therapists. More often they will pursue jobs that require them to supervise and train family therapists. This sequence is envisaged as a culmination of the student's clinical career at Purdue. It offers the student advanced training in the skills "meta" to therapy. In addition, it grounds the student in the theory, literature, and conceptual and research issues of the burgeoning field of supervision. Once again, theory, research, and practice are integrated.

The content track is met through a seminar that meets for two hours each week. Activities include the following:

1. Students prepare outlines and critiques of the major readings on supervision published during the past five years.
2. They write brief papers in response to a series of ten questions about supervision. This helps them to articulate their theory. For example:

    Question 2: What is the relationship between your theory of therapy and your theory of supervision? What are the implications of supervision? What are the implications of operating from a specific theoretical framework versus an eclectic approach?

    Question 6: What are the relative advantages and disadvantages of live supervision, case conferences, and the other modes of supervision?

    Question 9: Develop a plan for the assessment of your supervision. It should include methods for assessing your supervisory errors as well as strengths.

3. Students are asked to make an oral presentation on the theory and practice of the supervision of two of the faculty members in the department. This is completed after several weeks of observation of the faculty.
4. Students present their own goals as a supervisor, using the Goal Attainment Scaling format. These goals, developed early in the semester, are then used to evaluate progress at the end of the term.
5. Participants prepare a worksheet that a supervisor could use to help a therapist to increase his or her supervisory skills. One published model is by Schwartz (1981). For example, one student developed a worksheet to facilitate learning circular diagramming. Another prepared one on teaching positive connotation. Alternatively, students may develop a form for supervisory note taking, such as the one published by Heath (1983).

For the clinical track, two supervisors-in-training (students) are assigned to a supervisor-of-supervisors (faculty member). The supervisors-in-training are assigned to one of the practica at the on-campus Marriage and Family Therapy Center, which typically meets from 2:00 to 9:00 P.M. The supervisors-in-training and the supervisor-of-supervisors meet at the beginning and end of this time to discuss the progress of the therapists, specific issues that have arisen during the process of supervision, and group process (Constantine, Piercy, & Sprenkle, 1984). During the remainder of the time, the supervisors-in-training conduct the presession meetings with therapists, the live supervision of cases, and posttherapy feedback sessions. In addition, they typically meet with the therapist before supervision begins to establish a relationship, discuss the therapist's overall goals for supervision, and ascertain how the supervisor-in-training can be helpful. As cases progress, they also meet individually with the therapist as needed.

The supervisor-of-supervisors keeps the contact with the therapist to a minimum, and works through the supervisors-in-training. The supervisor-of-supervisors is not in the therapy room during the pre- and postsessions but, rather, remains in the observation booth to monitor the work of the supervisors-in-training. The supervisor-of-supervisors may, however, call in to make suggestions or provide support for the supervisors-in-training. The supervisors-in-training answer all such calls to ensure that there is little direct contact between therapist and supervisor-of-supervisors (Constantine, Piercy, & Sprenkle, 1984).

The Purdue faculty learned through somewhat painful experience the importance of maintaining appropriate hierarchical boundaries. As supervisors-of-supervisors, we initially made frequent direct suggestions to the therapists and undercut the supervisors-in-training. This undercutting took the form of making call-ins without consulting with the supervisors-in-training, interrupting and sometimes leading pre- and postsession conferences, and so on. That is, we extended our rather direct, active, and complementary role as supervisors to what should more appropriately be a more removed role of supervisor-of-supervisors. Not only did we undercut the supervisor-in-training, but we also confused the therapists, who had to cope with multiple layers of feedback (Constantine, Piercy, & Sprenkle, 1984).

Our training program is even more complex in that students who have completed the supervision sequence as described can enroll for training as a supervisor-of-supervisors. In this case the faculty member (an AAMFT-approved supervisor) supervises the advanced student supervising the supervisor-in-training. If this sounds extraordinarily complex, it is! Suffice it to say, however, that doctoral graduates may well be placed in administrative positions where the supervision-of-supervision will be an integral part of their job description.

CONCLUSIONS

The degree-granting program in family therapy is an idea whose time has come. The growth explosion of the past five years is likely to continue. While there are obstacles to the development of these programs, their expansion seems assured by the growth of family therapy itself as a unique professional identity. As long as this general trend continues, universities will offer programs that capitalize on this popular professional movement.

The more difficult question is whether the university programs will assume a position of leadership in the field. One issue I have struggled with is why so few prominent family therapy thinkers are on the faculties of the degree-granting programs. Do these current faculty members only respond to the professional ferment that is "out there," or could they be its catalyst?

One might argue that the conservatism of academia makes these settings less attractive. "Nonscholarly" theoretical publications on family therapy may be accorded low prestige in some settings, and may figure less in merit increases of salary than empirical articles in scholarly refereed journals (which tend not to engender fame as a family therapist!). "Big names" in the field may also find academic salaries and limitations on consulting unattractive.

Yet even when one uses a criterion of prominence that would seem to favor academicians—namely, citations in the Social Science Citation Index—current faculty are generally not well known. In the most recent prominence study (Textor, 1983), only the 33rd and 37th place (on a list of over 50 of the most frequently cited authors) were held by faculty members from the degree-granting family therapy programs. One might be tempted to argue that while academia encourages publishing in general, perhaps it does not encourage publishing in family therapy because the field is still "too unscientific." Yet many of the names in the top 20 (e.g., Gerald Patterson, 1; Alan Gurman, 5; Neil Jacobson, 7; Bernard Guerney, 17; and James Alexander, 19) work in other (not MFT degree-granting) academic settings.

The most logical (and perhaps gracious) explanation is the relative youth of these programs and their faculties. All but two of them have been in existence, in their present form, a decade or less. Current budgeting restrictions will not allow the hiring of established senior persons from other settings or programs. These people, without generous offers, are understandably reluctant to move. Only time will tell, then, whether the assistant and associate professors who dominate the MFT degree programs will become major contributors to the field.

The maturity of the field itself will also determine the extent to which their contributions are valued. So long as the most prestige is accorded to charismatic clinicians whose wizardry at workshops and glibness at the typewriter is prima facie evidence of their effectiveness, these young scholar/clinicians will appear to be lightweights. Their work will, perforce, be less flashy, more tentative, slower, and less likely to breed discipleship.

In the long run, however, these same limitations contain the seeds of promise. The maturity of family therapy as a discipline, and its place in the mental health field generally, will depend on its ability to move beyond the pronouncement of true believers to authenticate its efficacy (Schwartz & Breunlin, 1982). The university programs are giving people the tools to carry out this task. Perhaps it will be decades before it bears fruit.

At the level of theory, not being "true believers" of one theory poses another challenge for these programs: Can they avoid the opposite role of assuming a wide-eyed eclecticism (Liddle, 1982)? As Piercy (1984) reminds us, "if eclecticism means just mixing together various theories, the result can be an intellectually indigestible stew of half-baked ideas" (p. 21). While encouraging students to examine critically the various theories, these programs must also encourage them to develop a coherent theory of change, which can serve as a lens through which to view the therapeutic process. If that lens is too fragmented, nothing can be seen clearly and the trainee stumbles.

These struggles, then, around the interfaces of research, theory, and practice are what the degree programs are all about. If clinical supervision is synonymous with training, then let these programs die. Students can see more clients and have more time for supervision elsewhere. The other demands of the curriculum will only get in the way.

If, on the other hand, the basic assumption of these programs is true, the eventual result will be exciting: family therapy theory that is grounded and relevant, family therapy research linked to both theoretical principles and application, and family therapy practice guided by both a coherent rationale and objective assessment (Sprenkle, 1976).

Acknowledgment

The author wishes to express appreciation to Nicholas Aradi for his assistance in the research for this chapter.

References

American Association for Marriage and Family Therapy. (1981). *Marriage and family therapy annual on accreditation.* Washington, DC: Author.

Bloch, D., & Weiss, H. (1981). Training facilities in marital and family therapy. *Family Process, 20,* 133-146.

Broderick, C. B., & Schrader, S. S. (1981). The history of professional marriage and family therapy. In A. S. Gurman & D. P. Kniskern (Eds.), *Handbook of family therapy.* New York: Brunner/Mazel.

Constantine, J., Piercy, F., & Sprenkle, D. (1984). Live supervision-of-supervision in family therapy. *Journal of Marital and Family Therapy, 10,* 95-98.

Everett, C. (1979). The master's degree in marriage and family therapy. *Journal of Marriage and Family Therapy, 5,* 7-13.

Garfield, R. (1979). An integrative training model for family therapists: The Hahnemann master of family therapy program. *Journal of Marital and Family Therapy, 5,* 15-22.

Hall, R. (1968). Professionalization and bureaucratization. *American Sociological Review, 33,* 92-99.

Heath, A. (1983). The live supervision form: Structure and theory for assessment in live supervision. In B. Keeney (Ed.), *Diagnosis and assessment in family therapy.* Rockville, MD: Aspen.

Henry, P. (1983). *The family therapy profession: University and institute perspectives.* Unpublished doctoral dissertation, Purdue University.

Joanning, H., & Castle, S. (1983). *AAMFT directory of marriage and family therapy graduate programs and training centers.* Washington, DC: AAMFT.

Kiresuk, T. J., & Sherman, R. E. (1968). Goal attainment scaling: A general method for evaluating comprehensive community mental health programs. *Community Mental Health Journal, 4,* 443-453.

L'Abate, L., Berger, M., Wright, L., & O'Shea, M. (1979). Training family psychologists: The family studies program at Georgia State University. *Professional Psychology, 10,* 58-65.

Larson, M. S. (1977). *The rise of professionalism: A sociological analysis.* Berkeley: University of California Press.

Liddle, H. (1978). The emotional and political hazards of teaching and learning family therapy. *Family Therapy, 5,* 1-12.

Liddle, H. (1982). On the problems of eclecticism: A call for epistemologic clarification and human-scale theories. *Family Process, 21,* 243-250.

Liddle, H., & Saba, G. (1982). Teaching family therapy at the introductory level: A model emphasizing a pattern which connects training and therapy. *Journal of Marital and Family Therapy, 8,* 63-72.

Nichols, W. (1979a). Doctoral programs in marital and family therapy. *Journal of Marital and Family Therapy, 5,* 23-28.

Nichols, W. (1979b). Education of marriage and family therapists: Some trends and implications. *Journal of Marital and Family Therapy, 5,* 19-28.

Olson, D. (1976). Bridging research, theory, and application: The triple threat in science. In D. Olson (Ed.), *Treating relations.* Lake Mills, IA: Graphic.

Peterson, J. (1968). Marriage counseling: Past, present and future. In J. Peterson (Ed.), *Marriage and family counseling: Perspective and proposal.* New York: Association Press.

Piercy, F. (1984). The true believer and the eclectic. *The Family Therapy Networker, 8,* 21.

Piercy, F., & Sprenkle, D. (1983). Ethical, legal, and professional issues in family therapy: A graduate level course. *Journal of Marital and Family Therapy, 9,* 393–402.

Piercy, F., & Sprenkle, D. (1984). The process of family therapy education. *Journal of Marital and Family Therapy, 10,* 337–349.

Schwartz, R. (1981). The conceptual development of family therapy trainees. *American Journal of Family Therapy, 9,* 89–90.

Schwartz, R., & Breunlin, D. (1982). Why clinicians should bother with research. *The Family Therapy Networker, 7,* 22–27.

Sprenkle, D. H. (1976). The need for integration among therapy, research, and practice in the family field. *Family Coordinator, 24,* 261–263.

Sprenkle, D., & Piercy, F. (1984). Research in family therapy: A graduate level course. *Journal of Marital and Family Therapy, 10,* 226–240.

Textor, M. (1983). An assessment of prominence in the family therapy field. *Journal of Marital and Family Therapy, 9,* 317–320.

Winkle, C. W., Piercy, F., & Hovestadt, A. (1981). A curriculum for graduate-level marriage and family therapy education. *Journal of Marital and Family Therapy, 7,* 201–210.

15

Born Free: The Life Cycle of a Free-Standing Postgraduate Training Institute

FREDDA HERZ
BETTY CARTER
The Family Institute of Westchester, Mt. Vernon, New York

During the 1960s and 1970s family therapy training increased dramatically. The number of postdegree training institutes more than doubled in 20 years, indicating a widespread impulse in the field for independence from the constraints of more traditional educational facilities. This trend mirrors the thrust of family therapy as a "new" method of treatment, designed to transcend the limitations of more conventional techniques. Yet despite this remarkable growth, the number of unallied programs still remained less than half that of programs connected to institutions, such as universities, clinics, and hospitals (Bloch & Weiss, 1981). Given the challenges such a venture presented to the authors and others when they founded the Family Institute of Westchester (FIW), this smaller number is understandable. However, since FIW did ultimately prove to be a viable means to further our own professional growth, and that of the next generation of family therapists, we believed it worthwhile to examine the obstacles we encountered, and to offer some insight into the predictable crises in the life cycle of a free-standing family therapy training institute.

WHY DO SUCH INSTITUTES DEVELOP?

What do such institutions offer their founders that institutionally based programs do not? Why do their numbers remain relatively small? In any area of life, there are always people unhappy with the status quo, who because of their own inherent needs feel pushed by outside circumstances to press beyond the limits of that which has already been established. These people are looking for something else, and, as often happens, find it in themselves. Ours is a culture with a very recent pioneer history that has valued individuality and the spirit of entrepreneurship.

One answer to the above questions lies in the tendency in a field such as family therapy to be creative, and in a desire to be unfettered by the strictures and structures of bureaucracy. Founders of family training institutes are generally entrepreneurial types who wish to seize the opportunity to make traditions instead of being constrained by them, and it seems that most postgraduate centers grow out of the strong need of talented professionals to escape the limitations of mental health bureaucracies where family

249

therapy is, at best, a fringe activity, and at worst an anathema. Thus, new centers are established as much for the trainers as for the trainees. Certainly FIW is an example of this, since it developed mostly from the professional and personal needs of the founding group.

While the desire to be free of institutional constraints often motivates the founding of a new training business, it is certainly not sufficient cause in and of itself. Another key ingredient is the founders' willingness to take risks with their time and money. Founders are a peculiar breed of people who are able to ignore the actual costs of establishing a new venture because they view it as an important opportunity. They believe they have something—a product or a service—peculiar to themselves. They gamble with financial and personal resources because it is important to their personal and/or professional sense of self. This lack of focus on money seems to be necessary to begin such a business, and a major reason for the demise of so many of them. With the old adage "time is money" being so true in a profession where one's major source of income is related to the number of client-hours billed, and or based on a 40-hour week in a salaried position, the two factors are naturally intertwined. It therefore seems appropriate to address the issue of resources in a dollars-and-cents framework, even in the context of social services, where money is a closet topic.

Money tends to be a disreputable subject among all mental health professionals, family therapists included. The business world, which measures success by money, tends to be disparaged by our field. Part of the disrepute of money and business evolved logically from the focus on "helping" in the mental health professions. Historically, it has been viewed as difficult and, at times, immoral to charge for helping. Those (mostly women) with a background in social work—a field of service steeped in the tradition of Jane Addams and Hull House—may be even more susceptible than either psychiatrists or psychologists (mostly men) to this way of thinking. Since family therapy includes a great many social workers, this influence carries a great deal of weight.

The disrepute of money and business for family therapists also derives from another factor; that, in spite of male leadership, we are mainly a women's profession. Women's work has traditionally been underpaid and undervalued by working women themselves and others, and unpaid or underpaid work by women is a major factor in the viability of most family institutes. These factors combine to unfocus the money and business aspect of establishing an institute. However, the issue of money (i.e., financial solvency) quickly rears its head and becomes *the* ongoing central dilemma. The failure to think through and resolve this issue is the major reason for the failure of new programs.

How to do quality training and research while remaining financially solvent was the major ongoing dilemma cited by respondents to an informal survey of free-standing institutes. The exact definition of solvency may vary, but generally the cost of running the training program must be offset by the income produced. Institutes reported a variety of income-producing tactics, each with its own assets and liabilities. Only four institutes balanced this equation solely with income from training. The others had to devise other methods to offset costs through such means as clinic fees, grants, and/or other forms of fund raising. The liabilities and encumbrances of each of these methods may lead to the failure of the system. The reliance on training as the major income source limits the ability of the program to grow, because every attempt to increase the size and the quality of the product increases costs. However, it does keep finances clear and simple. Counting on clinic fees also involves increased costs in terms of space and supervision and often increases the overhead costs far above the net profit. Grants increase income without increasing costs; however, it is dangerous to seek financial stability from grant money because such money is difficult to secure and hard to maintain.

So while money may not be the initial reason for establishing a training business, it is the central issue in maintaining one. The money issue must be addressed in such a way as to establish a viable organization with clearly defined jobs and membership rules, and adequate rewards for work performed. An organization without these elements may survive, but it will do so without achieving the very freedom initially sought by the founders. Instead, it will tend to become a closed system with few new ideas or creativity, no turnover at the top, and burnout and endless turnover in junior positions.

This chapter presents a model for understanding the evolution of an institute from an idea about freedom from bureaucracy into a business that, by becoming both financially solvent and well organized, ultimately frees its staff to do training and other professional tasks. Toward this end, the authors will discuss the life cycle of a free-standing institute and the development and marketing of its product: family therapy training.

LIFE CYCLE OF AN INSTITUTE

We have come to believe that free-standing institutes have a predictable life cycle with definable phases and tasks. Like every system, a training institute must evolve an organization and financial structure that is flexible yet structured, and that permits the entry, growth, and departure of members (both trainees and faculty).

There is a tendency for new training organizations and their founders to function more like a family than a business. In fact, they function much like a family business. While the pioneer spirit may be sufficient to cause people to join forces, it is very much akin to the phase of "falling in love," which establishes a new family-of-origin for future generations. Love is grand, but you can't live on it. And if a new system is born out of ideals, it is money that keeps it together, or creates the issues that may destroy it. Indeed, difficulties throughout the course of the life cycle of an institution seem to evolve from the failure to acknowledge and deal with the differences between a family and a business organization in terms of goals, structures, operational procedures, and boundary mainte-nance. It is important to elaborate these differences as they form the fabric of the training institute life cycle.

The Family and the Business

While families are in the business of caring for and developing people, businesses have as their primary goal the production of some task, product, or service for financial profit. Historically, part of the confusion of educational programs, training institutes included, has been that, while businesses, they also have not-for-profit goals that are also oriented toward the development of people. Excessive focus on people and relationships bogs down a business with concern for personal issues, preventing necessary business decisions. On the other hand, a business that loses sight of nonfinancial values also loses business because of low employee morale (Pasquale, 1978). The founders' emphasis on personal relationships, therefore, may hinder the movement of the system toward defining organizational goals and operational procedures. Furthermore, if the founders are already personally connected, and if the group is small, there is even greater difficulty in deciding the organizational hierarchy and enforcing competence as the requirement for membership.

Although, increasingly, businesses are giving attention to the quality of life of their employees, the goal of such activities is measured in greater productivity. But when the "product" is the functioning of trainees, and their eventual influence on the functioning of clients, how does one define "more and better," and how is this definition related to profit-and-loss statements?

Competence is a major determinant of membership in a business; that is, if one cannot do the job, one is fired or is not hired. However, in organizations that function more as enmeshed emotional systems or families, consideration of competence becomes difficult and the ability to hire and fire is impaired. In such organizations, the criteria for maintaining membership are not explicit, and loyalty and trust glue the structure together. In a business-like organization, the ability to expand or decrease membership on the basis of shared goals and competence of the members is of utmost importance. In fact, the similarity of goals among the founders will enable them to pull together to do "more than their share" in the early phases of business development. Founders are generally colleagues who share relationships based on mutual interests that may extend into their personal lives. They empathize with each other by virtue of similar complaints and parallel situations. They may have been trained in the same setting. More important, they are midwives to the same birthing process, and have the benefit of common experience to bind them together. As professionals, they may also be at the same life cycle stage in their careers.

To the degree that a free-standing institute is based on personal relationshps and goal congruence of the founders, the more likely it is that the institute will function as a family (Pfeiser & Wooten, 1983). Similar to the problems presented in a family by the marriage of offspring and the need to integrate spouses of children, there are basic differences between the founders and anyone else who might wish to join at a later time.

During the first three years, it is possible for the enthusiasm and spirit of "family" to hold the organization together. During later phases of business development, however, a lack of congruence between the goals of the founders and those of new members often creates another set of problems. Once the organization achieves some initial success, the pioneers tire, and the day-to-day grind of running the organization sets in. Now it is likely that the founders' mode of operation will begin to be questioned by newcomers, and the honeymoon of the pioneers' relationships comes down to earth. At that time, the congruence of goals, both personal and professional, will be called into doubt. It is only later, depending on how this crisis is handled, that a real organization develops. The authors have delineated three phases that we believe describe the movement of a training organization from its founding "family" stage to a stage of some stability and viability: (1) the pioneer phase—The work of idealists; (2) keeping the system going—The dawning of reality; and (3) moving on—becoming an organization.

THE PIONEER PHASE

To understand something about the start-up of any organization, it is important to consider the tasks that must be accomplished. When these are considered, it becomes clear why relatively few begin such an enterprise, and why even fewer continue it over a long period of time. There is no direct relationship between the size of the planned training organization and the number of tasks or the amount of work necessary to establish it. Start-up tasks are numerous, and include the development of a product, the procurement of space and equipment, financing start-up and operating costs, public relations, marketing, and office work connected with the above. The work in each of these areas depends partly on the initial circumstances. For instance, if the training program grows out of the private practices of a group of therapists, then finding space may not be a major concern. Certainly, unless people have been teaching or practicing together for a long time, the amount of work necessary to put together a product (the training program) agreeable to all is immense. In comparison, other tasks at first may appear relatively easy. For instance, the initial pool of trainees can be recruited from the supervisory groups and professional contacts of the founding faculty. However, some attention must be paid to public relations and marketing if there is to be a continuing pool of applicants.

The development of curricula, recruitment, and most of the work in this phase is conducted according to an unbalanced efficiency model. It is interesting to consider the working assumptions of our own beginning at FIW.

Seven of us began the Family Institute of Westchester (FIW) in 1977, with $800, much idealism, and a tremendous amount of energy. Several ideals guided our initial formation. The first was that we would only teach and participate in the training program to the degree that we wanted. This meant that we would have a program the size of which was dictated by our interests, not by financial need. Another corollary of this assumption was that we would not work to support the organization; rather, the organization would exist to support our work. Our organization's goal was to foster our own professional development. In terms of budget, we functioned for most of this phase without one. We had decided that none of us would receive a salary, but each would receive an hourly teaching fee instead. We believed that we could keep financial burdens small and prevent individual financial dependency on the organization, with faculty free to come and go as they wished. The third rule about finances also served to re-inforce the democratic spirit of the founding group. We decided that everyone would receive the same hourly fee for teaching, and we didn't allocate any fee for administrative work.

Most new businesses are financed by capital from the owner/founder(s), and their friends and relatives (Churchill & Lewis, 1983), and ours was no different. During this phase, the strategy is simple and short-term: to stay alive (Churchill & Lewis, 1983). The owner/founder(s) of the business perform all the important tasks and provide all the energy, direction, and capital. The spirit of the pioneer phase can be characterized as voluntary cooperation. In the case of FIW, this meant doing what needed to be done toward the common goal of establishing a place for training. There is little time available for considering how the organization should run in terms of its structure, nor is there any long-term planning in the area of guidelines or policies and procedures. Business practices, including a budget, are nonexistent. Decisions are often made by an informal process among founders.

For instance, at FIW, we had a quasi-organizational structure, an executive committee, which was responsible for the day-to-day operations. But overall we still thought of ourselves as peers, and decisions were made by consensus. There was no such thing as payment for organizational jobs well done in the first phase. The keynote of making a new business go is *sacrifice*, personal and financial. The founders of FIW struggled to make ends meet, not paying themselves appropriately and working twice as hard in their clinical practices to make up for the loss of income from so many "free" hours. Often, the families of the founders found them unavailable and preoccupied with their colleagues and the business. A frequent joke was that the "free" in free-standing stood for "free labor." While the organization was initially intended to promote the professional growth of the founders, it was impossible to promote growth when so much effort was being expended in survival. It is not until much later in organizational development that an organization can promote the founders' growth.

KEEPING THE SYSTEM GOING: THE DAWNING OF REALITY

The second phase of organizational development occurs when the business breaks out of "resource poverty" and onto a plateau of success (Pfeiser & Wooten, 1983). During this phase a developmental dilemma may occur: now the business either moves ahead or remains stable and profitable (Churchill & Lewis, 1983). In small retail, service, or manufacturing businesses, how this phase is managed may depend largely on the personality of the founder, or the balance of personalities of a group of founders. Partners are faced with internal changes, such as the need to integrate new employees, or find larger facilities. They also encounter external changes, such as the shifting market for their product or service, or the fluctuating cost of borrowing money. The enterprise having proved viable, decisions made at this point usually mark the attempt of the small business to break away from the "just making a living" mind set. Without a solid organizational structure, they become vulnerable to the slightest error in calculation.

The parallel situation in a nonprofit training institute may be the choice between a continued push versus merely staying afloat. Partners may begin to quarrel over goals or means, or one founder may experience burnout or a personal or family crisis which then directly affects the others, who have very little leeway in their busy schedules for emergencies. Symptoms appear in the organization and its relationships. With communication channels clouded by the myth of togetherness, and no firm structure to handle change, poor business decisions are likely. Most businesses are lost during this phase because of the failure of the founder(s) to handle power and responsibility appropriately in the conflicts and issues that inevitably arise.

Conflicts in nonprofit organizations are similar to difficulties encountered in professional associations of lawyers, physicians, and dentists, but may be magnified by virtue of economic strains. With the continued downplay of material rewards in favor of service among the founders, it becomes hard to find competent new professionals to expand the ranks. At the same time, the fervor of the founders' original vision may have cooled with the reality of long hours and minimal pay.

The "third-year crisis," as we've come to call it, heralds the need for system change, development, and reorganization. To keep the system going, more than the spirit of "voluntary cooperation" is necessary. For a free-standing training institute the tasks are to establish operating principles and structures to deal with the internal and external changes of the system.

External Changes. In considering the question of the third-year crisis for training institutes, the larger fields of mental health and family therapy cannot be ignored. Many family therapy training programs, free-standing institutes included, began during the 1970s, the heyday of family therapy. During that decade, there were few wrong decisions one could make in expanding training programs. Large conferences and workshops could always recruit trainees and increase the financial solvency of the sponsoring organizations. The 1980s ushered in a decade of settling down. No longer a therapy fad, family therapy had become a small field attracting only those interested in pursuing serious training. At the same time, the mental health field as a whole was receiving less government support, and training was severely curtailed by funding cutbacks. Thus, with broad enthusiasm waning and limited government funds, the competition for trainees was increasing. These external changes increased the stress on young institutes, and for FIW they added our own growing financial concerns, which reached crisis proportions when we were forced to seek new housing.

Internal Changes. Although the internal pressures experienced by FIW were specific (e.g., the necessity of finding new offices), we believe their effects to be typical enough that readers can extrapolate the general picture of how internal pressures affect similar training institutes.

By the end of our third year, the founders were tired and were looking for someone else to help in the routine tasks of running the organization. The need for new faculty was obvious. Since the organization had functioned mainly as a family, however, the question of how new members could join became an issue. Newcomers to an established organization have greater expectations of what they can gain from it than what they can give to it (Churchill & Lewis, 1983; Pfeiser & Wooten, 1983). Often, the pioneers, whose motto had been, "Sacrifice," viewed this as a flaw in the newcomers' attitude rather than in the organizational structure. The real problem was that without a clear organizational structure, and a more effective decision-making process, there was lack of clarity about jobs, levels of responsibility, and status within the organization. Thus, when new faculty or staff joined, they were supposedly peers—equal participants in all aspects of the organization. The difficulty was that they were not peers in terms of commitment, willingness to "sacrifice," and professional experience. They typically began to feel "abused" whenever they received less, or were asked to give more, than they had expected.

When the rules for new member participation in a professional organization are not clear, the new faculty are often unwilling to stay once they find out what is expected of them. Furthermore, if the founders' expectations for their involvement remain in the unspecified spirit of "voluntary cooperation," the new members may never understand why the connection didn't work out. As the issues of workload, membership, and hierarchy rear their heads, the myths of the early organization begin to tremble and fall.

The idealism of the founders falters. The original goal of the institute, that the founders be able to grow and develop professionally, is submerged under the need to make the organization run and remain financially solvent.

During this phase, the FIW founders attempted to keep the organization going by dealing with each crisis as it arose. Little attention was paid to the more serious structural or organizational issues that created the crises. The *modus operandi* was the same as in the first phase—*summon up more energy, more enthusiasm, and more cooperation* to deal with the crisis at hand. We didn't realize that the crises, themselves, evolved from the need to shift into a different mode of operation. The solutions during this phase were *first-order attempts at resolving problems*; more of the same—temporary solutions. They postponed the deeper shifts in organizational structure that were needed. The following list, though not exhaustive, explores typical first-order solutions found in small businesses and attempted by our own and other institutes.

First-Order Solutions. If the crisis focuses on power issues that challenge the leader(s), the "troublemakers" may be expelled after an intense struggle. In this situation, the system will usually close down to prevent a similar threat in the future. If the crisis involves a power struggle among fairly matched sides, fueled by strong emotions or hurt, a situation akin to divorce occurs. The split is intense and bitter and sometimes disguised as "ideological." The intensity of the split is directly related to the intensity of the original idealization of the founders' relationships. Such splits usually result in two separate systems, which then start the life cycle anew, but with a strong tendency to remain closed and self-protective. Development may be arrested at the "Mom and Pop" or "cult" structure, resembling those training centers started by the "masters" and their disciples. These institutes are usually small, authoritarian, and often subject to contained power struggles for second or "favorite son" position. The cult structure is quite stable during the lifetime of the master, but will experience a severe crisis at the time of his or her death or retirement. The family therapy training field is relatively young, and therefore has experienced only a few retirements/successions. One such occurred early on with the death of Nathan Ackerman. The institute that bears his name continues to function partly because a well chosen board of trustees was able to provide continued financing, and partly because Ackerman's successor, Don Bloch, had the vision to assemble a creative and talented faculty. Ackerman had put in place an organizational structure that is surviving him.

The second succession of note occurred recently, with Salvador Minuchin's retirement from the Philadelphia Child Guidance Clinic. Because his organization was embedded in a larger hospital structure, it, too, survived administratively when he left. The transition was made smoother through a gradual "leave taking," until Minuchin finally relocated in New York City. He certainly groomed a number of people to take over his position at the Child Guidance Clinic. It will be interesting, however, to see over the coming years whether the Philadelphia Child Guidance Clinic is able to hold its prominent place in the field without him.

If an organization's crisis focuses mainly on financial issues, the group will often pull together in an effort to forestall an organizational collapse. Special fund-raising efforts, seeking grants, reducing or delaying fees—these are all first-order methods by which a group tries to buy time and delay further crisis development.

Both the origins of FIW's financial problems (in our excessively democratic decision-making process) and our method of handling the financial crisis (to cease paying faculty for the rest of the year) heralded the need for reorganization. The founders took the nonpayment in stride, but new faculty members were dismayed, and not up for cheerful self-sacrifice as the price for membership. Reorganization undoubtedly would have occurred at this point, except for the eviction notice, which postponed the internal crisis by pulling the group together to face the outside threat to survival. The founders went back into high gear looking for a new home ("more of the same").

MOVING ON: BECOMING AN ORGANIZATION

An organization may persist for several years in a state of crisis before any significant change occurs. The need to move from "more of the same" solutions to new ones becomes clear after a few years of heroics. A change in structure, a *second-order solution*, becomes necessary. The creation of an organizational structure with a clear hierarchy, an efficient decision-making process, operational procedures in the form of policies, roles with clearly defined tasks and rewards, and rules for membership, entrances, and exits— all these permit the members to function more productively and with less tension. The alternatives enumerated below involve various changes to the organizational structure of an institute. Each has its own costs and benefits. The process of this reorganization is the major task of this phase.

One alternative is the establishment of a board of trustees, which has the purpose of fund raising. This alternative frees the director and faculty from financial woes so they can attend to the work of training. Since most free-standing institutes are founded and run by mental health professionals who are often neither adept nor interested in fund raising, they may see a board as giving them valuable time to perform preferred professional duties. Paradoxically, the time and energy necessary to recruit a board are immense, and the director may now spend most of his or her time dealing with the board. Another possible cost of this alternative is a triangle involving the board, the director, and the staff, where issues center on who is to control the destiny of the organization—professional staff or board, with the director usually caught in the middle.

Some free-standing institutes affiliate with a larger organization, such as a hospital or university. This solution solves some of the financial and workload issues, but it usually ends the free-standing status of the institute. The price tag is that the institute now becomes one subunit of a larger organization, subject to its rules and parameters. This solution benefits a founding generation that is either worn out or that has reached its goal in terms of personal and professional growth. As the competition for trainees and money increases, and as the need for legitimate family systems research continues, mergers between larger organizations and free-standing institutes begin to have more potential benefits for both.

The third and most difficult solution involves restructuring the system in ways that move it toward a hierarchical yet democratic organization, with (1) enough rules for stability; (2) enough flexibility to attract competent, self-motivated staff with energy to create income; and (3) enough openness to permit easy entry and exit to and from the system. Such a solution, in whatever form it takes, must deal with the financial, power, and workload issues equitably. The FIW developed one form of this alternative during our sixth year of operation (see Table 15-1), following three years of pioneering and three years of crises.

RESTRUCTURING THE FAMILY INSTITUTE OF WESTCHESTER

The key to our reorganization was our final letting go of the myth of "peers" and recognizing that we were, in fact, a hierarchical group. We reinvented the "grandfather clause," deciding that we, as founders, could agree among ourselves about our own membership rules, but everyone else who had joined since the founding, or would join in the future, would be *required* to rent office space in the building for two days a week at a very moderate rate. This rule allowed the founders to continue their "uneven" but satisfactory methods of financial contribution to the organization, while *requiring* an even contribution from the postfounding members. This rule relieved the newer members of the anxious feeling that "something more" was always expected of them but was never enough.

The reorganization also gave our old administrative titles full power for the first time, and transferred the decision-making process from the now mythical "group of peers" to the reconstituted executive committee under the leadership of the director. The new membership rule gave us a functional financial structure for the first time since the eviction and change of offices, which had dramatically increased our overhead. The business of the organization returned to the director, the administrator, and the executive committee. This permitted the group as a whole to return to the professional meetings and projects we had enjoyed in our first years. The narrow title of "faculty" was redefined as "staff," so that researchers, clinicians, and creative experimenters could join the organization without a teaching requirement or concern about theoretical orientation. This distinction also allows faculty to take a sabbatical or quit teaching without having to leave the organization. The faculty are now drawn from the staff at the invitation of the director of training. It was made easy to start any project of interest (as long as funding could be self-generated). It was also made easy for newcomers to "try us" for a year before commitment, and for old members to leave without guilt about the institute's survival. Almost as soon as our financial and membership issues got settled, there was an influx of new staff, who have contributed greatly to the general spirit of vitality that prevails. Full staff meetings became interesting again, and the smaller faculty group arranged to meet separately to continue the task that has always been our main interest—development of quality training for family therapists. Integrating the principle that quality training does *not* pay for itself allowed us to develop an organizational structure that supports training rather than attempting to have training support the organization.

The net effect of the structural changes has been immense. The administrators get paid a little something and have the authority as well as the responsibility in their designated areas. Faculty are paid for teaching at a higher-than-average rate per hour, and all our staff have a forum to exchange ideas, as well as a sponsor for projects they wish to conduct. Morale appears high, and staff members are energetic and creative. Our overhead is carried by office rentals (36%), trainee tuitions (34%), clinic patient fees (13%), fund raising (11%), special seminars (4%), and grants (2%).

TABLE 15-1. Family Institute of Westchester Table of Organization (1983–1984)

Director: *Betty Carter, MSW
Director of Administration: Lillian Fine, BA

Director of Training:
*Fredda Herz, PhD
Assistant to the Director of Training

Faculty

Intensive Training:
Fredda Herz, PhD
Demaris Jacob, PhD
Elliott Rosen, EdD
Judy Stern Peck, MSW
Natalie Schwartzberg, MSW
Pamela Young, MSW

Faculty Supervisors:
Fredda Herz, PhD
*Monica McGoldrick, MSW

Extern and Advanced Faculty:
Betty Carter, MSW
Fredda Herz, PhD
Monica McGoldrick, MSW

Director of Clinical Services:
Judy Stern Peck, MSW

Director of FIW Clinical Projects:
Adele Holman, DSW

Staff Projects:

Research Consultant: Demaris Jacob, PhD
Staff-at-Large: Vincent Androsiglio, MSW
    Henry Berger, MD

Delayed Launching Study:
Director: *Kenneth G. Terkelsen, MD
    Jennifer Manocherian, MS

Divorce Mediation Project:
Director: Jennifer Manocherian, MS

Postdivorce Treatment Study:
Director: Judy Stern Peck, MSW
    Jeniffer Manocherian, MS
    Monica McGoldrick, MSW
    Betty Carter, MSW

Holocaust Survivors Study:
Director: Fredda Herz, PhD

Family Business Project:
Director: Pamela Young, MSW
    Fredda Herz, PhD

Computerized Genogram Project:
Director: Randy Gerson, PhD
    Monica McGoldrick, MSW

Child Abuse Project:
Director: Natalie Schwartzberg, MSW

*Remaining founders.

259

In December 1984, one of the founders retired, knowing her job would be continued by new staff members. Since then two of the original founders have also retired, with their roles and functions being readily carried on by new members. Although the remaining founders, two of whom (the authors) hold key positions (director and director of training), have not retired, our plan is to arrange an orderly transfer of power that will permit the organization to continue. Until that actually occurs, we cannot be said to have achieved full organizational stability.

Once the place of training was defined in our overall structure, there followed a more rapid and focused development of the training program. Furthermore, once the training program was no longer the possession of the founder(s), it became everyone's responsibility. The director of training experienced a new sense of responsibility to develop training and, since their participation was more clearly defined, the faculty also had a renewed sense of commitment. The very definition of who the teachers were began to change once staff members did not have to teach to remain connected with the institute. Those who were interested in teaching and who were asked to do so by the director of training became more actively involved in refining our product: the training program. While a free-standing institute means the freedom to be creative and innovative in teaching and learning, the paradox that develops is that without a clearly defined organization structure, such freedom does not exist.

Development of a Product: A Family Therapy Training Program

The major challenge for a free-standing institute is deciding what to offer trainees. Few small businesses have such a problem; a plant store obviously sells plants. Defining goals and objectives in education, particularly when personal growth is involved, is an arduous task for which mental health professionals are ill prepared. It is much easier to be a family therapist than to decide how to train others to be family therapists. It is even harder to decide how to do this as a group, trying to reach some consensus on objectives and how to accomplish them. In the field of family therapy the task of defining goals and objectives has often been bypassed, partly because of the newness of the field and partly because most of the training programs have developed on the basis of a major theorist's model. However, without faculty concurrence in the training objectives and teaching model, trainees often become disgruntled and unclear about what they are expected to do with families. Not only does training take longer when a dependable progression of knowledge and skills is not made explcit, but also faculty are often frustrated in their teaching and supervision by a lack of clarity and focus. Such a lack of clarity often leads to tension, and eventually uproar, in either the trainee or the faculty group, and usually has a ripple effect on recruitment if either of these groups remains displeased. We cannot emphasize enough that the time spent on this effort is essential to the organization's survival.

Establishing training objectives for the development of knowledge, clinical skills, and the use of self can be approached in many ways. The current literature has defined a few methods that elucidate the process of training (Falicov, Constantine, & Breunlin, 1981; Liddle, 1980; Tomm & Wright, 1979). Each teaches a model of family treatment that integrates various theories and focuses on the development of clinical judgment in the trainee. The need for integrated models has evolved in part from the AAMFT criteria for postgraduate institutes and partly from the focus in the field on clarifying similarities and differences between various models (Sluzki, 1983).

At FIW the process of writing objectives was made easier because all of us had worked together at training before and were in general agreement about our ideas. Objectives needed to be written, evaluated, and revised periodically for them to be clear to trainees, and later to new faculty. Writing objectives and evaluation tools began in earnest in our second year. The objectives covered five components of the process of family therapy: engagement, assessment, treatment planning, treatment, and termination and/or referral.

The length and structure of a training program become clearer when one begins by elucidating goals and objectives. Still, some areas may need to be defined by trial and error. We learned by what did or did not work for us in our own training. We constructed programs that built on its good points and made it better. Details of a program, such as the size of the supervision groups, the amount of supervision, the ratio of supervision to didactic presentation, and the ratio of individual to group supervision, are often factors that are decided by the "what works" principle. For instance, at FIW, experimentation taught us that a supervision group of five is optimal, but that a group of four (but not six) can also work. We also found that trainees need almost an even amount of time in supervision and theory. This may result in part from the level of experience and training of the trainees, and we are continuously rethinking and altering ideas based on trainees' learning needs.

When a program is based on the commitment and investment of the total faculty group, rather than on the model or fame of *one* teacher supervisor, it often seems to fare better in terms of program development. Each faculty member is committed to developing a program that functions well, not just to carrying out a model developed by others. The abilty to be creative typically spreads to areas other than the training program. With a clearer sense of purpose, faculty are free to develop other clinical interests, and have them become a part of the training endeavor. In our experience, a wide range of projects can be developed, the potential of which for assisting recruitment and funding is very impressive.

The Market Trends and Marketing

Over the past several years overall attendance at large conferences has decreased, as the field moves from the "fad" phase to a phase of serious interest in family therapy supervision and training. At the same time, successful conferences have been held for those who apply systems theory to nontherapeutic work with clients, for instance, family physicians and business consultants. Since recruitment to training programs was once done through large conferences, this change necessitates new recruitment strategies and training curricula.

Without an organizational structure that supports training (rather than burdens it), there is little possibility for a free-standing institute to ride the wave of these trends by preparing curriculum or conferences to meet it. Faculty need the creative freedom and organizational support to develop program(s) to meet the changing needs of the field.

Furthermore, having the financial leeway to experiment is of the utmost importance. Such leeway is absent when a training program carries the burden of supplying the main income source.

Public Relations and More Marketing Skills

One measure of a successful and high-quality program is the ability to recruit trainees. This measure correlates with another measure, the satisfaction of current trainees, graduates, and faculty. The tensions that surface in organizational development can impede the recruitment (and retention) of trainees. Since the core of training takes place in small supervisory groups, it is easier for the tension to be communicated to trainees, directly or indirectly, than it would be in large teaching seminars. Once trainees feel triangled into the organizational issues, it becomes impossible to resolve these issues without having fallout in the training program. It is our experience that energy devoted to keeping issues and tensions within the appropriate organizational level, or between the appropriate individuals, is energy well spent in terms of satisfied trainees and future recruitment.

Trainee satisfaction depends largely on whether or not trainees feel they have received valuable training. Although subjective, one measure of value is the degree to which the trainees see positive changes in the way they work with families. Thus the mark of a good program is its ability to affect a trainee's practice. Faculty who have a genuine interest in the development of supervisory techniques to help trainees learn to think, analyze, and collect data in a systems framework are the major asset of a quality program. Faculty should be offered as much support as possible in their ongoing work with trainees. Small groups for supervisors, where they exchange supervisory difficulties and assist each other in dealing with them, are helpful.

Faculty who are supported and encouraged to develop as supervisors, and trainees who value their efforts, are excellent recruitment sources. When possible, the faculty should conduct the application interviews, as they best represent the product the trainees are considering. Another useful technique is to allow a "test drive"—potential consumers can derive great benefit from observing training groups. And there is no advertisement like the endorsement of a satisfied customer.

Word of Mouth versus Advertising

In considering how to market the training program, it is important to remember that "students choose family therapy programs in the way they choose an electrician" (*Family Therapy and Research Newsletter*, 1984); on the basis of "word of mouth." Word of mouth describes the informal or indirect method of verbally rating a training program (or supervisor) by either a friend's or a colleague's recommendation. The term can also be stretched to include hearing a presenter at a workshop.

The electrician theory suggests the items that trainees look for in choosing an institute: "who is good; who works the hours or the days compatible with a busy schedule; the proximity of the electrician to the home; whether the electrician has an opening for their work; and how much the electician charges" (*Family Therapy and Research*

Newsletter, 1984). Mental health professionals look for ways to get quality training without adding to their already overloaded schedules and budgets.

After an institute is well established, these factors may not be the most important ones in consideration of the program by potential applicants. Since it is now rare for agencies to give either time or money for advanced training, applicants are concerned about getting "quality" training for their money. Programmatic issues frequently raised by trainees include the theoretical model utilized, the balance of theory (didactic) to experiential training, the experience and training of supervisors, and whether families are available. To address these issues, we stress the importance of establishing early in the founding phase clear objectives, structure, and methods of training.

Advertising

A small number of programs have been able and will continue to draw trainees because of their name or the name of the founder. However, with the continued proliferation of programs, most programs need to be able to meet stiff competition for applicants.

Word-of-mouth recommendations, faculty presentations and publications, and the interview process are low-cost marketing devices. It is also important to have formal public relations such as advertising and brochures that make the institute visible to the professional community. The value of an attractive brochure is immense in stimulating new interest in the program, particularly in the beginning phase. Although underwriting the cost of such an item may be no small matter on a shoestring budget, it is always worth the investment.

Securing Space and Equipment

For some lucky groups, securing space to conduct a training program is not a problem. Either these people already have space in which practice and/or supervision was being done, or they live in an area where space is readily available at a cost which is not prohibitive. For others, securing training space becomes a major occupation (or preoccupation), and often an obstruction to packaging a program in the manner in which it was planned. Most institutes need as a minimum enough space to conduct live supervision of at least one supervision group at a time, and video playback equipment in several formats. The reality of financing such facilities comes early in the development of a free-standing institute. Failure to be realistic about the needs of the program—the cost of space and equipment—and how such costs will be handled, leads to disaster later on, and may even cause permanent damage to the reputation of the program.

CONCLUSION

We have generalized from our personal experience what to expect during the evolution of a free-standing institute. FIW started as a group of "foxhole buddies" (split from another institute) and grew to a stable, established organization. Some groups might start as a proper organization and then journey toward the loyalty, affection, and respect that we began with. Whichever way the process moves, there will come (around the third year) a crisis over money, workload, and/or power that will give the group three options: (1) go under, (2) beat the system to death (make first-order changes), or (3) reorganize the structure.

In the isomorphic way of systems, we have found that the clearer and more open the organizational structure, the more creative and enjoyable the work of training. And when it happens for a free-standing institute—one that it is not only born free, but actually survives, thrives, and comes of age—then look for the kind of creative, serious work and fun that training should be all about.

Finally, paradoxically, while we would no longer define our organizational goal as "fostering staff development and relationships," that is what is happening. As in real life, happiness at work is a by-product, not a goal.

References

Bloch, D., & Weiss, H. (1981). Training facilities in marital and family therapy. *Family Process, 20,* 137–147.

Churchill, N. C., & Lewis, V. L. (1983). The five stages of small business growth in growing concerns. *Harvard Business Review, 61*(3), 30–39.

Falicov, C., Constantine, J., & Breunlin, D. (1981). Teaching family therapy: A program based on learning objectives. *Journal of Marriage and Family Therapy, 7,* 497–506.

Family Therapy and Research Newsletter (Boston, Winter 1984).

Liddle, H. A. (1980). On teaching a contextual or systemic therapy: Training content, goals and methods. *American Journal of Family Therapy, 8,* 55–69.

Pasquale, R. T. (1978). Zen and the art of management. *Harvard Business Review, 56*(2), 153–162.

Pfeiser, R. B., & Wooten, L. M. (1983). Life cycle changes in small family businesses. *Business Horizons, 26,* 59–65.

Sluzki, C. (1983). Process, structure and world views: Toward an integrated view of systemic models in family therapy. *Family Process, 22,* 469–476.

Tomm, K., & Wright, L. (1979). Training in family therapy: Perceptual, conceptual and executive skills. *Family Process, 18,* 227–250.

16

Family Therapy Training in Psychiatry

LEE COMBRINCK-GRAHAM
Institute for Juvenile Research, Chicago

Family therapy has had a hard time gaining acceptance in psychiatry, even though many of the pioneers in family therapy were or are also psychiatrists. Many who traveled the road from traditional training in psychiatry to the discovery of family therapy tell a story of an enlightenment and, in many cases, a turning away from the traditional background.

Family therapy's problems in psychiatry are manifold. Sugarman's review of the state of family therapy in psychiatry training (1984) lists a number of controversies that complicate training. First among these is the definition of family therapy—is it a modality or an orientation to psychotherapy? Second, should it be elective or required in a residency program? The AMA Residency Review Committee required family therapy training in all residency programs (1979), and a survey of general psychiatry residencies reported that the majority of these programs offer some experience of family therapy, averaging about 300 hours over the course of the residency (Sugarman, 1981). A third area of controversy, according to Sugarman (1984), relates to the curriculum content. What school or schools of family therapy should be taught? At what point in the training should family therapy be taught? Who should teach it? As recently as 1981, there were no residency training directors who felt qualified to do a family therapy presentation at the annual meeting of the American Association of Directors of Residency Training (Henderson, 1981). It has been necessary, therefore, to rely on nonmedical personnel to teach family therapy, a situation that, not providing appropriate professional role models, is almost bound to lose the interest of most residents (see also APA Task Force report, 1984).

Further controversy arises out of the ferment in psychiatry itself. This is a field struggling with its identity in the broader fields of mental health and medicine. More than any other professional discipline, psychiatry straddles both fields (Brodie, 1983), but this balancing act is not without its costs. One such cost is that many psychiatrists are confused about who they are and what professional role they should fill. Finding that most of the psychotherapeutic roles can be filled by non–medically trained professionals, many psychiatrists turn, for a unique identity, to the biological aspects of their field. This trend has raised the question of the value of psychotherapy training in psychiatric residencies. The same movement toward the more biological aspects of the field has also placed a greater demand for scientific proof of efficacy on psychiatrists doing psychotherapy. Like all psychotherapies, family therapy has not yet conclusively demonstrated its areas of effectiveness or its areas of potential harm, and thus does not immediately attract the outcome-oriented psychiatrist.

FAMILY SYSTEMS THEORY AND PSYCHIATRY

Family therapy is new to psychiatry, even though the recognition of the importance of family influences on health has been a part of the very basis of medical and psychiatric practice. What is new for psychiatry as a mental health specialty is what is new about family systems theory for all of the mental health fields—the systemic approach. Ecosystems epistemology is a fundamental way of observing and organizing data, one that understands information as patterns and events as recursive. It is new and fundamentally different from traditional mental health thinking, with the potential to revolutionize the field.

Many distinguished psychiatrists have raised the issue of the importance of a systemic orientation to psychiatry and medicine. The author of the biopsychosocial model, George Engel, began by studying the family contexts of patients with ulcerative colitis, making a memorable entry into the linkage between family context and illness as early as 1959 (Engel, 1959). Continuing his work on the medical–psychiatric interface, Engel presented to both psychiatry and medicine an innovative conceptual approach. This was an antidote to what he called the "biomedical" model, which in his view was linear and reductionistic. The new model includes the observations and experience of the biomedical model and is called the "biopsychosocial" model. This model conceptualizes relationships between parts and wholes at different levels of hierarchy. For example, the endocrine system can be described as a functionally discrete system. The adrenal glands, which can be isolated as separate organs, are a part of the endocrine system, which in turn is a part of the organism, called the individual, which in turn is a part of a system called a family, and so on. Thus any whole is composed of parts, and is also a part of another whole (Engel, 1977, 1980).

While Engel's model suggests the importance of social context, this is not emphasized in his work. Social psychiatrists, however, have made important observations about the effects of a patient's context on his or her state of health. For example, an individual's involvement with his or her family in relation to mental illness, hospitalization, and subsequent treatment is one area of investigation (Ferber, Kligler, Zwerling, & Mendelsohn, 1967). Several studies about the relationship between the richness of a person's interpersonal system and the incidence of illnesses of all kinds have been presented, with the conclusion that illnesses are more likely to occur and be more serious in individuals whose social network is impoverished (Pattison, 1977; Greenblatt, Recerra, & Serafetinides, 1982; Wilkinson & O'Connor, 1982).

Finally, there are those in psychiatry who contend that psychiatry is the area of medicine that integrates the biological, psychological, and social perspectives. These people write that the systems approach may be the only sensible way for modern psychiatry to think (Marmor, 1983). It is from this perspective that the current discussion of family therapy training in psychiatry will be oriented. What family therapy training offers to psychiatry is the systems orientation the applications of which in psychiatry are broader than the practice of family therapy. Because of these kinds of explorations, psychiatry is a field in which "family" systems theory really transcends the family in the richness of its implications.

In elaborating the systems epistemology, many writers have highlighted important attitudes about the nature of system behavior, integrity, and organization. Traditional views of such concepts as developmental lines, outcome studies, and natural courses of illness all are questioned in light of the systemic views of equipotentiality (that many causes can be related to one outcome) and equifinality (that many outcomes can occur from a single event). The notions of recursive phenomena and repetitive sequences present new ways of understanding reality—in fact, they bring up the question, "What is reality?"

Though it has long been recognized that the family has an important effect on its individual members, and that the family environment has an important effect on the expression of psychiatric symptoms, early attempts to respond to the family's influence were to isolate the patient from the family. This was probably effective in a time when there were institutions where patients could remain long enough to be adopted by the institution, and in which the relationship aspects of the program provided active corrective alternatives to the family relationships. Several things have happened to change this practice. First, patterns of health care have changed so that it is not likely that a patient will be able to be adopted by a healthy institution for a sufficiently long time. Furthermore, therapists are much more mobile than they were, so that the adoption process would become more like a series of foster parents for the patient. Finally, whereas it was formerly assumed that families could not be changed, we now believe that families can change. In fact, it is likely that family systems can change their interactions more readily than individuals can change in individual treatment.

The ideas that systems cannot malfunction; that they are what they are (Dell, 1982, 1985); and that systems have their own self-healing and self-correcting mechanisms (Elkaim, 1981) lead to a drastically altered role for the psycho-healer. Once, the therapist was thought to be essential to the process of psychic reconstruction. The systemic psycho-healer has moved to a new position, that of facilitator. In this role the ecosystemic psychiatrist is facilitator of healing not only at individual and family levels, but at all levels of the hierarchies described in Engel's biopsychosocial model, and at the interfaces of these levels.

If he or she can achieve an ecosystemic awareness and acquire some skills in working with systems, the psychiatrist can assume a critical position in medical and behavioral scientific ecology, with an opportunity to enter the biopsychosocial continuum at many of its human system levels. Trained in biology, the psychiatrist understands neurotransmitters, neuroanatomy, and neurophysiology, and can investigate the effects of these microsystems on the macro-effects on behavior. Trained in psychology, the psychiatrist understands the interplay of experience and behavior. Trained in systems, the psychiatrist will understand the relationship between interpersonal variables in the patient's life and the other levels described. An important aspect of this will be the psychiatrist's awareness of his or her own place in the ecology of patient care. A systemically trained psychiatrist who winds up at the top of the mental health hierarchy is likely to have an enormous impact on the mental health field.

A distinction between the "ecological" and "interdisciplinary" approaches to treatment was made by Auerswald (1968). The latter, he points out, may actually be a way of taking a patient apart. In specialty outpatient clinics a patient may spend several days a week going, for example, to a cardiac clinic, a diabetes clinic, a vascular clinic, a podiatry clinic, or a psychiatry clinic. The only means of communication the physicians in these clinics will have with each other is through the chart or an occasional phone call. This is the most fragmented form of interdisciplinary medical care. The ecological approach would gather these medical problems together under one coordination and planning system. In addition, the patient's resources for home care, disposition for healing, and other related life experiences would be integrated into the treatment plan. Psychiatrists, again, are the most appropriate physicians to coordinate an ecological planning system.

FAMILY THERAPY TRAINING

Considering the foregoing observations about the role of family systems thinking in psychiatry, the specific tasks of family therapy training in psychiatry training should be:

1. To orient the physician toward looking for and eliciting resources within patient systems.
2. To teach the interactive relationships between levels of system functioning in the biopsychosocial continuum.
3. To teach the physician about the ecosystemic versus the interdisciplinary approach to working with patients in mental health, medical, social, and biological contexts.

With these tasks in mind, the remainder of this chapter will examine the state of psychiatric residency training and the problems inherent in trying to introduce an ecosystemic approach.

SEQUENCE OF TRAINING

A brief outline of the typical sequence in psychiatry training will orient the reader. Most psychiatric residencies begin in the first postgraduate year (PGY-I) with an experience that combines psychiatry and primary care medicine, such as 6 months of psychiatry and 6 months of general medicine or pediatrics. The PGY-II focuses primarily on inpatient work, where the resident meets the most difficult, disturbed, and chronic patients. In the PGY-III the resident develops outpatient skills through continuing the follow-up outpatient work with patients begun in the inpatient year, and begins to work with better functioning outpatients. PGY-IV offers the opportunity to continue treatment initiated in the second and third years, and to conduct research or find specialized training in an area of interest. In some programs the PGY-IV year allows the resident to begin analytic training; in others the resident focuses on research or chooses to develop skills in marital and couples work; in still others, residents may take a year of training in work with children, perhaps in preparation for a fellowship in child psychiatry.

THE TRAINEES

One set of obstacles to the introduction of systems thinking comes from the way medical students are oriented to their responsibilities as doctors. Physicians right out of medical school enter psychiatry with the burden of their training, which, currently more than ever, focuses on the complex biological technology of the medical model. As Engel (1977, 1980) noted, the biomedical model is essentially reductionistic. Students trained in the art of differential diagnosis are forced to focus on a process of identifying one-to-one relationships, and to eliminate possibilities, so as to establish the causes of a particular disorder.

Evidence of this orientation, is provided by a group of the Beth Israel Hospital in Boston who attempted to interest students in the biopsychosocial perspective during their first in-hospital clinical rotations. Even at the end of an experience elected by the students, which was to be explicitly oriented toward the biopsychosocial continuum, students continued to request additional data on biologic information and did not ask for more psychological or social information (Silverman *et al.*, 1983). How is it that despite an increasing shift toward a systems epistemology in physical and biological sciences, medical training still favors such reductionism? Silverman and colleagues speculate that the failure of their experiment reflects widely on medical practice. They make several suggestions on the basis of their findings, as follows.

1. The answer may not be to have more psychiatrist-precepted clinical sessions; possibly students simply tolerate the psychosocial input rather than to embrace it.

2. There seems to be a need for more explicit study, and presentation to students, of the governing conceptual models of medical practice. Specifically, a considered and researched presentation of contrasting biomedical and biopsychosocial viewpoints could help the students take a meta-view of themselves in the medical context. In addition, one program's experience with parallel care given by the same physicians and students to medical and psychiatric patients on the same ward helped to expand the students' awareness of the importance of psychosocial factors and the similarities of the medical and psychiatric patients (Shemo, Ballenger, Yazel, & Spradlin, 1982).

3. The roots in medical theory and philosophy of the so-called dehumanized, defensive medical practice may not yet have been addressed. The reference here is to another interface of biomedical science and society, that with the legal system. Defensive medicine is practiced by the doctor who is compelled by law to offer treatment, but who is also fearful of malpractice suits. One observation is that there is a cycle of escalation whereby the more effective medical treatment becomes, the greater the demands placed on the practitioner become to perform more and more extraordinary feats, but at greater risk (Sider & Clements, 1982). This same combined responsibility and caution may lead the physician to leave no question unasked, no lab study unordered, no observation unrecorded, in his or her effort to cover himself or herself in the practice of conventional (or consensual) medicine. The psychosocial material, not being so relevant, takes a second place.

A clear outcome of medical school training that is another obstacle to the acquisition of a systemic perspective is that the burdens of decision-making responsibilities quickly fall on the physician. Graduating medical students, though not thoroughly expert in their chosen specialties, are prepared to assume these responsibilities and are immediately placed in positions where they must exercise these skills. This leads to the absurd situation on a medical ward where a nurse with 20 years of experience caring for patients asks the intern in his or her first week of clinical practice what to do. How these nurses manage to keep training young physicians year after year is a major question. A perceptive intern will realize that the nurse is a resource and ask what the nurse thinks should be done, or what is usually done. In this rare instance, the intern will have had an early experience in collaboration and in searching for resources in the system—an experience that could lead to a more profound examination of the system's operations and to more skillful blending of them. The majority of interns, alas, believe that it is the physician's responsibility to make the decisons. So, if a consultation is necessary, they will call the resident, fellow, or attending physician, or, as a last resort, another intern. Thus, physicians are socialized to ignore important nonphysician sources of data regarding the patients' treatment contexts.

Young physicians who have chosen psychiatry as a specialty usually have acknowledged the importance of psychological data, although they may not connect this with somatic experiences except in those conditions delineated as psychosomatic illnesses. The beginning psychiatrist, being biomedically trained, will wrestle with the dichotomies of *psyche* and *soma*, and of nature and nurture; will attempt to establish a diagnosis, determine the precipitating factors, develop a treatment plan specifically for this illness, select specific drugs for specific effects; and, when treatment yields improvement, will attempt to isolate the effective factors. All are worthy inquiries, but all tend to operate on only a few of the levels available for work in the biopsychosocial continuum. Fortunately, psychiatry has a significant contingent of "retreads"—primary care physicians who enter psychiatric training for a career change. These physicians often choose psychiatry specifically because their experience has taught them that psychosocial factors play a large role in illness and medical care. They have learned that a medical practice has a large group of consumers who can be designated the "worried well." A good mix of these experienced physicians with the recent medical school graduates is desirable in a residency group.

If the program is to institute a systems orientation, it is necessary to recognize that it is a rare resident who has a natural interest in systems, and that it is most common for residents to have a heavy burden of responsibility for patient care and for coordinating and directing treatment. These doctors believe that their patients rely on them for their health, and, in some cases, for life itself. They are dedicated; they often virtually abandon their own personal lives and families to develop the skills to manage their responsibilities. Thus it becomes difficult for physicians to examine seriously or accept any nontraditional ideas that might involve extra effort or risk.

TRAINING IN SYSTEMS

Since the opportunity for studying systems is available at every level of the psychiatrist's experience, it is necessary to develop a sequence of training in systems work that orients the psychiatrist not only as therapist, but also as a member of the therapeutic ecology in inpatient units and in working with chronically ill, in community settings, and in child and adolescent units. Because the young psychiatrist has been trained to take responsibility for patient care—to function at the pinnacle of the medical hierarchy—training must include a delicate mixture of building on already acquired skills and attitudes and shaping new ones.

For child psychiatry trainees to evolve from working with individuals to thinking about systems, the following sequence was proposed (Combrinck-Graham, 1980). The trainee already knows how to conduct an assessment interview and to draw some conclusions about the individual, so the first task of systems training is to reformulate individual intrapsychic dynamics in terms of intrafamilial processes. In the second stage the trainee is to include other family members in his or her understanding of the process, but to continue to diagnose each family member, and to attribute separate motivations to each one. In the third stage the trainee learns to describe the interaction among family members in such a way that feedback loops and symptomatic cycles could be conceptualized. Only at this stage will the trainee be able to formulate the way a systems thinker does. In the fourth stage the trainee learns to intervene in a systemic way. This proposed reorientation of the child psychiatry trainee is a gradual process that builds from the resident's prior experience to an increasingly comprehensive grasp of systems.

The Systemic Residency

Psychiatry programs rarely have much input into the 6 months of primary care of the PGY-I. Ideally, these 6 months would be spent in a general medicine or family practice setting, so that the young trainee could work with the more mundane medical problems of a primary care setting rather than the esoteric and puzzling diagnostic problems presented to the tertiary care facility. The house officer should have plenty of opportunities to meet with the families of the patients with no other task but to talk with them and to hear their stories. This will increase the resident's comfort with being with families, and it will help him or her to recognize the family's role in the health of all of its members.

The organization of the 6 months of psychiatry in PGY-I varies from program to program. Some programs offer this experience on inpatient units, while others offer it in child and adolescent facilities. In any case it is an opportunity to begin systems training. A skilled systems-oriented psychiatrist should conduct a case conference or family interview on a weekly basis throughout the year. This teacher could interview families of both medical and psychiatric patients, with the intern then assigned to the case. Such an experience offers a psychiatrist role model who elicits important information about the family system and relates it to the intern's work with the identified patient. This kind of experience could well continue throughout the 4 years of training. As the residents become more experienced they can become more active in these interviews, as a cointerviewer or cotherapist, and finally conduct them alone, with the mentor and colleagues observing.

The PGY-II is usually an inpatient year where the opportunities for systems learning are manifold. There is now an increasing body of research demonstrating the beneficial role of family work in the treatment of severely and chronically disturbed patients. Such work has been done with families of patients with schizophrenia, affective illness, borderline conditions, substance abuse disorders, handicaps, and psychosomatic conditions. (Family therapy for these conditions has been described in many contexts. For an overview see Lansky, 1981.) Information regarding this work would be integrated into the primary teaching of assessment and treatment of these disorders. Thus a basic course on psychopathology would include (1) criteria for diagnosis (using the *Diagnostic and Statistical Manual of Mental Disorders*, third edition, revised, or DSM-III-R); (2) important historical information about the illness (the content of current thinking about the condition); (3) how to assess the condition in the patient (interview and mental status exam); (4) what family information is available; (5) how to assess the families of these patients; (6) what the relevance is of family interactional data to the expression of symptomatology (family context of the condition); (7) what the natural history of the illness is, and what role the family is known to play in this process; and (8) the treatments and the interplay between treatment and context. In this way family data are included in basic learning about the phenomenology of psychiatric illness.

The other major level of systems experience in PGY-II occurs in the complex relationship between the resident and the rest of the hospital staff. Some hospitals have a therapeutic community in which all staff and patients interact. These communities may have difficulties with hierarchies, but involvement in efforts to establish and maintain a therapeutic community focuses the resident on the ecology of the hospital unit. The resident must learn to see himself or herself in the context, for example, of a decision to increase a patient's medication. A nonsystemically oriented resident will believe that this decision is being made on the basis of the patient's condition. A nurse may ask a resident to evaluate a patient's agitation. The resident will see the patient, look for the agitation (and, having been affected by the nurse's concern, the resident will undoubtedly find it), and then rationally adjust the medication. The systems-oriented resident, however, will see the nurse's observation of the patient's agitation as information about the unit— about the nurse, the composition of patients and how well they are doing, how successful the staff feels about their work with this particular patient, whether or not they like the patient and the patient's family, the relationship between the nurse and the doctor, and that between all the nurses and all the doctors. A suitable text for this learning is Stanton and Schwartz's *The Mental Hospital* (1954), while many of the practicalities of applying a systems approach in a psychiatric hospital are reviewed in Combrinck-Graham (1985).

A clinical seminar linking these two levels of experience (clinical assessment of a patient and assessment in context) could be modeled after a seminar that ran at the Philadelphia Child Guidance Clinic for about seven years. The object of the seminar was to teach assessment in context. It was a teaching seminar designed primarily for the child psychiatry fellows and medical students, but all of the inpatient staff was invited, and the experience was most effective when professionals other than psychiatrists were also present. The format of the seminar was simple. Each week a resident presented a case, at first in a rather classical way: identifying information, chief complaint, relevant history, family history, mental status on admission, treatment, course in the hospital, and questions for the seminar. Following this, questions about the family context and the inpatient context were explored. The process of the group during this discussion provided further information about context and about the patient. Finally the patient was interviewed by the resident, with the others observing through the one-way mirror. Occasionally the seminar leader would join the interview for some period. Observers were asked to watch both the patient and the interviewer. What did the patient do to their colleague? What did the interviewer do to the patient? In the case of a youngster who acted stupid, the interviewer talked to the 13-year-old boy in the loud, clear, deliberate tones used for a very young or very deaf person, or one who didn't speak English. When this was observed behind the mirror, a volunteer was selected to see if it were possible to talk with the boy in another way, and what the boy would do. Three separate interviewers entered the room and were inducted into talking with the boy as if he were retarded. When the seminar leader succeeded in talking to him differently, the boy became very irritated and left the room! This was a dramatic experience of how interviewers' behaviors and subsequent impressions are shaped by patients. After each interview there was a discussion of these observations and their relevance both to the difficulties experienced by the child and the staff and to the treatment plan.

Harbin (1980), in describing his inclusion of family therapy training in a psychiatry residency, gave each resident a family therapy supervisor as one of four supervisors (the other three are for assessment, ward management, and child and adolescent therapy). He noted that just this addition to the inpatient resident's experience has been associated with greater than 87% of inpatients being treated conjointly with other family members. Ongoing family therapy supervision would be an essential part of the program proposed here as well.

PGY-III is usually an outpatient year. Residents in this year of training often do consultation and liaison work in the hospital and acute care in the emergency room (the latter may have begun in PGY-I), in addition to their work in the outpatient clinic. By providing, as Harbin did, one family therapy supervisor for each resident, and requiring ongoing treatment of at least one family or couple in the outpatient clinic throughout the year, the program offers the resident strong input in systems work in psychotherapy. This experience should be supplemented with weekly seminars in family therapy, where family therapy as a psychotherapeutic approach is highlighted. The background and the various schools and techniques of family therapy would be topics of this year-long seminar.

The psychiatrist-in-context is the focus of the systemically oriented consultation and liaison work. As with the inpatient work, a patient is the original object of interest. Here, however, the patient is in a medical rather than a psychiatric milieu. As with the psychiatric inpatients, their families and hospital personnel contribute to the well-being and adjustment of the patient (some would also say to the healing, as well), so the psychiatric consultant cannot limit the assessment to the patient alone. Meeting with the nursing staff, gossiping with the ward clerk, observing the other patients in the room and on the ward, discovering that the house officer has lost three patients in the last month— all will provide significant information in addition to the interview with the patient and family. Sometimes it is possible to have a resident rotate on one service for a period of time so that he or she can become assimilated into the ward context. This experience can be strongly enhanced by weekly ward conferences involving a systemically oriented staff psychiatrist. Such conferences are primarily for the benefit of the staff caring for the medical patients. They are invited to present the cases of patients about whose psychosocial adjustment they worry. The process of the conference is to explore the available information about the patient and the feelings of the staff, and to offer suggestions for intervention based on these findings. The systemically oriented psychiatric consultant rarely intervenes directly with a patient or takes a patient into treatment. An example of this kind of intervention came up on rounds on a children's oncology service when the attending oncologist observed that they had run out of treatment for little Susie, who required platelet transfusions every day because of hypersplenism. The psychiatrist observed that the physicians had debated for weeks about whether to take out her spleen or irradiate it. The psychiatrist wondered what was going on. The attending physician said that Susie's mother wasn't prepared for Susie to die, even though it was clear that the proposed treatment could only prolong the child's life a short while. The psychiatrist wondered whether it was Susie's mother or the hospital staff who was less prepared for Susie's death. The physician thought about it and talked that day to Susie's mother about her daughter's condition. The child died peacefully the next day, *everyone* having accepted it. In this case, the psychiatrist not only had not met with the patient or her mother, but had not even conducted an official consultation; rather, an intervention came from the psychiatrist's observations of the system.

In PGY-IV the resident can elect time in marital and family therapy or in other areas where a systems approach will enhance the psychiatrist's contributions to the work being done in his or her professional and training context. Some of these areas in which residents elect time during this training year include student health, school consultation, halfway houses, drug and alcohol abuse, rehabilitation, hematology–oncology (that is, work with the terminally ill), and research. The training program should offer continued family therapy supervision and an advanced family therapy seminar that addresses the application of ecological orientations to some of the specific contexts in which the residents are working. In addition, problems that psychiatrists commonly face should be addressed, including antisocial problems; legal involvement and testimony; and study of mental health laws, such as right to treatment, commitment requirements, and professional responsibility.

In summary, the psychiatric resident's training in ecosystems orientation and family therapy occurs throughout the four years, with the simultaneous presentation of the psychotherapeutic modality and use of systems concepts in the conduct of professional tasks at each level of training. In this way the psychiatrist will learn to work within professional contexts developing an "ecological" rather than an "interdisciplinary" approach to the resources within the interpersonal systems in which he or she and the patients will be.

PROBLEMS WITH IMPLEMENTATION

There are many problems with implementing such a program for residents, although what is conceivable today was not conceivable 10 years ago. In fact, Harbin (1980) points out that most of the family therapy supervisors in his program were social workers at first. At the time of publication of his article, 11 family therapy supervisors were psychiatrists—many of whom had graduated from his program. In addition, he points out, there was a substantial increase in the numbers of cases treated in conjoint marital and family therapy. This experience confirms the relevance of the systems model to residents— provided that it is offered in the right way. What is required?

First, good teachers are needed. Although Harbin's experience demonstrated that teachers from another profession can succeed as supervisors of family therapy, the other experiences proposed here must be done by psychiatrists, both as role models and as physicians trained in the cross section of medicine and psychotherapy. There has to be more than one systems-oriented psychiatrist, both to share the load and to offer the residents enough diversity to demonstrate the application of a model with a great deal of breadth. At the moment, outside of Harbin's program, there are scarcely enough properly trained psychiatrists to go around.

Second, the residency training director has to be convinced of the value of this approach. This is not likely to happen in more than a few exceptional programs until family therapy and the systems orientation are more widely recognized as valuable conceptual approaches in psychiatry. What we have proposed includes training in all the traditional subjects in psychiatry, but adding a systems flavor.

Many of the ideas proposed by the systems-oriented teachers will appear to come into conflict with ideas taught by the more conventional members of the department. An example was a problem experienced by a resident who had been encouraged by her family-oriented supervisor to see a very maladjusted young woman and her husband. The young woman was diagnosed by others as having a borderline personality disorder. The resident presented the case at a conference where she was questioned about the advisability of seeing such a "sick" patient in "couples therapy." The concern of the more conventional psychiatrists came from their conviction that the first order of business in the treatment of borderline disorders is in the one-to-one relationship with the therapist in which the patient can integrate the "splitting" that is a *sine qua non* of the condition. The family therapy supervisor, hearing of the resident's experience in the case conference, assured her that the patient could be treated either way, depending on how the resident formulated the issues and planned the treatment approach. In relationship to her husband, many of the patient's peculiarities could be understood as responses to complementary peculiarities of his. The resident had a choice—to treat the woman in the context of the therapeutic relationship, or to treat her in the context of her own marital relationship. The resident continued to see this woman with her husband, although she did choose to treat other cases individually and was supervised by other individually oriented supervisors. Residents like this one usually develop a good sense of their training contexts so that they can get from each teacher the best of what that teacher offers. The job of sifting through and integrating these different and seemingly conflicting teachings usually falls to the resident. The systemically trained supervisor, however, like the one in the example, can help the resident to develop a perspective that clarifies the choices to be made.

It is clear that the product of a training program like the one proposed would be very unlikely to retreat to a private office practice of psychoanalysis, because classical psychoanalysis, in order to be effective, requires an exclusion of real context. A psychiatrist finishing a program like the one described would be too aware of patient contexts to be able to block them out, and would have acquired some skills in effecting changes in extrapatient contexts. Thus this graduate will be prepared to contribute to many of the areas in which psychiatry should, but often does not, play a role—such as care of the chronically mentally ill, the handicapped, and the poor or socially disrupted.

A third requirement for implementation of such a program is a pragmatic outlook. Many residents enter psychiatry with a dream of transforming troubled individuals through the power of psychotherapy. The pragmatic approach presented here might not be accepted by these idealists, who would seek out more traditional programs. This is important because the family therapy model changes the role of the psycho-healer from chief to collaborator—from one who cures to one who facilitates healing.

It should be noted that the elements of the program proposed were not invented for the purposes of this chapter; all have been implemented at different times and in different contexts of psychiatric training with enough success that at least one out of four residents in one training program who had been exposed to these kinds of experiences chose to do further training in family therapy.

CONCLUSIONS

Psychiatry is a field that operates at the interface of the biopsychosocial continuum. From within psychiatry there is increasing interest in the systems orientation as a way of managing the integrative role of the psychiatric professional. What is needed from a systems orientation, however, is not merely family therapy, but an ecosystemic grasp of all of the work of the psychiatrist. A program for training psychiatrists has been presented (with the understanding that complete implementation remains for the future).

In the earlier part of this chapter it was noted that psychiatrists had been major contributors to the development of family therapy theory, and that many psychiatrists support a systems overview. A psychiatrist developed the biopsychosocial model, which is a most promising framework for incorporating the vast wealth of biomedical experience into the larger contexts of healing. Psychiatry does not need to shed its reductionistic, linear ways; it needs to adapt these methods to the varieties of areas in which psychiatrists may work. A systems approach appears to be the best way currently available to orient this work.

Acknowledgment

This article was written when the author was the director of the Master of Family Therapy Program, Hahnemann University.

References

AMA Residency Review Committee. (1979). Requirements in psychiatry.
APA Task Force on Family Therapy and Psychiatry. (1984). *Family therapy and psychiatry*. Washington, DC: APA.
Auerswald, E. A. (1968). Interdisciplinary versus ecological approach. *Family Process, 7*, 201–215.
Beels, C. C., & McFarlane, W. R. (1982). Family treatments of schizophrenia: Background and state of the art. *Hospital and Community Psychiatry, 33*(7), 541–549.
Brodie, H. K. H. (1983). Presidential address: Psychiatry—its locus and its future. *American Journal of Psychiatry, 140*(8), 965–968.
Combrinck-Graham, L. (1980). The role of family therapy in child psychiatry training: Why and how? In K. Flomenhaft & A. E. Christ (Eds.), *The challenge of family therapy* (pp. 109–124). New York: Plenum Press.
Combrinck-Graham, L. (1985). Hospitalization as a therapeutic intervention in the family. In R. L. Ziffer (Ed.), *Adjunctive techniques in family therapy* (pp. 99–124). Orlando, FL: Grune & Stratton.

Dell, P. (1982). Beyond homeostasis: Toward a concept of coherence. *Family Process, 21,* 21-41.

Dell, P. (1985). Understanding Bateson and Maturana: Toward a biological foundation for the social sciences. *Journal of Marital and Family Therapy, 11*(1), 1-20.

Elkaim, M. (1981). Non-equilibrium, chance and change in family therapy. *Journal of Marital and Family Therapy, 7,* 291-297.

Engel, G. L. (1959). "Psychogenic" pain and the pain-prone patient. *American Journal of Medicine, 26,* 899-918.

Engel, G. L. (1977). The need for a new medical model: A challenge for biomedicine. *Science, 196,* 129-136.

Engel, G. L. (1980). The clinical application of the biopsychosocial model. *American Journal of Psychiatry, 137,* 535-549.

Ferber, A., Kligler, D., Zwerling, I., & Mendelsohn, M. (1967). Current family structure: Psychiatric emergencies and patient fate. *Archives of Genetic Psychiatry, 16,* 659-667.

Greenblatt, M., Recerra, R., & Serafetinides, E. A. (1982). Social networks and mental health: An overview. *American Journal of Psychiatry, 139*(8), 997-984.

Harbin, H. T. (1980). Family therapy training for psychiatric residents. *American Journal of Psychiatry, 137*(12), 1595-1598.

Henderson, P. (1981). Personal communication.

Lansky, M. R. (1981). *Family therapy and major psychopathology.* New York: Grune & Stratton.

Marmor, J. (1983). Systems thinking in psychiatry: Some theoretical and clinical implications. *American Journal of Psychiatry, 140*(7), 833-838.

Pattison, E. M. (1977). A theoretical-empirical base for social system therapy. In E. P. Foulkes, R. M. Winthrob, J. Westermeyer, *et al.* (Eds.), *Current perspectives in cultural factors in psychiatry* (pp. 217-253). New York: Spectrum.

Shemo, J. P. D., Ballenger, J. C., Yazel, J., & Spradlin, W. W. (1982). A conjoint psychiatry-internal medicine program: Development of a teaching and clinical model. *American Journal of Psychiatry, 139*(11), 1437-1442.

Sider, R. C., & Clements, C. (1982). Family or individual therapy: The ethics of modality choice. *American Journal of Psychiatry, 139*(11), 1455-1459.

Silverman, D., Gartrell, M., Aronson, M., Steer, M., & Edbril, S. (1983). In search of the biopsychosocial perspective: An experiment with beginning medical students. *American Journal of Psychiatry, 140*(9), 1154-1159.

Stanton, A., & Schwartz, M. (1954). *The mental hospital.* New York: Basic Books.

Sugarman, S. (1981). Family therapy training in selected general psychiatry residency programs. *Family Process, 21,* 147-154.

Sugarman, S. (1984). Integrating family therapy training into psychiatry residency programs: Policy issues and alternatives. *Family Process, 23*(1), 23-32.

Wilkinson, C. B., & O'Connor, W. A. (1982). Human ecology and mental illness. *American Journal of Psychiatry, 139*(8), 985-990.

17

Nursing and Family Therapy Training

LORRAINE M. WRIGHT
University of Calgary

MAUREEN LEAHEY
Holy Cross Hospital, Calgary,

In the past few years nursing theory has made a dramatic shift from focusing on the individual to focusing on the family. Nursing now considers the family as one of the primary units of health care. The nursing literature is replete with such terms as "family centered care" (Cunningham, 1978), "family nursing" (Friedman, 1986); "family-focused care" (Janosik & Miller, 1979), "family conferences" (Wiley, 1978), and "family interviewing" (Wright & Leahey, 1984). These terms are also evident in many components of undergraduate and graduate nursing curricula, especially in the area of community health.

The involvement of families in nursing is interesting because it has come full circle. Although family nursing has always been part of nursing, until recently it was not labeled as such. Because nursing was first practiced in patients' homes, it was natural to involve family members in providing care. With the transition of nursing practice from homes to hospitals during the 1930s and 1940s, the family was excluded from involvement. Nursing is once again, however, inviting families to participate in both home care and hospital treatment. One example of this trend is the large number of fathers now involved in all aspects of maternity care. Family nursing has come to mean nursing care of the well and sick, and health counseling for all members of the family.

Despite the statement that *family-focused care* is widely accepted within the discipline of nursing, it should be noted that *family therapy* is less widely accepted within nursing. Nursing educators have incorporated family therapy into their mental health nursing programs only as one more treatment method, rather than as a different orientation to human problems.

Some possible explanations for this phenomenon can be offered. First, the majority of nurses are highly committed to maintaining their professional identity within the nursing profession, and therefore have been hesitant to enter into the mainstream of family therapy. Nurses are keen to do "family work," but do not want to be considered family therapists. This difference in professional identity between nurses and family therapists has been further accentuated in recent years by the recognition of family therapy as a distinct profession. Second, there is a dearth of family therapy role models within the nursing profession itself. There are few nurse educators/clinicians who specialize in the practice of family therapy. Therefore, most nurses have to go outside of their profession to receive family therapy training. Nursing students often rely on psychologists, social workers, and other professionals to serve as prototypes of family therapists. When students are not trained by or do not observe a competent *nurse* engaged in family therapy in a *nursing context*, the likelihood that they will associate the significance of family therapy within the discipline of nursing is lessened. Thus, it can be stated that many nurses are interested in family nursing but few have received specialized training in family therapy.

Perhaps a more compelling reason for the hesitancy of the nursing profession to embrace family therapy is that nurses are often made to feel that once they have specialized in family therapy, they must make a choice between identifying themselves as either nurses *or* family therapists. Our experience has been that *our* identity varies according to the professional context in which we find ourselves. That is, at times we identify ourselves as nurses with special training in family therapy, and at other times as family therapists who have a background in nursing. We believe that a more satisfactory solution to this professional identity dilemma would be the clear distinction of two levels of expertise in nursing with regard to family work: generalists and specialists. The purpose of this chapter is to discuss the issues involved in training both generalists and specialists in family work in nursing. Attention will be given to distinctions between training nurses in family nursing (generalists) and training nurses in family therapy (specialists).

TRAINING ISSUES

To clarify and compare the training of nurses in family nursing and in family therapy, the following issues will be discussed: context of training, education levels, faculty, curriculum, goals of training, supervision methods, and facilities for training. Each will be addressed separately.

Context of Training

Most nurses have an innate "family-mindedness," and some have been taught a conceptual base for family work. Many, however, find it difficult to apply their conceptual model in actual clinical practice. Part of the difficulty is that nurses, understandably, place emphasis on families with health problems.

Interest and emphasis on families with health problems is idiosyncratic to nursing and other health care professions. It has, however, implications for training. Nurses readily pay attention to family members with health problems, whereas family therapists without a nursing background tend to ignore or be uninformed about health issues. Nurses are taught to use a holistic approach in their clinical work, and emphasize *both* the biophysical and psychosocial aspects of health care. Because their orientation is primarily toward physical care, nurses tend to be more aware of the biophysical than the interpersonal aspects of an illness. They easily recognize the impact of the illness on the individual's functioning, but require more training to assess the impact of the illness on *all* family members.

Another significant implication for training is that nurses, because of their employment context, are required to learn first about the physical aspects of illness and only secondarily about the interactional aspects. For example, in working with a family with cancer nurses must be knowledgeable about both cancer as an illness and its management within the family system. Family therapists, on the other hand, are not expected to know about such physical aspects as colostomies or medication side effects. It is thus a challenge for nurses to try to integrate a family systems approach with their nursing education.

Education Levels

We recommend that the education of a nursing student in family therapy be provided only at the graduate or postgraduate levels, while the training of a student in family nursing may be provided at the undergraduate and/or graduate level (Wright & Leahey, 1984).

GRADUATE AND POSTGRADUATE EDUCATION

Graduate nursing master's or doctoral programs and postdegree institutes specializing in family therapy provide heavy emphasis on family assessment, models of family therapy, and the necessary skills to practice family therapy. Extensive clinical supervision, preferably live, of students' skill development (perceptual, conceptual, and executive) is provided by educators/clinicians. In North America, only a few graduate nursing programs or postdegree institutes offer family therapy courses taught by *nurse* educators (e.g., the Oregon Health Sciences University, Portland, Oregon; the University of Washington, Seattle, Washington; and the Family Therapy Institute, Holy Cross Hospital, Calgary, Alberta). Also rare is the supervision of nursing students in their clinical family therapy practica by *nurse* educators/clinicians.

We will briefly describe two graduate nursing programs that do offer family therapy courses and clinical supervision. These are examples of attempts to incorporate family therapy training into nursing programs. The first is the master's program, Faculty of Nursing, University of Calgary, Calgary, Alberta, Canada. The program is designed to prepare clinical nurse specialists. Students entering the program who desire to specialize in family therapy are able to focus on this area of interest within their clinical practica. Two elective courses are also offered: "Family Therapy Models: Structural, Strategic and Systemic"; and "Families and Illness." The predominant assessment model used is the Calgary Family Assessment Model (Wright & Leahey, 1984), while the predominant intervention model is an integration of the systemic–strategic approach. Live supervision is provided by two nurse educators/clinicians who themselves have specialized training in family therapy. The graduate nursing students also have opportunities to observe their professors interviewing families. Families interviewed by the graduate students are seen at the Family Nursing Unit at the University of Calgary (Wright, Watson, & Duhamel, 1985).

Another example of a graduate nursing program that offers family therapy courses and clinical supervision is the master's program at the University of Washington. This program offers a course entitled "Theoretical Models of Family Analysis and Intervention." The structural family therapy approach is presented in the clinical practica, although students are given the opportunity to select other approaches as well. Students are fortunate to have live supervision provided by a nurse educator/clinician who has specialized training in structural family therapy.

UNDERGRADUATE EDUCATION

At the undergraduate level, many nursing programs teach family nursing within the community health or mental health part of the curriculum. An example of this type of baccalaureate program is the School of Nursing at the Oregon Health Sciences University, Portland, Oregon. At the undergraduate level, appropriately, it is not the goal to prepare nursing students to be *family therapists*. Rather, these programs provide theory and skill development in family assessment and intervention. They prepare generalists with adequate skills in *family nursing*. Specifically, these nurses are able (1) to conceptualize human needs and problems in families using systems/cybernetics/communication concepts, (2) to assess normative events using a family assessment model, (3) to intervene with such normative family events as the birth of a child, and (4) to use direct and straightforward interventions such as recommending that parents read a particular book on child rearing. Undergraduate nursing students normally receive supervision of their family interviewing through case discussion and/or audiotape or videotape supervision. Rarely do undergraduate nursing students have their work with families viewed directly.

Many practicing nurses, especially those graduated before 1970, are also interested in continuing education courses in family nursing. Even though these professional nurses received little if any training in family nursing, they are eager for this type of knowledge and training. They seek opportunities for learning family nursing both in their own agencies or institutions and through continuing education courses in academic settings. An example of such a continuing education program offering an introduction to family nursing is the Post-Basic Mental Health Nursing Certificate Program at Mount Royal College, Calgary, Alberta.

Faculty

As mentioned earlier in this chapter, one of the primary obstacles at present to providing more extensive family therapy to nursing students and professional nurses is the lack of sufficient role models. There are very few nurse/educators who bridge the two disciplines of nursing and family therapy.

Although there are few nursing educators who are practicing family therapists, there are several nurses who have expertise in family theory and research, having received their own graduate education in child and family development or family studies. These educators provide leadership in family nursing, and are establishing ties with other health professionals to foster family-focused care. For example, at the annual National Council on Family Relations (NCFR) meeting in 1983, a special interest group for nurses and family health professionals held their first meeting.

The emphasis on the importance of nursing role models is not meant to disqualify the increasing use of interdisciplinary faculty. As a nursing student develops family therapy skills, there are times when it would be highly desirable for the student to receive supervision from other members of the helping professions. At the early stages of graduate training, however, competent role models within nursing are vital and critical if family therapy is to become more accepted within the discipline of nursing.

Curriculum

An examination of the curricula taught to students in family nursing, and to students specializing in family therapy in nursing, reveals three trends that serve to limit the extent to which family therapy can become an integral part of the nursing discipline. The first trend is that family nursing and/or family therapy courses are seldom identified as such. This trend is idiosyncratic to nursing. Within undergraduate curricula, family nursing is often hidden or embedded in other courses. For example, a course called "Clinical Nursing" can contain a significant amount of material concerning the family. Yet the title of the course does not reflect the family focus. Even at the graduate level, courses dealing with family therapy are frequently identified by such general titles as "Special Topics in Health Care." This reflects, we believe, nurse educators' ambivalence about a systems perspective and their lack of articulation of the levels of expertise in family work. However, as more nurse educators adopt a systemic perspective to health problems, this articulation should be reflected in the nursing curricula, with family-oriented courses more readily identifiable.

A second trend in nursing is the adoption of a wide variety of family assessment models (Clark, 1978; Friedman, 1986; Grace & Camilleri, 1981; Horton, 1977; Wright & Leahey, 1984). These models tend to be eclectic, and to incorporate a few family therapy concepts along with many concepts from nursing and sociology. The following statement from Janosik and Miller's work (1979) perhaps best identifies the beliefs of the nursing profession about the need for an eclectic framework. They state that

> focusing on one aspect of family life reveals that aspect but may ignore others of equal or greater importance. To adopt a single framework is unnecessarily restrictive, because it discounts the multiple aspects of family life and confines itself to a reductionistic point of view. Every conceptual framework is advantageous in some respects, but consigning all observations into one theoretical framework results in emphasizing some details at the expense of the others (p. 14).

This belief in eclecticism has enabled nursing to maintain an interest in family theory, but has limited its ability to develop theoretical models integrating family therapy and nursing. There are no specific models of family therapy associated with the nursing discipline. Rather, nurses have generally selected specific concepts (e.g., pseudo-mutuality, double-bind) from a wide variety of family therapy models. Rare mention is made in the nursing literature of the newer family therapy approaches, such as the strategic approach or the systemic (Milan) approach.

One book, *Nurses and Families: A Guide to Family Assessment and Intervention* by Wright and Leahey (1984), does attempt to integrate the most useful concepts from nursing and family therapy. The authors have presented a systematic family assessment model and have offered guidelines for intervention. The assessment model is the Calgary Family Assessment Model (CFAM), which is a multidimensional framework consisting of three major categories (structural, developmental, and functional). The model is based on a systems/cybernetics/communication theory foundation. Although the model has been primarily adapted from the family assessment framework developed by Dr. Karl Tomm and colleagues at the Family Therapy Program, Faculty of Medicine, University of Calgary, it integrates the work of Carter and McGoldrick (1980), Epstein, Bishop, and Levin (1978), and Minuchin (1974). In their guidelines for intervention, Wright and Leahey have integrated the work of Bateson (1979), Hoffman (1981), Haley (1977), Keeney (1982), and the Milan group (Selvini-Palazzoli, Boscolo, Cecchin, & Prata, 1980; Tomm, 1984a, 1984b). Other nursing authors who have taken on the challenge of bringing together significant concepts from nursing and family therapy include Friedman (1986) and Clemens and Buchanan (1982).

A third trend that can be noted in the nursing curricula is the lack of emphasis on family intervention. Despite the proliferation of family assessment within nursing curricula, little emphasis has been given to family intervention and the processes by which change takes place. Sound interventions are based on sound assessments and clear identification of problems, but most nursing texts stop at this level. Very few nurses consider what types of interventions are appropriate for various types of families with problems. The specific "how-tos" of family intervention are seldom discussed, either in family nursing literature or in family therapy training in nursing. One recent contribution to the literature is the three-volume *Family Nursing Series*, which emphasizes assessment *and* intervention for specific health problems (Leahey & Wright, 1987a, 1987b; Wright & Leahey, 1987). Until recently, nurses were limited in their ability to be innovative or devise interventions because they were entrenched in a medical hierarchy where they were expected to carry out physicians' orders. The majority of nurses who are employed in traditional hospital settings still find themselves unable to take as much initiative as they would like. However, with the advent of more and more nurses prepared with strong clinical skills at the masters level (e.g., family nurse practitioners and clinical nurse specialists), nurses are seeking opportunities to provide not only sound clinical assessment but intervention as well. An example of this is the Family Nursing Training Program, established at the Holy Cross Hospital in Calgary, Alberta, where nurses on the inpatient psychiatric units receive live and videotape supervision on their family interviewing from a family clinical nurse specialist. Many such clinical nurse specialists have already been integrated into and esteemed by other hospital and community health settings. Master's-prepared nurses are taking the lead in recognizing the interactional domain as a significant and legitimate aspect of nursing.

Goals of Training

The primary goal of training both family nurses and family therapists in nursing is to develop strong *conceptual, perceptual,* and *executive* skills. To *conceptualize* health care at the family level, students must recognize the impact of illness on the family and the influence of family interaction on the "cause" or "cure" of illness (Wright & Bell, 1981). To do so, both undergraduate and graduate nurses should use a systemic approach to conceptualize needs and/or problems in families.

Perceptual skills include the ability to make accurate observations, and to abstract from those observations the repetitive patterns of interactions among family members (Goren, 1979). Janzen (1980) emphasizes that the beginning nursing student already has intuitive perceptual/conceptual skills learned in other life experience. Because the student may not be aware of many of these skills, they need to be emphasized during training.

Executive skills are required to carry out therapeutic interventions in an interview. Students skilled in family nursing will be able to assess and intervene with normative events in families with the use of direct interventions. Students taking family therapy training in nursing will be able to assess and intervene in both normative and paranormative family events using an identifiable intervention model. Their interventions may be straightforward, or may be more complex and indirect (e.g., use of rituals or reframing). Both family nurses and nurses who have specialized in family therapy will conclude treatment with a therapeutic termination. Nurses skilled in family nursing would most often refer families if further treatment was indicated.

Since nurses more than other health professionals have frequent contact with families, particularly in hospital and community settings, they need to possess strong interpersonal skills to be effective. Family therapy offers many skills that are useful in relating to families. Examples are engagement skills, taking a "one-down position" when dealing with symmetrical families, and maintaining neutrality. Regardless of the level of expertise, all nurses need skills that are unique to work with families.

Supervision Methods

The predominant focus of supervision in nursing is on the development of skills (psychomotor and interpersonal), and not on the personal development of the nurse. The methods used to supervise family nursing and family therapy training in nursing appear to be going through a clearly identifiable, evolutionary process. There is an increasing emphasis on direct observation of the nurse's work. In the past, verbal and written process recordings were used heavily. We believe this method of supervision is the least effective method for aiding the development of therapeutic competence (Wright & Leahey, 1984).

The next evolutionary step, audiotape recording, was important in correcting the distortions of traditional verbal and/or written content. However, the major disadvantage of this type of supervision is that it omits extremely valuable data concerning nonverbal behavior. It is unfortunate that most students engaged in family nursing receive, at best, supervision only on their audiotaped interviews.

Although direct observation has been a common method used for the development of the nurse's psychomotor skills, live supervision of interactional skills has not been pursued as vigorously. The underuse of live supervision can be attributed, in part, to a lack of one-way mirrors in many facilities. Educators, however, can use other methods of direct observation. Supervisors can sit in on the actual interviews and participate minimally, or preferably not at all. Live supervision provides guidance predominantly in the development of executive skills (Wright, 1986).

Training Facilities

To the best of our knowledge, appropriate and well equipped facilities for training nursing students in family nursing or for specialization in family therapy are rare in North America. One excellent facility is the Family Nursing Unit (Wright, Watson, & Duhamel, 1985) at the Faculty of Nursing, University of Calgary. The training facilities have been used predominantly by graduate students and, to a lesser degree, by undergraduate and continuing nursing education students. The architectural design of the physical space and the use of technical equipment have a significant influence on the nature of training. The suite of five interviewing rooms and one large observation room provide a high degree of flexibility for the use of one-way screens, telephone intercom, and videotape equipment (Figure 17-1). Each room has a one-way mirror so that the interview can be observed and supervised. In addition, three rooms can be viewed not only from the observation room but also from adjoining rooms. All of the rooms are equipped for videotape recording. Remote-control color cameras are available in one of the large rooms and are concealed within triangular oak "bookshelves" in three corners of the room. All rooms are connected with an intercom system. A technician in the central control room does all of the recording.

Families seen at the Family Nursing Unit[1] normally receive the benefit of a team approach; graduate (master's) nursing students conduct the interviews, while a supervisor (nursing faculty) and three or four other graduate students observe. All team members have input into both assessment and interventions (Wright, Miller, & Nelson, 1985).

CONTRIBUTION OF NURSING TO FAMILY THERAPY

Nursing can make two unique contributions to the family therapy field. First, nurses can help family therapists become more aware of the health issues with which families cope by making them cognizant of the interrelationship between biological and psychological issues (Leahey & Wright, 1985). Nurses, for instance, are not intimidated by families

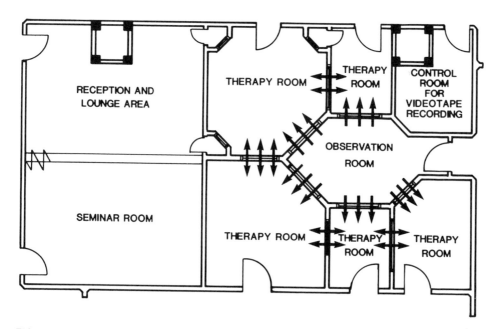

FIGURE 17-1. The Family Nursing Unit, University of Calgary.

dealing with life-threatening illnesses such as cancer, or chronic illnesses such as multiple sclerosis. They are knowledgeable and sensitive about stresses involved in dealing with specific types of chronic illness such as diabetes mellitus, which fluctuates daily, and arthritis, which varies little from day to day. In contrast to family therapists, who may lack knowledge about health problems, nurses automatically tend to include these issues in their family assessment. For example, a family may present with a 5-year-old diabetic boy who is irritable and unmanageable, especially before supper time. Recognizing that hypoglycemia can manifest itself behaviorally as transient irritability, anxiety, or confusion (McArthur, Tomm, & Leahey, 1976), a nurse would more naturally assess this connection between the physiological and behavioral aspects of the presenting problem. Adjustment of the eating schedule or the insulin dosage are appropriate interventions that could be suggested by a nurse to family members (Tomm, McArthur, & Leahey, 1977).

A second contribution of nursing to the family therapy field is the potential for a great influx of family interviewers. There are over 1.6 million practicing nurses in the United States. More than most other professionals, nurses have unique opportunities to work with families because of the number and variety of contexts in which nurses provide health care, such as in hospitals, homes, and occupational health settings. As nurses increase their conceptualization of the family's role in the formation and/or mainte-nance of symptoms as well as the impact of illness on the family, more families will receive the benefit of a systemic approach to health problems. One of the hoped-for consequences of nurses adopting a new epistemology of health problems is that they will be able to make more accurate and thorough family assessments. In so doing, they will make better judgments as to whether or not family intervention is indicated or desirable (Leahey & Slive, 1983).

Is family therapy open to accepting the contribution of the nursing profession? Particularly, is family therapy ready to address the interrelationship of biophysical and interactional factors in family functioning? There does seem to be a burgeoning interest in the family therapy field in helping families with health problems. The relatively new *Family Systems Medicine* journal is one sign of interest in this area.

Whether the family therapy field is ready to accept *nurses* becoming more in-volved with families remains to be seen. Within most hospitals and health care settings the issue of territoriality is alive and well! It is our experience that other traditional disciplines, namely social work, psychiatry, and psychology, have difficulty accepting nurses doing family therapy. How a "family problem" and how a "health problem" are defined in a particular work setting can fuel the controversy, because the definitions involve issues of identity and professionalism. If nurses (working with a patient who has had a recent colostomy) invite the spouse to come for instruction on how to assist in changing the colostomy bag, are the nurses treating the family or treating the health problem?

If nursing and family therapy are to bridge camps, then the definition of whether a problem is a nursing or a family issue is a question of semantics. Ideally, the best person to intervene in a situation is the one with the most ready access to the system level in which a problem manifests itself. Nurses may have an advantage over other professionals in sidestepping territorial issues; by a simple reframing they can invite whole families to participate in nursing care rather than family therapy to minimize territorial issues. In this way they can avoid conflict with other professionals, such as social workers, psychologists, and psychiatrists, who may believe that nurses should not work with families. Reframing can also facilitate initial engagement with families. Experience has shown us that families are more receptive when invited for a *family nursing* meeting than for a *family therapy* session.[2]

RECOMMENDATIONS FOR TRAINING NURSES

The following recommendations are based on our seven years of experience in teaching over 1,000 practicing nurses about family assessment and intervention. In addition, it is based on our experience in teaching nursing students in a certificate program, a bachelors program, a master's in nursing program and a family therapy institute. Because we have also taught physicians, social workers, and psychologists, we are aware of the different issues involved in educating nurses.

First, we recommend that trainers be aware of nurses' sensitivities to the discrepancy between their educational level and that of their colleagues. Practicing nurses are aware of the fact that they may not have a master's or even a university degree, and yet may deal with the same types of patients and their families in the same setting as professionals from other disciplines. Thus, nurses may sometimes feel very insecure and unskilled in comparison to other team members, while at other times they may feel very resentful because they are expected to deal with these patients and their families on a day-to-day basis, and they often cope as well as or better than other health professionals.

Second, we recommend that training be offered in the nurses' context using *their* families, *their* presenting problems, and *their* language whenever possible. Nurses respond very well when family interviews are conducted in their own work setting (e.g., the hospital or community health agency). We have gone to acute care hospitals, auxiliary hospitals, and home care and community health agencies to interview families with which the nurses are already working; because the presenting problems were health-related, the nurses were quite able to apply family therapy concepts to situations with which they were already familiar. When problems less familiar to the nurse must be addressed, this can be done by translating the problem into language familiar to the nurse. For example, we have had success in teaching nurses how to deal with "leaving home" issues by presenting a family interview in which this issue was connected with the young adult's chronic illness, which the parents thought should prevent him from establishing his independence.

CONCLUSION

Family therapy in nursing is an evolving new specialty. This specialty fits well in the practice of nursing because of the existing emphasis on the family as one of the primary units of health care. Nursing also has the advantage of providing 24-hour hospital care, which allows nurses to utilize opportunities afforded by family visits (Wright & Bell, 1981). Family therapy can be compatible within nursing if there is more openness within *both* disciplines, and if one doesn't attempt to consume the other.

However, in order for a family therapy specialty to be appreciated and recognized within the nursing profession, more nurses need to obtain training in family therapy both at the master's and doctoral level. Initially some nurses may obtain this training outside the nursing discipline. For others it will, one hopes, be obtained in *nursing* graduate programs. As more nurses possess specialized training in family therapy, and thus are able to teach and train other nurses, the family therapy specialty will become more valued. We see a strong trend in this direction.

Notes

1. The Family Nursing Unit, directed by Dr. Lorraine M. Wright, offers families assistance when one or more family members are experiencing difficulties with a physical and/or emotional illness.

2. The decision to use the name Family Nursing Unit for the training facility at the University of Calgary was a very deliberate and conscious one to avoid potential territorial and engagement issues.

References

Bateson, G. (1979). *Mind and nature.* New York: E. P. Dutton.

Carter, E., & McGoldrick, M. (Eds.). (1980). *The family life cycle: A framework for family therapy.* New York: Gardner Press.

Clark, C. (1978). *Mental health aspects of community health nursing.* New York: McGraw-Hill.

Clemens, I. W., & Buchanan, D. M. (Eds.). (1982). *Family therapy: A nursing perspective.* New York: Wiley.

Cunningham, R. (1978). Family-centered care. *Canadian Nurse, 2,* 34–37.

Epstein, N., Bishop, D., & Levin, S. (1978). The McMaster model of family functioning. *Journal of Marriage and Family Counseling, 4,* 19–31.

Friedman, M. (1986). *Family nursing: Theory and assessment.* New York: Appleton-Century-Crofts.

Goren, S. (1979). A systems approach to emotional disorders of children. *Nursing Clinics of North America, 14,* 457–465.

Grace, H., & Camilleri, D. (1981). *Mental health nursing: A sociopsychological approach* (2nd ed.). Dubuque, IA: William C. Brown.

Haley, J. (1977). *Problem-solving therapy.* San Francisco: Jossey-Bass.

Hoffman, L. (1981). *Foundations of family therapy.* New York: Basic Books.

Horton, T. (1977). Conceptual basis for nursing intervention with human systems: Families. In J. Hall & B. Weaver (Eds.), *Distributive nursing practice: A systems approach to community health* (pp. 101–115). New York: Lippincott.

Janosik, E., & Miller, J. (1979). Theories of family development. In D. Hymovich & M. Barnard (Eds.), *Family health care: General perspectives* (2nd ed.) (Vol. 1, pp. 3–16). New York: McGraw-Hill.

Janzen, S. (1980). Taxonomy for development of perceptual skills. *Journal of Nursing Education, 19,* 33–40.

Keeney, B. (1982). What is an epistemology of family therapy? *Family Process, 21,* 153–168.

Leahey, M., & Slive, A. (1983). Treating families with adolescents: An ecological approach. *Canadian Journal of Community Mental Health, 2,* 21–28.

Leahey, M., & Wright, L. M. (1985). Intervening with families with chronic illness. *Family Systems Medicine, 3*(1), 60–69.

Leahey, M., & Wright, L. M. (1987a). *Families and life-threatening illness.* Springhouse, PA: Springhouse Corporation.

Leahey, M., & Wright, L. M. (1987b). *Families and psychosocial problems.* Springhouse, PA: Springhouse Corporation.

Minuchin, M. (1974). *Families and family therapy.* Cambridge, MA: Harvard University Press.

McArthur, R. G., Tomm, K. M., & Leahey, M. (1976). Management of diabetes mellitus in children. *Canadian Medical Association Journal, 114,* 783–787.

Selvini-Palazzoli, M., Boscolo, L., Cecchin, G., & Prata, G. (1980). Hypothesizing–circularity–neutrality: Three guidelines for the conductor of the session. *Family Process, 19*, 3–12.

Tomm, K. M. (1984a). One perspective in the Milan systemic approach: Part I. Overview of development, theory and practice. *Journal of Marital and Family Therapy, 10*, 113–125.

Tomm, K. M. (1984b). One perspective on the Milan systemic approach: Part II. Description of session format, interviewing style and interventions. *Journal of Marital and Family Therapy, 10*, 253–271.

Tomm, K., McArthur, R. G., & Leahey, M. (1977). Psychological management of children with diabetes. *Clinical Pediatrics, 16*, 1151–1155.

Wiley, L. (1978). Family-centered conferences for better trauma care. *Nursing, 8*, 70–77.

Wright, L. M. (1986). An Analysis of live supervision "phone-ins" in family therapy. *Journal of Marital and Family Therapy, 12*, 187–190.

Wright, L. M., & Bell, J. (1981). Nurses, families and illness: A new combination. In D. Freeman & B. Trute (Eds.). *Treating families with special needs* (pp. 199–206). Ottawa: Canadian Association of Social Workers.

Wright, L. M., & Leahey, M. (1984). *Nurses and families: A guide to family assessment and intervention.* Philadelphia: Davis.

Wright, L. M., & Leahey, M. (1987). *Families and chronic illness. Vol. 2: Family Nursing Series.* Springhouse, PA: Springhouse Corporation.

Wright, L. M., Miller, D., & Nelson, K. L. (1985). Treatment of a nondrinking family member in an alcoholic family system by a family nursing team. *Family Systems Medicine, 3*(3), 291–300.

Wright, L. M., Watson, W. L., & Duhamel, F. (1985). The Family Nursing Unit: Clinical preparation at the master's level. *The Canadian Nurse, 81*, 26–29.

18

Family Therapists Teaching in Family Practice Settings: Issues and Experiences

DONALD C. RANSOM
University of California, San Francisco

This chapter is addressed to family therapists who are teaching or thinking about teaching in family practice settings. Since the formal recognition in 1969 of family practice as the 20th specialty in medicine in the United States, opportunities for family social scientists and family therapists have grown steadily (Ransom, 1981). These new roles have not come easily or without controversy and some pain (see Doherty, 1986; Dym & Berman, 1985; McDaniel & Campbell, 1986; Merkel, 1983). We can now draw on almost 20 years of experience to lend a perspective that may be helpful to reflect on this line of interdisciplinary work.

The discussion is organized by answering a set of questions. Where does family therapy fit within family practice, and what is the purpose of family systems training? Where do the pitfalls lie, and what approaches to teaching have been successful? Why should family therapists bother to teach within medical settings, and what does the future hold?

THE PLACE OF FAMILY THERAPY WITHIN FAMILY PRACTICE

From the beginning, the modern specialty of family practice was built upon a platform that included an integration of medical and behavioral science, and emphasized the role of the family in health, illness, and care. But this does not mean what the average family therapist is likely to think it should mean; family practice is not to medicine as family therapy is to psychotherapy.

To the family therapist, family therapy is not simply another tool in the professional's kit. Family therapy refers to a variety of forms of therapeutic intervention, but most significantly to a conceptual orientation and approach to human problems. At a very important point in the history of psychotherapy, the early family therapists stood conventional individual approaches on their heads. The novel shift was the reversal from viewing individual pathology and primary social relationships in terms of the patient to viewing the patient's condition as a product of interaction with the social environment. Figure and ground became reversed. In time family therapy assumed the status of a movement in the field of mental health, and has gradually extended itself to all types of health and personal problems.

The stimulus for the emergence of family therapy came from observing that patients' otherwise strange behavior seemed to make sense when seen in the light of family interaction and family history. The nature of this observation supported the reemerging "epistemological" challenge of American pragmatic reasoning (contextualism) against all earlier mechanistic and reductionist approaches. Family therapy also reflected and became an emerging political force in the 1960s that championed the underdog, countervailed against blaming the victim, and legitimized the profession of psychotherapy for a wide range of practitioners by openly rejecting the medical model.

Family practice, on the other hand, had different practical, political, and intellectual roots. It emerged as a reform movement within mainstream medicine (Cogswell, 1981). Early supporters saw in family practice a corrective for fragmented, episodic, bureaucratic, impersonal, and technocratic care, as well as for an increasingly geographically maldistributed physician population.

Family practice was proposed as a discipline of synthesis, integrating a wide range of medical and personal skills into the practice of a single physician. In the early days, however, its intellectual roots were shallow. If anything, family practice was anti-intellectual and antiacademic. This attitude prevailed in spite of the discipline's and the profession's need to gain respectability and a firm position in the institutional training structure of medicine. It is instructive that in its first 20 years, the chief conceptual contributions to the emerging field of family medicine came from those inspired by the British general practice tradition and from social and behavioral scientists who have participated in the development of a new field.

In the debates of the mid-1960s there was controversy about changing the name from "general" to "family" practice. Although it has not been confirmed, word has it that it was a well paid New York–based public relations firm that insisted on the new name in the end. Their research confirmed that "family" is one of the warmest and most positively associated words in the English language.

The early emphasis on being different from general practice, and the promotion of an ambitious new model, which included social and behavioral dimensions, led to unanticipated but understandable effects. Persuasive rhetoric created an expectation that real *family* physicians would be produced. This idea took hold not just in the public mind, but in the minds of all those who threw in with family practice in the beginning, and in the minds of medical students who were to choose family practice residency training in increasing numbers because of what they were led to believe it was all about. This is the lofty legacy that has been inherited by all those who are currently involved in family practice training.

An illuminating observation provided by Stephens (1982) is that, in the formative years, those who spoke for family practice said more than they knew. They heard themselves speak a new language and grew accustomed to words like *wholeness, care, person, responsibility, continuity, comprehensiveness*, and, I would add, *behavioral science, culture, ethnicity, family*, and *community*. They glimpsed a new vision of what medical care can and ought to be, and they turned toward it. In the process, something of the meaning of these terms became known, but as I have heard many a veteran lament, far more was got than was bargained for.

It is useful for family therapists entering family practice settings to have some understanding of the differences in themes and historical backgrounds of the two fields in order not to make the mistake of assuming they hold too much in common, intuitively easy to do because of the shared term *family*. In particular, family therapists are often bothered by the lack of interest in the "new epistemology" and the low level of explicit focus on families as units of care shown by physicians who call themselves "family" doctors.

On the other hand, the two disciplines do have some things in common, even if these similarities are not immediately obvious. Both have formed "countercultures" in tune with progressive themes and changes in the culture at large; both stand out on patient advocacy; and both embody a style of working that is eminently practical and economical.

Summarizing the central purpose of a family therapist's training efforts in family practice is problematic because there is an underlying and unacknowledged lingering conflict over what family practice itself should be (Ransom, 1985b). Two views have been discernible from the beginning. They are approaches that are not necessarily incompatible, but which represent a different essential feeling, and different kinds of imagination at work. Family therapists fit usefully into both approaches.

One view is that family practice is a horizontal specialty in the tradition of other specialties, a discipline of synthesis. In this model family physicians exercise skills originating in other disciplines, which may learn and exercise them in greater depth. Added to this is a special appreciation of the patient as a person, and the patient's family, community, and culture. Insights and techniques from family therapy are useful in this approach because they both add to the physician's repertoire of skills and shed light on factors that otherwise obscure the process of diagnosis and interfere with optimum treatment.

Significantly, this approach leaves the biomedical model unchallenged and seeks, instead, to expand it and make it more complex. In contemporary terms, *psycho* and *social* are added to *bio*, but all are flattened out along the same logical plane in the data-gathering and reasoning processes. There are simply more variables to include and more skills to learn. Ironically, solutions are more esssentially technical than ever; even the humanistic dimension of practice becomes reducible to proper human engineering. Imaginations at work on this model ask basic questions, such as how effective family therapy is for certain diagnoses, before they include family therapy training in the curriculum. They seek further to decide how much family therapy a family physician should really do.

The second view follows from a different sense of what a generalist is (Carmichael, 1985). The premium here is not the breadth of horizontal reach nor even the synthetic integration, but the depth and skill with which one can understand what ails the patient and what the patient needs to get well, to feel well, or to suffer as little as necessary. The crucial distinction here is one of framing and detailing; the patient's aims and condition and the physician–patient–family–community relationship are hierarchically—logically—prior to and inform any technical exchange that might occur between physician and patient.

From this perspective the insights and methods of family therapy are valued, not as one more set of tools in the doctor's bag, as in the first model, but as a means to glimpse the subject of practice with new lenses and to increase one's understanding of the patient's condition in order to be more helpful. In this sense family therapists are seen as allies in the effort to transform the first view sketched out above, contributing to a reconstruction of the basis of primary care and to the development of new habits of physician thought and behavior.

TEACHING PITFALLS AND BREAKTHROUGHS

Few family practice programs set as an objective the training of residents to do family therapy. The teaching task is broader and in some ways more difficult than that found in family therapy training centers. Along with the basics of individual and family development, and the emotional and behavioral problems family therapists are familiar with a family curriculum must also deal with health-relevant issues of normal life transitions and family response to the stresses of acute and chronic illnesses. This is because families turn to family physicians for a much greater range of reasons than they turn to family therapists. In family practice, family therapy is required only a small percentage of the time, although many of the skills and the knowledge base of the family therapy are relevant most of the time.

This tension between "working with families" and "family therapy" has been a continual theme at annual workshops organized by the Task Force on the Family in Family Medicine of the Society of Teachers of Family Medicine. The exploration of this theme has led to an increasing recognition and understanding of the special training needs of family physicians.

A controversial issue has been the emphasis on pathology present in family therapy approaches, together with the difficulty everyday family practice has in adopting techniques that were invented for treating severely pathological situations. *Therapy*, in contrast with *counseling* or *working with*, deals with seemingly irrational or unchangeable problems through corresponding irrational or, at least, counterintuitive means, such as precipitating crises, and paradoxical injunctions. In addition to the problem of providing cortex scramblers and sledgehammers when a meaningful conversation would do, many of these methods, and the larger approaches from which they stem, simply do not graft well onto family practice. This is a source of potential conflict and confusion that any family therapist taking up teaching family physicians must recognize.

One proposed solution to this problem is the distinction drawn by Doherty and Baird (1983) between "primary care family counseling" and "specialized family therapy," which are where the two are distinguished as different levels of intervention. The distinction identifies a necessary and realistic role for family physicians that restricts them to being neither watered-down family therapists nor strictly biomedical practitioners who should leave all "psychosocial" aspects of health care to others. It also provides a perspective for the natural link between family physicians and family therapists for consultation and referral. Doherty and Baird (1986) have elaborated and further refined this framework by outlining a developmental sequence of five stages they have observed many physicians moving through as they increase their competence in family-centered care. The sequence seems to be from exchanging information, to dealing with affect, to assessing and altering social processes:

Level 1: Minimal emphasis on family
Level 2: Ongoing medical information and advice
Level 3: Feelings and support
Level 4: Systematic assessment and planned intervention
Level 5: Family therapy

Each level is described in terms of a knowledge base, personal development needed, and skills required. This scheme is helpful in setting program training goals and outlining general areas of curriculum development.[1]

Pitfalls

Many pitfalls await the family therapist who embarks on a training venture in family medicine. Three of the most common are the following.

1. The most serious mistake is the failure to appreciate the context of family practice. This is odd, considering that family therapy was built on the insight that a patient's condition must be understood in terms of that person's relevant life contexts; yet family therapists seem to view family physicians unempathically.

Hochheiser and Chapados (1985) develop this point persuasively in their critique of Bishop and colleagues (1984) and, indirectly, of McLean and Miles (1975). There are both practice style and personal and professional identity issues involved here. Hochheiser and Chapados suggest that "family physicians' versus family therapists' views of patients, of themselves, of the context of care delivery, of patient care objectives, of content base, and of actual care delivery methods—create two radically different frames of reference" (p. 479). Obviously, these differences must be understood and accommodated if training is to be successful and satisfying.

The personal and professional identity issues are complex, involving the differing territories of the physician's and the family therapist's authority, and the anxiety that accompanies the trainee's perceived necessity to venture out from the felt security of the biomedical model (Ransom, 1985a). The human body is undisputed, familiar ground, whereas engaging the family is pushing the limits of knowledge, even when working in the specialty called family practice.

Physicians, with few exceptions, are systems thinkers whose systems thinking is limited to physical processes and stops at the boundary of the skin. Social and symbolic relations lie beyond the pale. The old family therapy rallying themes of "circular versus linear" and "systems versus individual" thinking are less relevant here than the physician's difficulty in incorporating social and cultural reality and meaning in construing the patient. Information and intervention are located not only in tissue relations but in social relations. What is revealed in disease and illness as physical signs and symptoms can also be embodiments of social relations disguised as natural things (Taussig, 1980). This leap is difficult to make, and it is in dealing with these issues that teaching efforts can be most helpful (Stein & Grant, 1985).

2. A second pitfall is to approach the family therapist's role too literally—as if it had to do primarily with teaching family physicians to do family therapy or to treat psychosocial problems. Statistics show that many visits to family physicians are "non-

medically based." For better or worse, the greatest provider of treatment for mental illness in the United States is the family physicians. Family physicians should be trained to do this work properly, but this does not mean that ways of doing therapy by family therapists in family therapy settings can be carried over to family practice. Nor do I believe teaching therapy as such is where to begin. What is needed first is an approach that helps the family physician transform the whole of practice in a direction faithful to the aims of the proposed new role as expressed in the best of the descriptive rhetoric. Again, drawing on Hochheiser and Chapados, such an approach would make use of concepts and techniques from family therapy in order to "improve understanding of patients' family dynamics and their implications for health," and to "improve patient care in such areas as: patient compliance; patient education; patient family care assistance; diagnosis and treatment planning; family crisis intervention; more effective referrals—including general medical and mental health care referrals; management of long-term care; and family physician personal family functioning" (1985, p. 479).

3. A third common pitfall is to be flattered into taking on a "group therapist" or "organizational consultant" role in dealing wtih faculty and program process problems. This pitfall awaits any therapist who takes a regular faculty position. It is to be distinguished from taking on a group facilitator role in either resident personal and professional development or support groups, or leading a resident or faculty Balint group (discussed in the next section). I am referring to the temptation to play a central role in dealing with faculty-to-faculty or faculty-to-administration conflicts, or in mediating faculty–resident disputes.

In the eyes of family therapists, physicians are primitive in their ability to handle intragroup conflicts, and are relatively unsophisticated "communicators" given their degree of professional training and stature. It is both tempting to step in and "show them how," and easy to get "triangled" into conflict that is better left to the group to struggle with, or better still, left to be handled by whoever is at the helm. The result of playing therapist is usually not good, either for the program or for the pseudotherapist.

A sampling of other potential pitfalls, listed as a series of "complaints" by a family physician striving to collaborate with family therapists, can be found in the tongue-in-cheek but astute article by McDaniel and Campbell (1986). Family therapists may find this piece refreshing because it provides an equal number of complaints by a family therapist collaborating with family physicians.

Breakthroughs

The challenge of teaching in family practice settings is to resist the inclination to export family therapy training approaches wholesale in favor of drawing on them selectively to create new styles and methods that fit the family practice environment. What this means can be inferred from the "pitfalls" outlined above and from the following group of suggestions that have a record of success.

1. *Make your top priority to provide practical help with real patients.* Family approaches achieve credibility as they prove useful. Residents are always busy and usually stressed. They appreciate nothing more than help when they need it. It takes only a few meaningful exchanges to start the relationship that is necessary if real teaching and

learning are to occur. Things work best when the consultant fits into the resident's flow. If the family specialist accommodates to the demands of the physician's situation, the family specialist's approach is more likely to be assimilated.

2. *Get into the room whenever you can.* Do not pass up opportunities to observe residents and patients face to face. Family therapists know well that watching is almost always more useful than hearing a description. What goes together in the mind and makes a good presentation does not necessarily go together on the job.

Until family therapists entered the family practice training arena, it was the norm for physicians to pass through medical school and residency training and to enter practice without ever having been directly observed interviewing a patient outside the hospital. In family practice, where the doctor–patient relationship is key, this was a great weakness in training. Now the combination of direct observation and shoulder-to-shoulder collaboration has changed this for the better.

Direct observation and collaborative care also have the advantage of creating opportunities for family therapists to be observed working with patients by physicians. Modeling is an effective form of teaching. Just hearing a few novel questions being asked, or observing the "joining" process with family members present, can lead to a significant breakthrough in the resident's approach.

3. *Use videotape whenever practical.* In certain situations recording has advantages over being in the room or observing through a one-way mirror. Family visits can be taped at one time and reviewed at another. Videotape can be taken home and watched on the resident's own equipment. Particular sequences can be selected for later discussion. Observing oneself in action on tape creates a unique learning opportunity. Saving real examples also provides powerful material for training tapes or use in seminar discussions.

4. *Take advantage of and create additional conditions for residents to see families.* Seeing families in action and discovering new information about them firsthand is more persuasive than hearing lectures. Home visits can be particularly valuable because something can be learned from the family's home environment and one's own reaction to it.

5. *Be a presence in the hospital and go to the bedside often.* Even though family practice is an ambulatory care specialty, family practice residents spend upward of 60% of their time in the hospital during training. Although the general hospital may not be the most congenial setting in which the family therapist can teach, it certainly offers many opportunities, if only by dint of the sheer volume and variety of work with which residents are confronted there.

The hospital is a likely if inconvenient place to meet family members in times of crisis and transition. The patient's condition can rapidly be made more intelligible through contact with family members. Discharge planning, at times, cannot occur without them. Family crisis intervention and helping people deal with serious illness and death are most likely to occur in conjunction with a hospitalization. Further, the hospital is a fruitful ground for observing cultural, professional, and institutional "systems dynamics" as patient, family members, family physician, subspecialists, nurses, administrators, and third-party payment monitors all play out their roles (Ransom & Dervin, 1978).

Points of entry for the family therapist teacher are "morning report" and bedside rounds, returning to the bedside later for longer conversations, and participating in team meetings (when multiple personnel are all involved with a patient whose care is likely to become conflicted and confused without communication and coordination among those involved).

6. *Teach family interviewing and family assessment as routine clinical skills to be learned early.* There is some controversy in family therapy about whether assessment should be separated from direct work on the problem presented. In family practice, however, it is not always clear what the problem is, or even if there is a problem, since people often do not come in or get themselves referred in order to work directly on a problem in the way they do in therapy. Doing a good family assessment provides valuable background information, and makes more intelligible the strands involved in working toward any goal in family practice. Further, family assessment fits within conventional medical practice even while it expands it.

Similarly, teaching basic interviewing skills should not be skipped over in favor of teaching "pure" family therapy models and other technical methods. Asking useful questions, actively listening, staying with and drawing out relevant details, and learning to lead and follow a conversation for its psychological and interactional relevance, are all crucial to the eventual success of family practice physicians.

7. *Get a seminar going.* Avoid placing too much emphasis on noon conference "smorgasbord" lectures. People quickly forget what they cannot soon apply or actively reflect on. Seminars with small groups of residents that do not excessively strain hospital and clinic coverage during a regular time slot are a good way to cover many themes and practice skills relevant to family training. Such regular meetings provide a good structure for digging into basic texts such as Christie-Seeley (1984), Doherty and Baird (1983), Glenn (1984), Medalie (1978), and Sawa (1985). Family practice training would be much improved if it were more like graduate school, but this is a luxury it cannot afford for the time being.

8. *Create opportunities for focused reflection.* Responding to immediate needs in the heat of the moment is paramount, but a different kind of learning takes place when a situation can be reviewed and less obvious alternatives considered. For example, charts can be reviewed using a family-focused approach (Wolkenstein, Lawrence, & Butler, 1985).

9. *Organize personal and professional development groups, and support groups for residents and partners.* Family therapists make excellent leaders for such groups; they are able to work with the individual needs of residents without losing sight of the group process. Residency programs benefit from such components because their residents are provided a tangible means to reduce stress and interpret their training experience within a supportive and structured process. Difficulties can be handled before they become crises. Family therapists benefit from participating in such groups because they gain invaluable insight into the day-to-day struggles of residents who are deprived of sleep, overworked, and dealing with issues removed from what most family therapists are accustomed to (Addison, 1984).

10. *Learn to lead Balint seminars.* Michael Balint was a Hungarian-born psycho-analyst who emigrated to Scotland in 1939 and, after World War II, moved on to London, where he worked at the Tavistock Clinic. Balint (1957) has done more than any other behavioral scientist to influence the style of British general practice. His impor-

tance was in teaching general physicians how to think about patient behavior as meaningful, how to view the reality of the patient's condition and the clinical encounter as a social construction, and how to work with countertransference, a lost art for many family therapists (see also Stein, 1985).

In Balint's later years he moved steadily closer to the family system. His grasp of the social context of health and illness led him to describe the child as the presenting symptom, to observe that changes in one member of a family follow changes in the relationship with another, and to give a detailed account of the dynamics of what we now call "triangles" in the relationship between patient, physician, and consultant (Glenn, 1983).

WHY BOTHER?

Anyone reading this chapter through to this point probably already has at least some experience in training family physicians, or at least is thinking about the possibility. Nevertheless, the question can still be raised: Why bother to work in such an unfamiliar setting, one fraught with limitations and difficulties, and destined to be controlled ultimately by physicians? A sense of the poignancy of this question is captured in Doherty's (1986) wistful departing piece, "A Missionary at Work: A Family Therapist in a Family Medicine Department."

Apart from practical reasons, such as competitive salary structures and opportunities for referrals, there are challenging intellectual reasons for family therapists to work with family physicians. Here I will mention three. First, I recently raised the possibility that family therapy may need family medicine to save it from itself (Ransom, 1982a, 1983). As I saw it, family therapy was showing serious signs of suffering from the lack of a working dialogue with another discipline.

After 20 years of open development, with contributions from a diverse group of creative reformers, family therapy had turned excessively inward and was in danger of isolating itself. In the early 1980s much discussion seemed to alternate between trance-inducing self-congratulation and self-aggrandizing pseudopolemics. No other field in the health professions or social sciences could equal family therapy in hero-worshipping, showmanship, and flamboyant rhetoric. Rejecting other approaches out of hand, staging meetings that turned into performances, and insisting that the "new epistemology" was the only proper way to look at the world—all seemed imminently self-destructive to me.

Likewise, family therapy showed signs of needing contact with a discipline that places high regard on concrete, material reality and on empirical investigation as the basis for daily practice. New sources of data besides those obtained in tertiary care family therapy referral centers needed to be explored. A potentially useful corrective for these ills lay in working with the related and noncompetitive discipline of family practice.

Recently, leaders in the field have lamented the failure of family therapy over the years to influence the basic institutions that serve people in our society (Liddle, 1986; Minuchin, 1985). This observation introduces a second good reason for family therapists to bother with family practice. There is much that is useful in the family therapist's approach to problems, in particular the skills and perspective that allow a contextualization of the subject of concern. Instead of complaining about how others conduct their business, family therapists have in family practice a realistic and challenging opportunity to influence one of the most ancient and universal roles among the helping professions.

Finally, through working with family physicians, family therapists have an opportunity to test and refine their own techniques and ideas in novel settings. How easy to generalize are family therapy methods, and what is their scope? How do family therapy thinking and its attendant practices need to be adapted to fit within another discipline? Family practice makes it possible to observe and to work with a much greater range of families than was heretofore possible. How will such experience modify the ways family processes are conceptualized, and what difference will practical work in this setting make, in turn, on the family therapist's accustomed style?

In my own case, 18 years of experience working primarily in family practice centers has led to adopting a style that has been significantly influenced by the family physician's: working, at least initially, with all manner of problems and all age groups; seeing people off and on for years when the need arises, thus modifying greatly the traditional therapist's concern with termination issues; working with three generations and members of extended families; functioning as a go-between with community agencies and institutions on patients' behalf; and, above all, demystifying treatment and the understanding of psychological and family processes and working steadily to forge and reinforce a collaborative relationship. If there is one thing I have learned working with family practice patients, it is that the problem of "resistance" has been greatly overestimated by those family therapy writers who are referred only the most immovable people, and that patients resist the approach of their helpers as often as they resist whatever it is about themselves that keeps them from changing (Ransom, 1982b).

THE FUTURE

The future for family therapists interested in training family physicians looks promising for a number of reasons. The social and economic forces that have carried these disciplines into the mainstream of North American culture are, if anything, increasing. Expectations for further collaboration can be traced to the following sources.

1. The steady increase in the age of the population, and the incidence of chronic disease and illness related to life-style and stress, require that, if health care provider responses are to be effective, they must be increasingly informed by an understanding of the social and behavioral bases of these problems. Similarly, looking from the other direction, the increasing demands of high-tech medicine, together with the often dramatic effects and fallout from such treatments on patients and their families, require that, if modern medicine is to be responsible in the exercise of its power and effective in the long run, it must work with those whose lives have been so radically changed. Family therapists have much to offer in preparing health care providers for this work.

2. The role of the family physician within the health care system at large is changing in ways that make the kinds of approaches and skills that family therapists teach increasingly useful. Here I am referring to the family physician not only as the true generalist and the point of entry into medical care, but also as the "gatekeeper" in large health maintenance organizations and prepaid health insurance plans. In these arrangements family physicians are far removed from the insulation of independent and small

group practices, and must deal constantly with organizational constraints and systems processes. Communications skills and knowledge of interactional dynamics can be invaluable in these settings if structures of collaboration can be built in which this expertise can be modeled and taught (Bloch, 1984).

3. The Family Practice Residency Review Committee is becoming increasingly stringent in applying its basic requirements for programs to train residents in family development, family processes, and office counseling. Further, family therapy is on the elective end of the continuum of levels of physician involvement with families outlined by Doherty and Baird (1986). To fulfill the first need, family physicians are bringing family therapists in to teach in family practice centers; to fulfill the second, fellows in family medicine and experienced family physicians are taking courses, workshops, and special practica at family therapy training centers across North America.

4. The sheer volume and type of problems brought to family physicians, together with a more complex framework within which to think about and respond to patient needs, make it ever more likely that family physicians and family therapists will be working together in teams (Hepworth & Jackson, 1985). In addition to the teaching teams already mentioned, faculty practices are including family therapists in a variety of ways as the pressure to finance training programs from internal revenue increases.

Some community-based team practices are already sufficiently well developed to have been described in the literature (Dym & Berman, 1986; Glenn, Atkins, & Singer, 1984). Also, within new delivery structures, family practice–based health maintenance organizations are hiring family therapists as contract providers (Crane, 1986). The recently introduced *Working Together: A Collaborative Health Care Newsletter*, edited by Michael Glenn, is evidence of the increasing numbers of primary health care providers seeking a forum to explore these new developments.

This growth has not gone unnoticed by the professional organizations representing family therapy. In 1982 the American Family Therapy Association formed an enduring interest group on "Family Therapy and Family Medicine." Most of those who have attended the annual meetings in the past five years have been involved primarily in training. The National Council on Family Relations added a section on "The Family and Health" in 1983. This group is composed largely of those with research interests, and many are also involved directly in training in medical settings. In the fall of 1986 a task force on "Medicine and Family Therapy" met for the first time at the annual meeting of the American Association for Marriage and Family Therapy. The initial group is composed of several members whose main concern is training. Further evidence of professional growth is the founding in 1982 of the journal *Family Systems Medicine*, edited by Donald Bloch. Its focus, "the confluence of family therapy, systems theory and modern medicine," makes it no accident that the lion's share of references cited in this chapter were drawn from that journal. These are all valuable resources for any family therapist interested in training in family practice settings.

Note

1. Readers interested in obtaining further details for curricular goals, objectives, and content should consult the following sources.

- Accreditation Council for Graduate Medical Education. (1983). *Essentials of accredited residencies in graduate medical education.* Chicago: American Medical Association.
- Family Health Foundation of America. (1983). *MERIT project, a compendium of topics for curricular development in family practice.* Kansas City, MO: American Academy of Family Physicians.
- Society of Teachers of Family Medicine Task Force on Behavioral Science. (1985). *Core competency objectives in behavioral science education.* Kansas City, MO: Society of Teachers of Family Medicine.
- Stein, H., & Grant, W. D. (1985). *Behavioral science in family medicine: A program for second and third year family medicine residents.* Oklahoma City: University of Oklahoma College of Medicine. Distributed by the Society of Teachers of Family Medicine, Kansas City, MO.

References

Addison, R. B. (1984). *Surviving the residency: A grounded interpretive investigation of physician socialization.* Unpublished doctoral dissertation, University of California, Berkeley (University Microfilms No. 84-268-89).

Balint, M. (1957). *The doctor, his patient, and the illness.* New York: International Universities Press.

Bishop, D. S., Epstein, N. B., Gilbert, R., van der Spuy, J. I. J., Levin, S., & McClemont, S. (1984). Training family physicians to treat families: Unexpected compliance issues. *Family Systems Medicine, 2,* 380-386.

Bloch, D. (1984). The family therapist as a health care consultant. *Family Systems Medicine, 2,* 161-169.

Carmichael, L. A. (1985). A different way of doctoring. *Family Medicine, 17,* 185-187.

Christie-Seeley, J. (1984). *Working with families in primary care.* New York: Praeger.

Cogswell, B. (1981). Family physician: A new role in process of development. *Marriage and Family Review, 4*(1-2), 1-30.

Crane, D. D. (1986). The family therapist, the primary care physician, and the health maintenance organization: Pitfalls and possibilities. *Family Systems Medicine, 4,* 22-30.

Doherty, W. T. (1986). A missionary at work: A family therapist in a family medicine department. *The Family Therapy Networker, 1986, 10*(2), 65-68.

Doherty, W. T., & Baird, M. (1983). *Family therapy and family medicine: Toward the primary care of families.* New York: Guilford Press.

Doherty, W. T., & Baird, M. (1986). Develpmental levels in family-centered medical care. *Family Medicine, 18,* 153-156.

Dym, B., & Berman, S. (1985). Family systems medicine: Family therapy's next frontier? *The Family Therapy Networker, 9*(1), 20-29, 66.

Dym, B., & Berman, S. (1986). Family physician and family therapist in joint practice. *Family Systems Medicine, 4,* 9-22.

Glenn, M. L. (1983). Balint revisited: On the 25th anniversary of the publication of *The doctor, his patient, and the illness. Family Systems Medicine, 1,* 75-81.

Glenn, M. L. (1984). *On diagnosis: A systemic approach.* New York: Brunner/Mazel.

Glenn, M. L., Atkins, L., & Singer, R. (1984). Integrating a family therapist into a family medical practice. *Family Systems Medicine, 2,* 137-145.

Hepworth, J., & Jackson, M. (1985). Health care for families: Models of collaboration between family therapists and family physicians. *Family Relations, 34,* 123-127.

Hochheiser, L. I., & Chapados, J. (1985). Training family physicians to treat families: What is done and what is needed. *Family Systems Medicine, 3,* 476-480.

Liddle, H. A. (1986). Redefining the mission of family therapy training: Can our differentness make a difference? In F. Piercy (Ed.), *Family therapy education.* New York: Haworth Press.

McDaniel, S., & Campbell, T. J. (1986). Physicians and family therapists: The risk of collaboration. *Family Systems Medicine, 4,* 4-8.

McLean, P. D., & Miles, J. E. (1975). Training family physicians in psychosocial care: An analysis of a program failure. *Journal of Medical Education, 50,* 900-902.

Medalie, J. (1978). *Family medicine: Principles and applications.* Baltimore: Williams & Wilkins.

Merkel, W. T. (1983). The family and family medicine: Should this marriage be saved? *Journal of Family Practice, 17,* 857–862.

Minuchin, S. (1985). An interview with Salvador Minuchin. *The Family Therapy Networker,* 8(6), 21–31.

Ransom, D. C. (1981). The rise of family medicine: New roles for behavioral science. *Marriage and Family Review,* 4(1,2), 31–72.

Ransom, D. C. (1982a). *The development of a family perspective in health care.* Paper presented at the National Conference on Family Systems Medicine: Therapy of Families with Physical Illness, New York.

Ransom, D. C. (1982b). Resistance: Family—or therapist—generated? In A. Gurman, (Ed.), *Questions and answers in the practice of family therapy* (Vol. 2). New York: Brunner/Mazel.

Ransom, D. C. (1983). Random notes: On building bridges between family practice and family therapy. *Family Systems Medicine, 1,* 91–96.

Ransom, D. C. (1985a). Random notes: A sense of purpose for teaching behavioral science in family medicine. *Family Systems Medicine, 3,* 494–499.

Ransom, D. C. (1985b). Random notes: The unconventional future of family medicine. *Family Systems Medicine, 3,* 120–126.

Ransom, D. C., & Dervin, J. V. (1978). The family, the hospital and the family physician. In R. B. Taylor (Ed.), *Family medicine: Principles and practice.* New York: Springer-Verlag.

Sawa, R. J. (1985). *Family dynamics for physicians: Guidelines to assessment and treatment.* Lewiston, NY: Edwin Mellen Press.

Stein, H. F. (1985). What ever happened to countertransference? In H. F. Stein & M. Apprey (Eds.), *Context and dynamics in clinical knowledge.* Charlottesville: University of Virginia Press.

Stein, H. F., & Grant, W. D. (1985). *Behavioral science in family medicine: A program for second and third year family medicine residents.* Oklahoma City: University of Oklahoma College of Medicine. Distributed by the Society of Teachers of Family Medicine, Kansas City, MO.

Stephens, G. G. (1982). *Family medicine as a counter-culture.* In G. G. Stephens (Ed.), *The intellectual basis of family practice.* Tucson, AZ: Winter Publishing Company.

Taussig, M. T. (1980). Reification and consciousness of the patient. *Social Science and Medicine, 14B,* 3–13.

Wolkenstein, A. S., Lawrence, S. L., & Butler, D. J. (1985). Teaching "family": The family medicine chart review. *Family Systems Medicine, 3,* 171–178.

19

Academic Psychology and Family Therapy Training

MICHAEL BERGER
Atlanta Institute for Family Studies

> *For nothing is worthy of man as man unless he can pursue it with passionate devotion*—Max Weber, *Science as a Vocation*

In writing this chapter, I take for granted that any form of training is influenced by the context in which training is conducted (Berger & Jurkovic, 1984a; Liddle, 1978). This context includes both the particular organizational structure in which a given program is embedded and the traditions and practices of the professional discipline to which the program adheres. Since the purpose of this chapter is to discuss family therapy training in psychology, I shall begin by reviewing and discussing the current status of family therapy within psychology. (Because the bulk of family therapy training in psychology occurs in academic psychology departments, I shall limit my discussion to those settings.) Next, I shall consider a number of areas within psychology (social psychology, child development, ecological and comunity psychology, clinical child psychology, and behavior therapy) where connections between that area and family therapy theory or practice might easily be made. I shall then grapple with the central issue, namely what seems to me to be the most effective way to train therapists in psychology departments, noting also the difficulties involved in providing such training in this setting. Finally, I shall speculate on the future of family therapy, and on psychology's contribution to that future.

THE STATUS OF FAMILY THERAPY IN PSYCHOLOGY

Family therapy, at present, is a minor part of psychology in general, and clinical psychology in particular. The most recent study (conducted in 1977) of the acceptance of family therapy in doctoral-level clinical training programs approved by the American Psychological Association (the major professional and credentialing organization in psychology), indicated that, nationally, about 10% of clinical faculty identified themselves as being primarily family therapy–oriented, that 32% of the programs had no family oriented faculty, that 18% of all psychotherapy courses were family-oriented, and that 21% of the schools had no family therapy courses (Cooper, Rampage, & Soucy,

303

1981).[1] These findings, while not overwhelmingly supportive of family therapy, indicate a greater acceptance of family therapy in psychology than the results of earlier studies (e.g., Stanton, 1975). This increased acceptance, however, is probably more acceptance of family therapy as another treatment method than as an orientation to human problems (L'Abate & Thaxton, 1983; Liddle, 1978). Support for the view that family therapy as a conceptualization of human problems is not taken seriously in psychology is found in the article by Cooper and his colleagues cited above. They note with interest that the number of family therapy courses in the doctoral programs they studied correlated not with the program's rating of the importance of family therapy, but with the total number of therapy courses offered by the program. This, the authors argue, fits with the fact that the majority of the programs they studied defined themselves as having an "eclectic" theoretical orientation to therapy. "It would appear," Cooper and his colleagues comment, "that schools with a psychotherapeutic orientation are committed to a generalist training approach and offer courses in all areas" (Cooper et al., 1981, p. 157).

The most recent study of training opportunities for predoctoral psychology interns in marital and family therapy (Solomon, Ott, & Roach, 1986) does not paint a more optimistic picture. Surveying all of the internships listed in the 1983–1984 Directory of Internships in Professional Psychology, the authors found that 95% of the responding sites said that they offered some training in marital or family therapy, and 75% of these sites indicated that some involvement for the entire internship year was feasible. The average percentage of the intern's time devoted to marital or family therapy was 14%, a smaller percentage of time than that devoted to any major intern activity (e.g., individual therapy, testing and assessment, training and supervision, and group therapy) except group therapy. The mean amount of supervision offered per week in marital or family therapy was 2.9 hours; however, less than half of the training staff at the internship sites was involved in supervision, and by far the most frequent form of supervision involved interns reporting their own behavior in marital or family session. Only 31% of the reporting internship sites had any training staff who were clinical members of AAMFT, and only 26% of the sites had doctoral psychologists who were clinical members. Twelve percent of the sites had training staff who were approved supervisors in AAMFT, and 9% had doctoral-level psychologists who were approved supervisors. In an attempt to delineate training sites that offer a major emphasis on training in marital and family therapy, the authors list 11 sites that meet the criteria of having at least 25% of the intern's total time for the year spent in marriage and family therapy training, and of having at least half of the intern's supervision involving either videotape or live supervision. The authors also list 11 other sites that permit interns to spend at least 20% of their time in marriage and family therapy training, and that utilize some videotape or live supervision.

In addition, other studies (e.g., Dunne & L'Abate, 1978) have shown that neither families nor family therapy are more than barely mentioned in introductory psychology textbooks, the medium that defines the field for most people. It is also true that until quite recently, systemic or family therapy theory and practice was poorly represented as an interest group in the American Psychological Association.

The almost nonexistent status of family therapy in psychology should not be surprising. Traditionally, the major conceptual unit and research in psychology has been the individual, isolated from his or her context (Bronfenbrenner, 1979; Berger & Berger, 1985; L'Abate & Thaxton, 1983). Family or systemic therapy, which conceptualizes problems as occurring between people (in units as small as two, but usually larger) and which suggests that behavior in living systems cannot accurately be reduced to either individual perception or individual behavior (Scheflen, 1978, 1980; Spiegel, 1971), threatens the entire conceptual and research tradition of psychology as a discipline.[2] The acceptance of family therapy theory as a way of thinking in psychology would require changes in psychologists' basic unit of conceptualization, in their ideas of generally appropriate research methods[3] and questions, and in their thinking about what sort of discipline-important knowledge it is appropriate to impart to students training to become members of the profession. Jay Haley (1975) noted years ago that changes of such magnitude tend also to involve changes in status and definitions of competence within the discipline, and therefore rarely occur easily, if at all.

AREAS OF CONNECTION

Thus far, it is not clear how family therapy has become as much a part of psychology as it is at present. Family therapy seems to have entered the discipline through the interests of particular faculty and students (Liddle, 1978), and perhaps through its increasing acceptance in the general clinical zeitgeist as a permissible mode of treatment (Cooper et al., 1981). There are, however, a number of areas in academic psychology where connections with family therapy theory and practice might easily be made (L'Abate & Thaxton, 1983). These include social psychology, child development, ecological and community psychology, clinical child psychology, and behavior therapy. These connections are of two sorts. The first are connections that directly affect family therapy theory and practice; the second are connections that indirectly affect theory and practice, either through providing information about child, adult, and family development and processes, or through providing methods that may usefully be employed in the study of family therapy. (See the dialogue on this last point between family researchers and therapists in Framo, 1972.)

In the early 1950s and 1960s social psychologists, with their large amount of experience in studying group behavior, were seen as likely sources of theory, methods, and findings that might well apply to families, since families can be viewed as groups (Aldous, 1971; Framo, 1972). In the past 20 years, however, a number of arguments have been raised about the wisdom of generalizing from the usually time-limited, artificial groups studied by social psychologists in the laboratory to ongoing natural groups with a history, such as families. Two remarks should make this line of argument clear. The first is from Karl Wieck, a social psychologist speaking at a symposium on family problem solving. Wieck notes that he is discomforted by the very phrase "family problem solving" because it carries the connotation of a set of activities separate and set apart from other family activities. "The point," he says, "is that the phenomenon in which we are interested is probably very difficult to isolate. It is part of an ongoing stream of behavior when members interact with each other, and many problems undoubtedly get stated and solved without the outside observer even knowing that something was amiss or being worked on" (in Aldous, 1971, p. 9).

This point, Wieck continues, has several implications for the relevance of laboratory studies of family problem solving to the actual experience of families in their daily lives.

> For example, any laboratory group that is given a ready-made distinct problem and the task of solving it probably bypasses many of the crucial dynamics in family problems. They bypass such questions as how one comes to know that a problem exists, what it does to solution adequacy to be working on several different things *concurrently* with problem solving, what it's like to go about solving a felt, intuited problem rather than an explicitly stated, consensually validated problem which was made visible to all members at a specific point in time. (in Aldous, 1971, p. 9)

Wieck's comments, although they point to profound differences between the study of family problem solving in the lab and in daily life, do not suggest that it would be impossible for social psychologists to study the phenomenon of daily problem solving in family life in ways that would come closer to capturing this phenomenon. It was left for Jay Haley to say something very like that. Commenting at a symposium on family interaction involving family researchers and therapists, Haley noted that

> for many years all of us, myself included, began to treat families as if they could be studied as units in themselves, ignoring the context in which they were being studied. We assumed that a family in the home and a family in the testing situation and a family in therapy were the same family, and the question is whether we are contaminating our results by not differentiating between these contexts. Once you have seen the same family in these three settings, you think about a family very differently. (in Framo, 1972, p. 195)

These two sets of remarks point to several conclusions. Wieck's comments highlight the sharp limitations of laboratory research in illuminating the process of problem solving in natural groups with an ongoing history such as families. Interesting confirmation of this point can be found in the book by David Reiss (1981), a noted researcher of family process and problem solving in both laboratory and naturalistic settings. As one goes from the first part of Reiss's book, which contains his laboratory studies, to the second, which contains his theory of how "family paradigms" develop, are maintained, and change in the world outside the laboratory, one notices that the concepts that are relatively adequate to explain the laboratory findings have been either dropped or radically altered in order to construct plausible explanations of family behavior in more naturalistic contexts. Reiss's book is also consistent with Haley's remark that the context in which the family is studied alters what can be seen. When Reiss talks about families in their daily world, he focuses on, he sees, different things than when he studies the same families in his lab.

Although families studied by researchers are not in the same context as families in therapy, the findings of social psychological researchers to date can offer family therapy some interesting information about family behavior outside of therapy and some ideas that may prove useful in therapy. (See, for example, the use made of social psychological "attribution theory" in the recent theory and practice of functional family therapy [Barton & Alexander, 1981].)

Generally, the research tradition in child development has involved the study either of individual children or of processes such as cognition or development within individual children (Berger & Berger, 1985; Harris, 1957). In the past 20 years, however, more and more developmentalists have noted that children live and develop within families, and more sophisticated conceptions of how families influence children have, at least on a theoretical level, entered the field of child development. Bristol and Gallagher (1983) summarize this as a shift from a conception of family influence as geing unidirectional— that is, mothers influence the socialization of children (e.g., Bowlby, 1958)—to one in which mothers and children are seen as mutually interactive dyads in which each member affects the behavior of the other (e.g., Bell, 1968; Lewis & Rosenblum, 1974; Thomas & Chess, 1977), to one in which families are seen as containing pairs of mutually interactive dyads—that is, mothers and children and fathers and children affect one another (Lamb, 1978)—to a more systemic notion in which the effect of either parent on the child may either be direct or be mediated not only by the other parent, but by the relationship between the parents as well (e.g., Parke & O'Leary, 1976; Weinraub, 1978), to a more ecological notion in which the entire family is "seen as *one* of an interactive, interdependent *set* of systems "nested" within each other and in which the child affects and is affected by the family system as well as by other systems of which the family is a part" (Bristol & Gallagher, 1983).

While the more ecological or systemic conceptions of family influence on child development are not yet the dominant paradigms in the field, and certainly have been more influential theoretically than in terms of generating actual research, the increasing importance of these concepts suggests that child development is likely to be a fertile source of information for family therapists about the child subsystem and about child-focused issues (Rosman, 1979).

Even the information generated about child development, and developmental processes within children, from nonsystemic research traditions should be useful to family therapists. An understanding of child development can only enhance the therapist's ability to discriminate between "normal" and "abnormal" child behavior and processes, as well as increase the therapist's ability to use developmental facts, concepts, and metaphors in reframing. Note, for example, the frequency and brilliance with which Salvador Minuchin, one of the best and most knowledgeable observers of children on this planet, will use developmental metaphors in his reframings: "He may look like he is 18, but he is acting like he is 12 and needs to be treated like a 12-year-old. Now, if he is 12, you, parents, need to . . ."

The same is true for the information contained in the adult development literatures in psychology. (For a summary and critique of this literature, see Berger & Berger, 1985.) As with the child development literature, adult developmentalists are beginning to talk in systemic terms (though they do so in a less sophisticated manner than do their child development colleagues). However, the information provided in the literature about adult processes and development can only be helpful to the clinician in guiding his or her understanding of predictable developmental issues, in helping the therapist distinguish between "normal" and "abnormal" adult problems, and so on (Carter & McGoldrick, 1980; Haley, 1973).

As Bristol and Gallagher (1983) make clear, an ecological framework has recently entered the literature on child development and family life. To date, this framework is most prominently seen in *The Ecology of Human Development*, by Uri Bronfenbrenner

(1979). This work sets forth a conception of ecological context that attempts to take into account systems at levels as different as the intrapsychic and the total community, at the same time viewing these systems as interdependent and nested within one another. This view will be familiar to family therapists who are acquainted with the theoretical work of Dick Auerswald (1968, 1983); Albert Scheflen (1978, 1980); and John Spiegel (1971). Although Bronfenbrenner's work is too recent to have had much influence on research to date, it has stirred up discussion in the field and interest in conducting research that would be more ecologically valid. In terms of intervention, Bronfenbrenner's framework is relatively consistent with much work in community psychology, for example, the 20 years of work done by Nicholas Hobbs through his Project Re-Ed (Hobbs, 1983). Hobbs's conception of children's problems and their treatment rests on a nicely ecological notion that problems develop when there is a lack of "fit," either between the child and one of the major systems in which the child was involved—for example, between the child and his or her parents, or between the child and his or her school—or when there is a lack of "fit" between the different systems in which the child functions—for example, between home and school, or the welfare department and home. While Hobbs is curiously weak in his descriptions both of family structure and of interventions with families, and seems not to know that the family therapy literature exists, numerous examples of the work of family therapists that are consistent with his views can be found (see, for example, Berger, 1984a, 1984b; Berger & Fowlkes, 1980; Clark, Zalis, & Saccho, 1982; Foster, 1984; Jurkovic, 1984). There is, then, work in the ecological and community psychology literature that connects nicely with major movements and ideas in family. And, if ecological thinking continues in psychology, it is likely to generate research findings that will help family therapists better understand that complicated web of interrelationships between individuals, families, social agencies, and commuties. (For the need for such understanding, see Berger & Jurkovic, 1984b.)

Until the past decade, clinical child psychology was heavily influenced by the psychodynamic child guidance tradition, in which individual, intrapsychic assessment and therapy were seen as the requisites of appropriate clinical work with children. This is no longer true. Rather, the field is in the midst of redefining what a relevant clinical child psychology would now be like (Tuma, 1982). While it is not yet clear whether a generally accepted model will emerge shortly, it is apparent that interest in families and family therapy has grown in this field. It is therefore quite possible that clinical child psychology will be a useful area in psychology for family therapists. More will be said about this below. What is clear even now is that this field has a good deal of information about effective interventions with children to offer family therapists. Such information is helpful since, as Montalvo and Haley (1973) have noted, intervening with individual children is one form of family therapy. And if the family therapist wishes, for tactical reasons, to work individually with children, the interventions used should be effective.

The most direct connection between an area in psychology and family therapy is that between behavioral marriage and family therapy and the field of family therapy as a whole. Behavioral marriage and family therapy, many major figures of which are psychologists and teach in psychology departments, has become a major movement in the family therapy field, generating theory (e.g., Gordon & Davidson, 1981; Jacobson, 1981; Patterson, 1985), a large amount of research (indeed, the hallmark of the behavioral approach may be its emphasis on evaluating clinical work and on tying theory to empirical findings), a body of clinical knowledge, and its own journals (e.g., *Child and Family Behavior Therapy*). It is certainly the major kind of family therapy that is taught and practiced in psychology.

Many family therapists who do not consider themselves to have a "behavioral" orientation have questioned whether what is called behavioral family therapy is truly a family therapy. Such therapists would argue that "behavioral family therapists" neither conceptualize treatment issues in terms of families nor intervene at a family level; rather, issues are thought of and treated in terms of dyads (Foster, Berger, & McLean, 1981; Haley, 1981). It does seem significant that much of what is labeled "family therapy" in the behavioral literature consists of interventions to alter the pattern of interactions between mothers and children (typically called "parent training"), with no apparent regard for whether changes in such interactions will reverberate throughout other areas of the family system. It also seems significant that, until recently, the behavioral literature has been quite parochial, with behaviorists citing only other behaviorists. There has, however, been a recent interest in strategic therapy (particularly in the work of Haley and Erickson), though mainly in terms of using strategic techniques to maneuver clients so that they will carry out behavioral programs.

An interesting example of the difficulty of locating "behavioral" programs in the family therapy field is shown by the case of Functional Family Therapy. Developed by James Alexander and his colleagues, this system of family therapy, described by Alexander as representing a synthesis of systemic and behavioral concepts, was first viewed as behavioral, and was published in behavioral journals. Over the years, however, the theory has been viewed as either behavioral or strategic, and it is now unclear how to place it. Readers of the Gurman and Kniskern (1981) *Handbook of Family Therapy* will note the editors' inability to decide whether this is a truly behavioral therapy that includes systemic techniques, or a truly strategic therapy that includes behavioral techniques.

Still, the behavioral marriage and family therapists have contributed a number of useful ideas and tactics to the family therapy literature. They have also greatly added to the methodological rigor of the field, first in their admirable insistence on empirically testing clinical ideas rather than accepting them on faith, and second, as a result of their interest in developing and using new sorts of research measures and methods, such as single-subject design, to evaluate the effects of family treatments.

Before concluding this section on possible points of connection between areas of psychology and family therapy, I would like to make two final points. The first I owe to my colleague, Lauren Adamson. Because psychology departments are characteristically housed in colleges of arts and sciences, they are administratively situated so as to make it easy for students in psychology to study in other fields (e.g., anthropology, sociology) which contain theories, methods, and information relevant to the understanding of families and of therapy. And, while this is rarely done at present, the placement of psychology departments within colleges of arts and sciences makes it administratively possible for students to study in the traditional humanist disciplines (e.g., literature, philosphy, and history) which also contain knowledge about individual and family life that may help make therapists more humane, more able to think about what they are doing, and less willing and able to be mere technicians. The second point is that the importance of empiricism in psychology makes it likely that family therapists trained in psychology departments will, at the very least, be oriented toward worrying about the empirical status of their beliefs about therapy. Furthermore, they will, one hopes, be more likely to organize their practice around data rather than around pure intuition or the practices of their peers or mentors.

FAMILY THERAPY TRAINING IN PSYCHOLOGY—A MODEL

It is time now to take a clear stand on the question of the advantages and disadvantages of training family therapists in academic psychology departments. I think that academic psychology departments are admirable settings for the training of strategic therapists, therapists who understand that part of their job is to understand the organization of their own treatment or training context, and to learn to speak the language and accommodate to the beliefs of others in that context (Jurkovic & Berger, 1984). The fact is that to announce straightforwardly in a psychology department that one is teaching a new kind of conceptualization that will alter the way in which students will think about pathology, assessment, change, and intervention is to doom one's students, if not oneself and one's program, to destruction (Liddle, 1978). Hence, the more useful tack to take is a strategic one (Todd, 1984).

A good way to illustrate this is through a description of the history of the family program at Georgia State University.[4] The program was started by Dr. Luciano L'Abate in the late 1960s. L'Abate, who had been trained as a child clinician, set up the program beautifully from a strategic point of view. First, he moved slowly from directing a child clinical program to focusing on families, thus minimizing the extent of his shift, since it seemed reasonable for child clinicians to attend to families. Second, rather than terming it a family therapy program, L'Abate first called it a program in family studies and, later, one in family psychology. His nomenclature highlighted the research aspects of the program (research is highly valued among psychologists). L'Abate was also diligent about setting up a laboratory (a traditional and highly valued institution in psychology departments) and in using that laboratory as a setting in which he and his students carried out publishable research (generating publishable research is a good thing in psychology departments). L'Abate also focused on family assessment (assessment being a traditional and highly valued activity among psychologists). L'Abate was also exemplary in not challenging the other major therapeutic paradigms in the clinical program (an adult-oriented humanistic transactional analysis–gestalt program, and a behavior therapy program). Rather, he was consistent in his praise of these other programs, encouraging his students to take courses in them as well as in the family program. To summarize, then, L'Abate talked the language of his setting, stressed the commonalities between aspects of his program and highly valued aspects of the department and discipline as a whole, and avoided challenging the other therapeutic paradigms in the department (L'Abate, 1983).

Several idiosyncratic aspects of the Georgia State program permitted L'Abate to be as successful as he was. First, he entered the graduate program early in its history and as a full professor, thus entering the setting at a time when there were many resources to go around, and entering at a level high enough to enable him to gather these resources relatively easily (Sarason, 1972). Second, the Georgia State clinical program is different from most APA clinical programs in two important ways: it has a long-standing tradition of allowing students to specialize in one kind of therapy, rather than in training "generalists," and the clinical faculty have always been strongly committed to training therapists. These traditions provided support for L'Abate in developing a specialist program for training family therapists, a support that would have been lacking in most doctoral programs in clinical psychology. Even with the support of these traditions, however, it is unlikely that, say, five years later, L'Abate would have been able to set up a new program as easily because, at that later time, summoning the resources for a new program would have meant removing them from some other, already existing program.

While there are obviously aspects of the Georgia State context that are unique to that university, I would in general recommend L'Abate's strategies for individuals who wish to train family therapists in academic psychology departments. In particular, I would suggest that the easiest way for family therapists, both currently and in the near future, to thrive in psychology departments is to label themselves as clinical child psychologists.[5] Clinical child psychology has a long and respectable tradition in psychology; thus, labeling oneself as a clinical child psychologist does not call attention to oneself as a revolutionary, or even as the new therapist on the block. Also, psychologists who work with children are allowed to concern themselves with families; thus it is legitimate for clinical child psychologists to concern themselves with families. In doing so, they do not raise the specter of a radically new theoretical orientation. Finally, as noted earlier, the field of clinical child psychology currently lacks a paradigm and is quite interested in families. Thus, with a little judicious reframing, it should be possible to do systemic therapy without being viewed as deviant within the clinical child psychology field.

There are, of course, some difficulties in training family therapists in academic psychology departments. One difficulty is that because training occurs in an academic department, students are continually evaluated on two different sets of criteria the relationship of which is unclear: their clinical skills and their academic skills. Many students report that these two sets of demands are often confusing and contradictory to them. Since it is arguable whether therapists need to be competent in both sets of skills, attempts to separate the two sets of criteria have been made in what APA terms "PsyD" programs; programs that do not require a doctoral dissertation, and that define the traditional model of the scientist–professional as meaning that a student may be either a scientist or a professional, and that it is legitimate to train persons who will mainly view themselves as clinicians.

However, even these programs will not solve another issue for students, namely, what is their professional identity? Certainly, at present, there are strong prestige and economic reasons for thinking of oneself as a clinical psychologist rather than as a family therapist—clinical psychology is the higher status discipline and, in many states, licensed clinical psychologists can collect third-party payments while family therapists cannot. One solution (recommended by Jurkovic & Berger, 1984) is to cease talking of family therapy and to train students to think of themselves as systemic therapists who define themselves by their expertise in solving a client's problem by intervening at the most propitious level of the ecosystem. While this solution commends itself theoretically, it has pragmatic limitations: almost no one knows what a systemic therapist is, states do not license systemic therapists, nor do insurance companies pay them. In my view, there is no good solution for this problem at present. Currently, therapists base their professional identities on a variety of criteria of different kinds—for example, on theoretical orientation (e.g., strategic, Bowenian, Jungian, Adlerian), on the discipline in which the therapist received his or her degree (e.g., psychologist, social worker, psychiatrist), or on the treatment unit most characteristically seen by the therapist. Until we have a broad and coherent conceptualization of therapy that encompasses all therapists, trainees and trainers will continue to have the current sorts of confusion about professional identity, and the choices they make about their professional identity will, in the main, be made on pragmatic or ideological grounds.

THE FUTURES OF FAMILY THERAPY AND THE CONTRIBUTION OF PSYCHOLOGY

It is necessary to distinguish two uses of the term "family therapy." The first refers to a way of thinking about human problems and their solution; in this sense, "family therapy" is but one level of intervention based on systemic thinking (Auerswald, 1968; Berger & Jurkovic, 1984b; Montalvo & Haley, 1973). As a believer in the utility of systemic thinking for the resolution of human problems, I see a bright future for this family therapy. I am particularly encouraged by recent developments suggesting that family therapy, as a way of thinking, has become mature enough to abandon some positions it took in opposition to psychoanalysis (the dominant theoretical paradigm against which the great mavericks who created the field rebelled) and to notice the obvious—for example, that there are times when individuals are the relevant units to work with and to understand, or that all of the usual therapeutic units (individuals, dyads, families, social networks) are arbitrary cuts into the ecosystem, and that conceptualizations and interventions useful at each of these levels need to be integrated (Rosman, 1979; Scheflen, 1978, 1980).

As a psychologist, I must, however, be skeptical of my faith and demand that, as much as is possible at any given time, the therapeutic notions that derive from systems thinking be empirically tested in the spirit of critical inquiry that looks, however reluctantly, for the disproof of one's cherished theories. Here, psychologists can certainly be justly proud, since much of the conceptually and methodologically sophisticated empirical research to date in family therapy (e.g., the work of Alan Gurman, of James Alexander, of Gerald Patterson, and of Duke Stanton and his colleagues) has been conducted by members of our profession. Such work needs to continue. There are far too many books published on family therapy that describe dramatically successful cases without providing the data necessary to evaluate the author's claims for his or her therapeutic work.

The second use of the term "family therapy" refers to its meaning as a sort of brand name for a profession that, like all professions, claims to have its own relatively unique body of knowledge, modes of training, and means of evaluating and credentialing potential members of the profession (Hughes, 1958). I am less optimistic about family therapy as a profession than I am about it as a way of thinking. I know that the men and women who created this way of thinking and founded the field came to it both because of their discomfort with the limitations of the disciplines in which they were trained, and because they passionately sought to pursue a set of issues that did not and do not fit comfortably within the purview of any one discipline (Berger & Berger, 1985; Dollard, 1935). To the extent that family therapy is now a profession and a discipline, it is likely that the kinds of people who will be attracted to the field now and in the future will be very different from the brilliant, charismatic, and eccentric mavericks who founded the field. This is, I gather from studies of other professions (e.g., Hughes, 1958; Levine & Levine, 1970), a familiar story; indeed, Max Weber in his phrase "the routinization of charisma" implies that such is the fate of all movements founded by brilliant leaders who have new ideas.

I hope that Weber will be proved wrong and that the fate of family and systemic theory and therapy is not to be codified and rigidified, that it will not die but, rather, will continue to develop, nourished by the contributions of new generations of workers in this area. Speaking of the *tshuvah*, the "turning toward," the reconciliation with God, Rabbi Farfon comments, "One is free not to complete the task, but one is not free not to undertake it." For myself, the ideas of family theory and therapy, and their potential for helping human beings solve their problems, are too important for us not to continually undertake the tasks of testing and developing them.

Acknowledgments

This chapter is a product of ongoing conversations on training issues with a number of individuals. The first is with my friends and colleagues at the Atlanta Institute for Family Studies, Carrell Dammann and Greg Jurkovic. The second is with my brother, Stephen. The third is with my former graduate students at Georgia State University, particularly David Kearns. The fourth is with my wife, Sherrill Oliver Berger. Finally, I wish to thank Jim Kochalka, Martha Foster, and Greg Jurkovic for their comments on earlier drafts of this chapter.

Notes

1. It is distressing to note that a recent study (Vanderbos, Strapp, & Kilburg, 1981) shows that while only 1% of psychologists have formal training in marital and family therapy, the psychologists themselves say that 40% of their cases involved treating cases that are primarily marital or family problems.

2. L'Abate (L'Abate & Thaxton, 1983) notes that while many psychological theorists (going back to Kurt Lewin) have talked about person–situation interactions, and thus can be seen as approaching a systemic view that looks at the relationship between different levels of analysis, these theorists have tended not to address the family per se as a crucial environmental context. Further, their analyses are static, as if persons and situations remain constant over time and do not change one another (Jurkovic, personal communication).

3. Although Gurman (1983) has cogently argued that many of the traditional methodologies used by psychologists can be appropriately used to answer systemic questions.

4. As far as I know, this is the only doctoral-level program in clinical psychology approved by the American Psychological Association that offers a specialization in family therapy.

5. The family and clinical child programs at Georgia State University followed this tack for 18 months, merging to form a combined Child and Family Psychology Program. In an interesting recent development, L'Abate has written several papers indicating his lack of interest in family therapy and proposing the importance of family psychology. In line with this change in interest, the family therapy program at Georgia State has been abolished as a separate track, and the primary faculty person identified with that program (the author) has resigned from the university, while L'Abate is now directing a specialization in family psychology.

References

Aldous, J. (Ed.). (1971). *Family problem solving.* Hinsdale, IL: Dryden.

Auerswald, E. (1968). Interdisciplinary versus ecological approach. *Family Process, 7,* 202–215.

Auerswald, E. (1983). The Gouverneur Health Services Program: An experiment in ecosystemic community health care delivery. *Family Systems Medicine, 1,* 5–24.

Barton, C., & Alexander, J. (1981). Funcational family therapy. In A. Gurman & D. Kniskern (Eds.), *The handbook of family therapy.* New York: Brunner/Mazel.

Bell, R. (1968). A reinterpretation of the direction of effects in studies of socialization. *Psychological Review, 75,* 81–95.

Berger, M. (1984a). Family therapy in special education settings. In M. Berger & G. Jurkovic (Eds.), *Practicing family therapy in diverse settings.* San Francisco: Jossey-Bass.

Berger, M. (1984b). Social network interventions for families with a handicapped child. In E. Coopersmith (Ed.), *Families with handicapped children.* Rockville, MD: Aspen.

Berger, M., & Berger, S. (1985). Individual and family life cycle development. In L. L'Abate (Ed.), *Handbook of family psychology and psychotherapy.* Homewood, IL: Dow Jones-Irwin.

Berger, M., & Fowlkes, M. (1980). The family intervention project: A family network approach to intervention. *Young Children, 35,* 22–32.

Berger, M., & Jurkovic, G. (1984a). Introduction: Families, therapists, and treatment settings. In M. Berger & G. Jurkovic (Eds.), *Practicing family therapy in diverse settings.* San Francisco: Jossey-Bass.

Berger, M., & Jurkovic, G. (Eds.). (1984b). *Practicing family therapy in diverse settings.* San Francisco: Jossey-Bass.

Bowlby, J. (1958). The nature of the child's tie to his mother. *International Journal of Psychoanalysis, 39,* 350–373.

Bristol, M., & Gallagher, J. (1983). *Psychological research on fathers of young handicapped children: Evolution, review, and some future directions.* Paper presented at the NICHD Conference on research on families with retarded persons, Rougemont, North Carolina.

Bronfenbrenner, U. (1979). *The ecology of human development.* Cambridge, MA: Harvard University Press.

Carter, E., & McGoldrick, M. (Eds.) (1980). *The family life cycle.* New York: Gardner.

Clark, T., Zalis, T., & Saccho, F. (1982). *Outreach family therapy.* New York: Aronson.

Cooper, A., Rampage, C., & Soucy, G. (1981). Family therapy training in clinical psychology programs. *Family Process, 20,* 155–166.

Dollard, J. (1935). *Criteria for the life history.* New Haven: Yale University Press.

Dunne, E., & L'Abate, L. (1978). The family taboo in psychology textbooks. *Teaching of Psychology, 5,* 115–117.

Foster, M. (1984). Family therapy and the schools. In M. Berger & G. Jurkovic (Eds.), *Practicing family therapy in diverse settings.* San Francisco: Jossey-Bass.

Foster, M., Berger, M., & McLean, M. (1981). Rethinking a good idea: A reassessment of parent involvement. *Topics in Early Childhood Special Education, 1,* 55–56.

Framo, J. (Ed.). (1972). *Family interaction: A dialogue between family researchers and family therapists.* New York: Springer-Verlag.

Gordon, S., & Davidson, N. (1981). Behavioral parent training. In A. Gurman & D. Kniskern (Eds.), *The handbook of family therapy.* New York: Brunner/Mazel.

Gurman, A., & Kniskern, D. (Eds.). (1981). *The handbook of family therapy.* Nw York: Brunner/Mazel.

Gurman, A. (1983). Family therapy research and the "new epistomology." *Journal of Marital and Family Therapy, 9*(3), 227–234.

Haley, J. (1973). *Uncommon therapy.* New York: Norton.

Haley, J. (1975). Why a mental health center should avoid family therapy. *Journal of Marriage and Family Counseling, 1,* 3–13.

Haley, J. (1981). *Reflecting on therapy.* Chevy Chase, MD: Family Therapy Institute of Washington.

Harris, D. (Ed.). (1957). *The concept of development.* Minneapolis: University of Minnesota Press.

Hobbs, N. (1983). *The troubled and troubling child.* San Francisco: Jossey-Bass.

Hughes, E. (1958). *Men and their work.* Glencoe, IL: Free Press.

Jacobsen, N. (1981). Behavioral marital therapy. In A. Gurman & D. Kniskern (Eds.), *The handbook of family therapy.* New York: Brunner/Mazel.

Jacobsen, N., & Margolin, G. (1979). *Marital therapy: Strategies based on social learning and behavior exchange principles.* New York: Brunner/Mazel.

Jurkovic, G. (1984). Family therapy and the juvenile justice system. In M. Berger & G. Jurkovic (Eds.), *Practicing family therapy in diverse settings.* San Francisco: Jossey-Bass.

Jurkovic, G., & Berger, M. (1984). Conclusion: Implications for practice, training, and social policy. In M. Berger & G. Jurkovic (Eds.), *Practicing family therapy in diverse settings.* San Francisco: Jossey-Bass.

L'Abate, L., Berger, M., Wright, L., & O'Shea, M. (1979). Training family psychologists: The family studies program at Georgia State University. *Professional Psychology, 10,* 58-65.

L'Abate, L., & Thaxton, L. (1983). The family as a unit of psychological study and practice. *Academic Psychology Bulletin, 5,* 71-83.

L'Abate, L. (1983). *Family psychology: Theory, therapy, and training.* Washington, DC: University Press of America.

Lamb, M. (1978). The father's role in the infant's social world. In J. Stevens & M. Mathews (Eds.). *Mother/child, father/child relationships.* Washington, DC: National Association for the Education of Young Children.

Levine, M., & Levine, A. (1970). *A social history of the helping services.* New York: Appleton-Century-Crofts.

Lewis, M., & Rosenblum, L. (Eds.). (1974). *The effect of the infant on its caregiver.* New York: Wiley.

Liddle, H. (1978). The emotional and political hazards of teaching and learning therapy. *Family Therapy, 5,* 1-11.

Montalvo, B., & Haley, J. (1973). In defense of child therapy. *Family Process, 12,* 223-233.

Parke, R., & O'Leary, S. (1976). Father-mother-infant interaction in the newborn period: Some findings, some observations, and some unresolved issues. In K. Riegel & J. Meacham (Eds.), *The developing individual in a changing world: Vol. 2. Social and environmental issues.* The Hague: London.

Patterson, G. H. (1985). Beyond technology: The next stage in developing an empirical base for training. In. L. L'Abate (Ed.), *Handbook of family psychology and therapy* (Vol. 2). Homewood, IL: Dorsey Press.

Reiss, D. (1981). *The family construction of reality.* Cambridge, MA: Harvard University Press.

Rosman, B. (1979). *Developmental perspectives in family therapy with children.* Paper presented at the Annual Meeting of the American Psychological Association, New York.

Sarason, S. (1972). *The creation of settings and the futures of society.* San Francisco: Jossey-Bass.

Scheflen, A. (1978). Susan smiled: An exploration in family therapy. *Family Process, 17,* 59-67.

Scheflen, A. (1980). *Levels of schizophrenia.* New York: Brunner/Mazel.

Solomon, J., Ott, J., & Roach, A. (1986). A survey of training opportunities for predoctoral psychology interns in marriage and family therapy. *Journal of Marital and Family Therapy; 12*(3), 269-280.

Spiegel, J. (1971). *Transactions.* New York: Science House.

Stanton, M. D. (1975). Family therapy training: Academic and internship opportunities for psychologists. *Family Process, 14,* 433-439.

Thomas, A., & Chess, S. (1977). *Temperament and development.* New York: Brunner/Mazel.

Tuma, J. (1982). Proposal for a national conference on professional preparation of clinical child psychologists. *Journal of Clinical Child Psychology, 11,* 3-7.

Todd, T. (1984). The family therapist as administrator: Roles and responsibilities. In M. Berger & G. Jurkovic (Eds.), *Practicing family therapy in diverse settings.* San Francisco: Jossey-Bass.

Vanderbos, G., Stapp, J., & Kilburg, R. (1981). Human Service providers in psychology: Results of 1978 APA Human Resources Survey. *American Psychologist, 11,* 1395-1418.

Weinraub, M. (1978). Fatherhood: The myth of the second-class parent. In J. Stevens & M. Mathews (Eds.), *Mother/child, father/child relationships.* Washington, DC: National Association for the Education of Young Children.

20

Marriage and Family Therapy and Graduate Social Work Education

DONALD R. BARDILL
Florida State University School of Social Work

BENJAMIN E. SAUNDERS
Medical University of South Carolina

Since its inception, social work has been practiced in a broad interface with the family both as a social institution and as a primary site of human growth and development. Social work is an integrative profession in that it has always been involved in many diverse areas of practice, and has employed a variety of intervention methods. Social workers develop and implement social policy, conduct social and behavioral research, administer organizations, and broker and deliver a wide range of social services. They work in public and private social service agencies, hospitals, mental health clinics, political organizations, federal departments, schools, universities, private practice, court systems, industry, and so on. Throughout this broad spectrum of practice activity, however, involvement with families has been, and continues to be, a consistent and pervasive part of the professional domain of social work (Bardill & Saunders, 1983; Kadushin, 1978; Saunders, 1980; Siporin, 1980). Consequently, training in the area of marriage and the family long has been an accepted part of social work education.

The purpose of this chapter is to begin a serious discussion about some of the issues surrounding social work's relationship to family therapy. The presentation is organized around three main themes. The first involves a historical view of social work practice with families which provides a context in which to examine training issues. The second theme involves a report on the current status of marriage and family therapy training in social work education. Past surveys as well as new data are used to examine how schools of social work teach marriage and family therapy. Included in this section is a discussion that addresses several critical issues relevant to teaching marriage and family therapy in social work education. Some of these issues concern serious obstacles to successful social work training in marriage and family, while others involve important advantages. The last theme covers a proposed Master of Social Work degree curriculum that complies with the accreditation standards of both the Council on Social Work Education *and* the American Association for Marriage and Family Therapy.

SOCIAL WORK EDUCATIONAL STRUCTURE

A brief description of the structure of social work education may be helpful for the reader unfamiliar with such an education program. Today, social work education occurs at the bachelor's, master's, and doctoral levels. The university or college administrative structure delivering the training may be a professional school of social work or a department of a particular college in a university. The nomenclature of the degrees granted is somewhat mixed. Undergraduate degrees may be called the traditional Bachelor of Science, or the more specific Bachelor of Social Work (BSW). Master's degrees typically are the Master of Science in Social Work (MSSW), or the more common Master of Social Work (MSW). Doctorates in social work are denoted by Doctor of Social Work (DSW) or the more tradition PhD degree. Many social workers also use the professional designation ACSW, signifying membership in the Academy of Certified Social Workers. Some use LCSW, Licensed Clinical Social Worker, or a similar symbol of state licensure. These last two designations ordinariy imply graduation from an accredited school of social work, two or three years of successful practice experience, and the passing of either a certification or a licensing examination.

The accrediting body for professional social work education is the Council on Social Work Education (CSWE). This body accredits undergraduate and master's degree social work programs according to strict academic and professional guidelines (CSWE Commission on Accreditation, 1984). Doctoral programs are recognized but not formally accredited by CSWE. There are numerous unaccredited social work programs, just as there are many people in the social service field who call themselves "social workers" but who have never received an accredited social work degree at any academic level. This chapter will be concerned only with accredited social work education.

FAMILIES AND SOCIAL WORK IN THE PAST

A proper understanding of the place of family therapy in social work education cannot be gained without some awareness of the history of social work practice with families, a history that is not widely known and is frequently misunderstood. Social work training has traditionally been intertwined with practice, and this is particularly so with family work.

Since the beginning of the profession, social workers have been concerned with the family both as an important social unit and as a critical area for effective therapeutic intervention. Ackerman, Beatman, and Sherman (1961) stated, "Historically, the family has been the major focus of social work concern" (p. 1). Siporin (1980) concurred with this view and wrote: "Marriage and family therapy are traditional and basic social work services. Social workers have provided these services as part of the core of social work practice since the beginning of the profession" (p. 11). As a result of this concern for families, social workers have made substantial contributions in every stage of development of family therapy practice and training.

Early Pioneers

While the significant influence of many recent social workers on family therapy is universally recognized (e.g., Papp, Hoffman, & Satir) the work of the early family caseworkers in the last 19th and early 20th centuries has been largely ignored by modern family theorists and practitioners. Speaking of these early workers, Siporin (1980) commented, "Recent historical accounts, including those of social workers, of the development of this area of practice [family therapy] have been grossly inaccurate in denying, depreciating, or neglecting this rich tradition" (p. 11). Bowen (1975), Guerin (1976), Erickson and Hogan (1976), Okun and Rappaport (1980). Hansen and L'Abate (1982), and Nichols (1984) have all written histories with this bias. A notable exception is the work of Broderick and Schrader (1981). In their excellent, comprehensive history of family therapy, due attention is given to the early caseworkers, particularly the progressive contributions of Mary Richmond. They concluded, "It seems likely that their [social workers'] actual contribution [to family therapy] is much greater than present accounts give them credit for" (p. 7).

How did social work's early concern for families develop? The purpose and technology of the profession at that early time give some clues as to why families became such an important focus of intervention. Social work as a profession began in the late 19th century and grew primarily out of the charity movements in England and the United States. Most social workers at that time were concerned with improving the lot of the poor and impoverished of society. Of course, workers sought to meet basic human needs by providing life necessities such as food and shelter, but they also were concerned with relieving the emotional distress of their clients and with changing the forces that maintained their clients in the subclasses of society. Two important "practice methods" are associated with early social work, the friendly visitor movement and the settlement house.

The friendly visitor was exactly that, a social worker who visited the homes of clients in order to assess needs and provide help. These visits brought social workers into regular, intimate contact with families. Workers observed the day-to-day functioning and situational context of entire families, and literally experienced their problems. The friendly visitor quickly became involved in helping with family relationship problems, especially those concerning parenting and marital issues. (Moggridge, 1882; Sanborn, 1890; Tuckerman, 1832).

Workers at settlement houses had similar experiences. Settlement houses were centers for social relief located in distressed neighborhoods and staffed by social workers. Wilson (1976) described what settlement house workers encountered.

> Few clients came by themselves to settlement houses. Instead, they came in twos or threes or larger groups. Their motivation was based on curiosity, rumor from school or neighborhood, consciousness of perplexing problems, or desire for friendly visiting. In the beginning, the helpers just responded to what they faced. They did not say to themselves, "Ah ha, here is the structure of a natural group" (p. 3)

Many of the "twos and threes" were whole families seeking aid. And, like the friendly visitors, the settlement house workers became involved in the everyday life problems of their client families.

These workers were faced daily with crushing human problems and needs that unmistakably involved entire families, as well as the larger social system. Their practice methods and conceptualization emerged from their continuing experience with trying to help distressed people. Their goal was not science but successful change.

Training in the early years of social work consisted mainly of practical experience under the supervision of senior workers. However, as practice methods became more refined and a conceptual framework for social work practice began to take shape, training became more formalized. The New York School of Philanthropy was founded as the first institution offering formal education in what was then termed "charity work." Family casework was probably the most developed aspect social work training at the turn of the century because of the family-oriented nature of practice and the concommitant conceptual development. Indeed the first course taught by the first school of social work in the United States involved family treatment and was entitled "The Treatment of Needy Families in Their Own Homes" (Meier, 1954; Siporin, 1980).

Though the terminology of family systems theory employed today is not present, the early family casework literature contains descriptions of many practice techniques and concepts that sound strangely modern. For example, friendly visitors were instructed to interview both parents at the same time in order to gain a complete picture of a family's problems. Consequently, "conjoint sessions" were common. In a time when mothers were the symbol of family life, fathers were to be included as much as possible in all interventions, still a wise course according to modern research (Gurman & Kniskern, 1981). Parenting instruction was a core area of practice, a precusor to formal family life education. Mary Richmond described a system of "charitable cooperation" between individuals, families, and other organizations, which Siporin (1980) correctly identified as an early form of family networking.

The idea with the most strikingly modern ring often repeated in this literature, however, is the injunction that a client family must be considered and approached as a whole. Smith (1890) commented, "We deal with the family as a whole . . ." (p. 377). Mary Richmond (1917), in her classic work, *Social Diagnosis*, prescribed treatment of the "whole family" and cautioned against interviewing only individual family members. Clearly, the early caseworkers considered the family to be a unitary social unit in much the same way that modern family systems theory views families.

The work of Richmond best demonstrated the progressive conceptual development concerning families by social work at this time. Her early development of the concept of family cohesion is especially interesting. She defined it, in much the same manner as modern theorists (e.g., Olson, Sprenkle, & Russell, 1979), as essentially the degree of emotional bonding between family members. In her view "degenerate" families had low levels of cohesion and the "best type of united" family had a high degree of cohesion. Unlike many modern theorists, however, she did not speculate on the negative effects of extreme family cohesion, or "family enmeshment." Much of her practice methodology was based on this idea of family cohesion.

Richmond also refined the notion of viewing families as systems within systems. She recognized that families are not isolated wholes (Closed systems), but exist in a particular social context, which interactively influences and is influenced by their functioning (i.e., they are open systems). She graphically depicted this situation using a set of concentric circles to represent various systemic levels from the individual to the cultural. Her approach to practice was to consider the potential effect of all interventions on every systemic level, and to understand and to use the reciprocal interaction of the systemic hierarchy for therapeutic purposes. She truly took a systemic view of human distress.

The hierarchical, multilevel systems view of human functioning was not unique to Richmond. Indeed, one of the great ongoing debates of early (and current) social work practice was directly attributable to this paradigm. One faction of the profession argued for direct, "Micro" intervention with individuals and families, while a second faction believed that true change in the human condition was possible only through "macro" intervention at a higher level of the cultural system, such as, changes in social policies. One result of this debate was that social work as a profession attacked problems of the human condition at every level of the social system; individuals, families, organizations, communities, and government. Though members of the opposing factions would only grudgingly admit it, each had a strong appreciation for the work of the other and both shared the multilevel systems view.

Early Alliance with Psychiatry

Broderick and Schrader (1981) commented, "With these strong beginnings it seems possible that the field of social work might well have brought forth the fields of marriage and family counseling as mere subspecialities within the broader field of family casework" (p. 6). While social workers continued to contribute to the understanding and treatment of families, the strong family system orientation of the direct practice arm of the profession began to change during the 1920s. This change was due primarily to social work's alliance with psychiatry and the resulting strong influence of psychoanalytic theory on social work practice (Bardill & Saunders, 1983; Broderick & Schrader, 1981; Quarata, 1979).

The individual orientation of psychoanalytic theory, the development of the orthopsychiatric team approach, and the emerging mental health professional hierarchy all worked to alter social work's traditional view of the family as a whole. At that time, psychiatric social work developed as a speciality area treating a particular, circumscribed part of the human condition, dysfunctional behavior. Individuals, families, and treatment became fragmented, with each professional on the team (Psychiatrist, psychologist, and social worker) responsible for certain pieces of the patients, their families, and their treatments. Psychiatric social workers still worked with families, but now they were viewed as relatives of patients rather than whole systems. Often workers were concerned with a very narrow range of problems, rather than the wide variety of issues managed by the early pioneers. And, while home visits continued, they became a special technique of practice rather than the norm. Consequently, family concepts and practice methods inherited from the early pioneers were used less frequently, while the use of individually oriented psychiatric theory and terminology increased.

The development of family intervention by social work changed but did not stop in the 1920s and 1930s. Social work continued to claim the domain of family work, and to provide the majority of service through the 1940s and 1950s. However, the strong systems theory flavor of the work diminished, and, as Siporin (1980) pointed out, with a few notable exceptions, the interventive style of the early family caseworkers was nearly forgotten.

Modern Family Therapy

Nichols (1984) commented that most historical accounts of the development of modern family therapy in the 1950s take either a "great man" or zeitgeist (climate of the times) point of view. Most accounts, including that of Nichols, fail to acknowledge the contribu-

tions of social workers and other nonmedical professionals who worked with the revolutionary "great men" of the 1950s. (There are a few notable exceptions to this rule, such as
Bateson, Haley, and Satir.) Obviously, psychiatrists such as Bowen, Ackerman, Wynne,
Jackson, and Lidz contributed tremendously to the development of family therapy and
are properly identified as pioneers of the modern development of the field. The intent is
not to diminish the importance of their work, but rather to acknowledge that they did not
work alone.

The "great men" were in fact great teams, most of which included social workers.
For example, a paper authored by Bowen, Dysinger, Brody, and Basamania, presented at
the 1957 annual meeting of the American Orthopsychiatric Association and reprinted in
1978 (Bowen, 1978), is many times referred to as the formal debut of modern family
therapy. Betty Basamania was a social worker who collaborated with Bowen as a member
of a research team concerned with schizophrenia. She was an integral part of the team
and contributed much to the development of early family therapy thinking (e.g., Basamania, 1961; Bowen, Dysinger, & Basamania, 1959). In a like situation Frances Beatman
and Sanford Sherman were social workers associated with Nathan Ackerman's group,
and were leaders in the early development of therapeutic techniques (Ackerman, Beatman, & Sherman, 1961, 1967). Similar team situations were the norm. Many people were
involved in the development of family approaches to treatment, and many of them were
social workers.

The important contributions of social workers to family therapy in the 1960s, 1970s,
and 1980s are more evident. Of course, a comprehensive list of social workers important
to the maturing of family therapy is not possible, but several leaders stand out. For
example, in 1964 Virginia Satir, a social worker first associated with Don Jackson's team,
published the first widely distributed, comprehensive, integrated model of family therapy, *Conjoint Family Therapy* (Satir, 1964). Her further contributions to the field are
well known. Ray Bardill and a team at Walter Reed Army Medical Hospital developed a
unique approach to family therapy involving social work (Bardill & Ryan, 1973). Celia
Mitchell (1960) contributed much in the area of clinical technique. Frances Sherz (1962)
examined family diagnosis. Several social workers associated with the Ackerman group,
such as, Peggy Papp (1976, 1980) and Lynn Hoffman (1981), have contributed heavily to
family therapy theory and practice and have become leaders in the field. Aponte's (1976)
work with the Philadelphia Child Guidance Clinic is also well known.

Sociopolitical Activities

In the 1960s and 1970s, there were powerful moves within the social work profession to
abandon the psychoanalytic/psychiatry model as a central frame of reference for social
work practice. These decades saw the dramatic ascendence of the environmental side of
the person-in-the environment paradigm for social work. The social policy, social
advocacy, sociopolitical (or *macro*), side of social work pushed to be an organizing frame
that would emphasize the social change activities of social work. The profession of social
work found itself in an identity struggle.

Recent attempts to find a unifying practice conceptualization or frame of reference
for the profession of social work have been hampered because of positions that may be

characterized as "either/or" and "right/wrong" thinking. Organizing formulations have been extreme in either an individual focus *or* an environmental focus. The "social changers" seem fearful that the "people changers" are going to take over the social work profession; thus, any efforts to include social work attention to personal and family issues is seen with alarm by sociopolitical activists as outside the purview of social work. Likewise, the "people changers" see sociopolitical activities as turning social work into a movement rather than a profession. Given either of these extreme views, any social work educational efforts directed to individual/family formulations *or* sociopolitical formulations would be viewed with suspicion by advocates of the opposite extreme.

Added to this either/or perspective is an indignant sense of right and wrong on the part of the extremists. In other words, it is considered a violation of social work values and ethics to concentrate on either the person *or* the environment in the person–environment scheme, and thus it is *wrong* to include any depth of understanding for either person or environmental formulations (depending on which extreme one occupies) within the broad framework of social work. Acceptable professional functions, such as linking, mediation, or networking, often provide watered-down formulations that both extremes accept and try to use to promote their own real positions. Thus, social work's current failure to clarify just where family therapy fits into the scheme of practice and education reflects a profession in turmoil.

FAMILY THERAPY AND SOCIAL WORK EDUCATION

It is surprising that family therapy, with its multisystemic conceptual base, has not emerged as a rallying point for social work. As can be discerned from the foregoing account, throughout its history social work has taken a systemic perspective, although modern terminology was not used; for social work, systems thinking is not really new. Social work is the only profession with this simultaneous, environmental, contextual, personal, ecosystemic practice frame of reference.

An ironic factor working against an emphasis on family therapy in social work is the emergence of the advanced generalist perspective, which seems to be gaining ascendency in social work education. Once the domain of undergraduate social work programs, the generalist formulation of social work has moved into the master's level programs. Practice formulations that primarily focus on interactions and links between people and their social environments are designated as advanced generalist practice. Advanced generalist practice emphasizes neither the person nor the environment but, rather, the interaction between people and their various social systems. Case management activities represent the typical area of concern for the advanced generalist. Advanced generalist practice is in every sense a social work specialization area. Often, however, it does not make room for more than brief attention to marriage and family theoretical and practice content or field experiences.

While education in family intervention methods has always been a part of social work education (Siporin, 1980), the current status of marriage and family therapy training in social work programs is less certain. The Accreditation Commission of (CSWE) recently published new standards for schools of social work which give scant attention to families, and do not mention family therapy as an area of specialization for social work. The new standards require an enormous variety of foundation curriculum content relating to social environment, human behavior, and generalist-focused direct practice. The standards do provide for a variety of advanced specialization areas, but the requirements for a generalist foundation leave little room for specialization of any depth. Therefore, how adequate marriage and family therapy content can be placed within a MSW curriculum is difficult to see.

While much of the visible leadership in social work education seems to have ignored family therapy, there are factors that indicate a stable or increased emphasis in family therapy by both professional MSW social workers and student social workers. Student interest in family therapy remains strong in most schools. In 1975–1976 Siporin (1980) surveyed 76 of the then 80 graduate schools of social work in the United States. Of these 90% reported that some instruction in marriage and family therapy was given in their basic direct practice methods courses. In addition, 68% of the schools offered elective courses dedicated to family therapy, 33% offered electives in marital therapy, and 46% offered courses that somehow combined the two areas. Student demand for these courses was apparently high, with only 61% of the schools reporting that they were able to meet the demand for family therapy courses and only 41% indicating that the demand for marital therapy instruction was satisfied. Siporin concluded from these and other data that marriage and family therapy "remains a core element in graduate social work educational programs" (Siporin, 1980, p. 14).

Family Therapy Survey

In the fall of 1983, 94 schools of social work were mailed a survey designed to identify the extent to which family therapy content and supervision was a part of their graduate social work program (Bardill, 1984). Ninety of the 94 schools completed and returned the questionnaire.

Eighty-four of the 94 schools (93.3%) reported having one or more separate family therapy courses, a substantially greater percentage than that reported earlier by Siporin. When the reported "family therapy" course titles were reviewed, it became apparent that for some schools, the concept of family therapy is somewhat broad in nature. For instance, several schools listed among their family therapy courses such titles as "Social Work on the Behalf of Children and Adolescents," "Family Policy," "Individuals, Families and Groups." Sixty-one schools of social work (67.7%) had easily identifiable family therapy courses as part of their curriculum, a finding similar to that of Siporin.

Only six schools (6.7%) reported no courses in family therapy. All of the six schools clearly had a strong generalist perspective. Most of these schools reported that family therapy content is covered in practice courses with more general titles such as "Social Treatment" or "Advanced Individuals, Families and Groups Practice."

The presence of a nonrequired family therapy course in an overall curriculum does not provide assurance that all the students will be exposed to family content, nor does it give any indication of the extent of the school's emphasis on family therapy. In looking further at the survey data it was found that 24, or about 26%, of the schools required at least one family therapy course. About half of the 26% required more than one family therapy course, indicating a stronger emphasis on family therapy.

Only 19 schools (21.1%) offered a substantive area specialization in family therapy. Ordinarily, this means that the program offers one or more advanced level family therapy courses, and provides field internships that give the student experiences with family therapy cases. Twenty-one schools (23.3%) reported substantial internship exposure to family therapy types of situations. Only six schools reported field experiences with little exposure to family cases.

Five schools of social work stand out because of the variety and depth of family courses and quality experiences. All of the five programs had at least five courses in family therapy, and the field internships in these programs had a strong emphasis on family theory and practice.

The survey findings about family therapy education and training in social work are consistent with impressions gained from discussions with social work faculty from schools across the nation. Clearly, most schools of social work provide family therapy content and some exposure to family situations during the field internships. A number of schools reported a weakness in the quantity and quality of their family therapy theory and practice content. Three schools expressed a strong intention to strengthen the family therapy content in their programs.

The survey data indicate that the increasing emphasis on the advanced generalist model works against a strong family therapy emphasis. Schools seem to regard family therapy as a specialized practice area that competes with the advanced generalist specialization.

FAMILY THERAPY EMPHASIS

The recognition of family therapy as an area of specialization in social work is important for a number of reasons. First, social work has a historical interest and expertise in family life to include family therapy. Second, the systemic perspective of family therapy fits well within almost any known frame of reference for social work practice. Finally, state licensure laws dictate that social work must lay claim to one of its legitimate areas of specialization. Otherwise, another profession could capture the practice of family therapy.

The question of family therapy as one of the major mental professions, has emerged and persists as a domain issue, and social work may have waited too long to reclaim family therapy within its practice domain. Over the past 15 years, the American Association for Marriage and Family Therapy (AAMFT) has grown into a professional association of almost 12,000 members, over 20% of whom are social workers (Johnson, 1984). The AAMFT Commission on Accreditation has been recognized by the U.S. Department of Education as the accrediting body for graduate degree programs and clinical training programs in marriage and family therapy education. Marriage and family therapists, counselors, psychiatrists, psychologists, and pastoral counselors all have increased their claims on family therapy.

Given social work's past conceptual and practice involvement with families, it is surprising that over the past several years other professions have so easily moved to claim the family therapy domain. Ordinarily, moves by other professions to claim a domain occupied by another professional group would meet with considerable resistance. Given social work's identity struggles, there has been little resistance. Social work's struggle to find itself seems to have left little room, or time, to remain one of its most traditional and identifiable practice areas—family social work.

Model Curriculum

The current national standards of the AAMFT Commission on Accreditation for Marriage and Family Therapy Education are broad enough to allow a school of social work to receive accredited status for a well delineated, clearly defined degree program in marriage and family therapy. Given the extensiveness of the generalist requirements in the social work foundation curriculum in the 1984 social work accreditation standards, an MSW program seeking accredited status in marriage and family therapy would likely need to expand its master's degree program beyond the ordinary graduate program of two years.

The model curriculum that guides accredited marriage and family programs fits very well with the direct practice direction of social work. The model curriculum (1975) proposes six areas of study (AAMFT Commission on Accreditation).

1. *Marital and Family Systems:* 2–4 courses with a minimum of 6 semester hours or 8 quarter hours. Course content in this area provides the theoretical basis for family treatment strategies. Material from different areas of study, such as sociology or anthropology, may be used as long as it is clinically oriented. Social work programs with a strong clinical/direct practice orientation have a range of courses that provide the content necessary for the requirements of this area of study.

2. *Marital and Family Course:* 2–4 courses with a minimum of 6 semester hours or 8 quarter hours. Social work methods courses in marital and family therapy provide the necessary applied practice content. The applied practice is expected to cover a wide range of individual, couple, family, group, network, and transgenerational content. Slightly over half of the schools of social work responding to the previously mentioned survey clearly have the courses needed to meet this requirement.

3. *Individual Development:* 2–4 courses with a minimum of 6 semester or 8 quarter hours. This requirement is likely to be easily met in schools of social work. The required social environment and human behavior content must cover life cycle content along with other behavioral theory. Additionally, schools with a direct practice speciality offer courses in psychopathology and human sexuality. The AAMFT standards require an integration of human development content with systems concepts. Social work's strong emphasis on ecological or systems thinking is congruent with the requirements in this area of study.

4. *Professional Studies:* 1 course. This course is "intended to contribute to the development of a professional attitude and identity." Professional studies content is ordinarily interspersed throughout a social work curriculum. Specific content relating to marriage and family areas may need to be added to the social work curriculum.

5. *Research:* 1 course. There are strong research requirements in graduate programs of social work. Schools of social work are likely to exceed the AAMFT requirements in this area. Research relating to the family will need to be a part of the research content.

6. *Supervised Clinical Practice:* 1 year with 9 semester credit hours or 12 quarter hours. Graduate programs in social work exceed the credit hours requirement for super-

vised clinical practice. Social work traditionally has emphasized quality in the supervised field practice. The supervisors must be clinically experienced MSWs who are approved by the school of social work. Social work accreditation standards require that the school liaison faculty work more closely with the field practice supervisors.

However, a major addition to the field requisites for most schools of social work is likely to be the requirements that (1) students must be supervised by a member of AAMFT who is an approved supervisor and (2) a substantial portion of the cases carried by the student be marital or family problem.

7. *Electives*: 1 course, 3 semester or 4 quarter hours. The elective hours are included to provide support for a specialized area the student may select.

To meet AAMFT accreditation standards the graduate program must provide a total of at least 27 semester hours or 36 quarter hours from areas 1, 2, and 3 above. All the required areas of study are designed to give the graduate basic but firm conceptual and practice knowledge and understanding.

An AAMFT standard that requires the most careful attention states that "the institution must offer a master's degree program of at least two years duration, and/or a doctoral program in marriage and family therapy" (AAMFT Accreditation Manual). This standard requires a self-contained marriage and family therapy program that is on a level equal to other programs within the particular academic unit. The academic location of the program is not critical in meeting the standards. What is required is that the marriage and family program be specifically identifed administratively, and that all required courses clearly relate to marriage and family therapy. The AAMFT Commission on Accreditation does not recognize programs that place the marriage and family program at a subspecialty level. For a school of social work to reconcile the standards of CSWE and AAMFT, there must be detailed attention to the administrative and curriculum requirement of each accrediting body.

It is proposed that family therapy education in social work incorporate the social work knowledge about working with families that already exists with the newly developing theories and skills most relevant to family social work. The social work literature of the last four decades abounds in the collective knowledge and skills that can be applied to the solution of a full range of family problems. Social workers, by tradition, are well versed in personal/situational dynamics.

The frame of reference proposed here is a multisystemic model based largely in relational systems thinking. The model assumes a strong attention to the assessment process. The goal is to identify the level(s) of intervention (individual, marital, family, community) most suitable for the specific problem situation. From the core perspective of relational/systems thinking, the problem-solving process is directed to a methodology most appropriate to the particular people and situation needing assistance.

Social work education in family therapy, by traditional interest, will emphasize work with poor and disadvantaged families. The theory building and research efforts geared to funding the most effective means for helping oppressed people must continue. The marriage and family degree in social work will, of necessity, demand a blend of traditional social work values, ethics, knowledge, and skills with the body of expertise developed by non–social work experts in the family therapy field. Thus, both AAMFT and CSWE standards must be met. In one sense a return to the family therapy field for social work will enrich the nature and the range of services available to children, couples, and families in distress.

With careful planning, schools of social work may seek accredited status for *sharply delineated graduate programs in marriage and family therapy.* Such an effort by a school will require that all AAFMT and CSWE standards be met by the program. Table 20-1 is a proposed School of Social Work curriculum with a family therapy program.

TABLE 20-1. A Proposed Curriculum for Master's Level Family Therapy Education in Social Work.

Semester I	*Hours*
Human Behavior and Social Environment	(3)
Direct Practice with Individuals, Families and Groups	(3)
Research	(3)
Field Internship Generalist Social Work Practice	(6)
Semester II	*Hours*
Social Welfare Policies and Services	(3)
Family Therapy in Social Work	(3)
Elective	(3)
Field Internship Generalist Social Work	(6)
Summer Semester	
Field Internships (Marriage and Family therapy)	(6)
	(Full range of cases)
Group Supervision	(3)
Semester III	
Social Work Elective**	(3)
Family Therapy Elective***	(3)
Elective	(3)
Field Internships (Marriage and Family therapy)	(3)
Semester IV	
Social Work Elective	(3)
Family Therapy Elective	(3)
Integrative Seminar	(3)
Field Internships (Marriage and Family therapy	(6)
	Total of 69 semester hours to graduate

Possible Electives

**Social work Electives*
    Empirical Practice of Social work
    Theory and Practice of Psychodynamic Social Work
    Behavioral Approaches to Social Work
    Community Organization
    Family Planning
***Family Therapy Electives*
    Intensive Family Therapy (3)
    Marriage Counseling (3)
    Human Sexuality (3)

(*continued*)

TABLE 20-1 (*continued*)

Possible Electives	
Social Work/Marriage and Family Electives	
Clinical Practice with Black Families	(3)
Family Planning	(3)
Theory and Practice of Crisis Intervention and Brief Treatment	(3)
Psychopathology in Clinical Practice	(3)
Clinical Practice with Children	(3)
Alcohol Abuse and Treatment	(3)
Group Treatment Principles and Techniques	(3)

Note: All CSWE Commission on Accreditation standards must be met. The family therapy program must be a clearly defined program comparable in status to all other programs in the school. There must be an administrative structure which assures autonomy for the program. (This is an absolute requirement for an accredited marriage and family therapy program.) There must be sufficient AAMFT-approved faculty to meet Commission standards.

SUMMARY

The most characteristic feature of professional social work has been, and still is, the strong emphasis on a holistic frame of reference from which to find solutions to human problems. Family therapy offers a way of thinking, and a primary intervention technique, that always consider the multisystemic aspect of human existence.

Given social work's historical and present interest in the family, it is appropriate for graduate social work education to use family therapy's systemic perspective as an organizing frame of reference for the future profession of social work. Given the current political struggles between the "people changers" and the "sociopolitical activists" in social work, and the combined requirements of CSWE and AAMFT accreditation standards, a social work effort to reclaim its family heritage will not come easily. This chapter has proposed possible entry points for such an effort, and addresses the critical need for social work to fulfill its professional obligation to the family. Finally, for some schools of social work it may be possible to be accredited by the AAMFT Commission on Accreditation with only slight program modifications. For many social work students, the prospect of graduating from a program accredited by both CSWE and AAMFT is highly desirable.

References

AAMFT Commission of Accreditation. (1975). *Manual on accreditation*. Washington, DC: Author.

Ackerman, N. W., Beatman, F. L., & Sherman, S. N. (Eds.). (1961). *Exploring the base for family therapy*. New York: Family Service Association of America.

Ackerman, N. W., Beatman, F. L., & Sherman, S. N. (Eds.). (1967). *Expanding theory and practice in family therapy*. New York: Family Service Association of America.

Aponte, H. J. (1976). Underorganization in the poor family. In P. J. Guerin, Jr. (Ed.), *Family therapy*. New York: Gardner.

Bardill, D. R. (1984). *Family therapy in schools of social work*. Unpublished survey, conducted by the Office of the Dean, School of Social Work, Florida State University, Tallahassee, Florida.

Bardill, D. R., & Ryan, F. J. (1973). *Family group casework* (rev. ed.). Washington, DC: National Association of Social Workers.

Bardill, D. R., & Saunders, B. E. (1983). Services to families and groups. In J. W. Callicut & P. J. Lecca (Eds.), *Social work and mental health*. New York: Free Press.

Basamania, B. (1961). The family as the unit of study and treatment. Workshop. The emotional life of the family: Inferences for social casework. *American Journal of Orthopsychiatry, 31*(1), 74–86.

Bowen, M. (1975). Family therapy after twenty years. In. S. Arieti (Ed.), *American handbook of psychiatry* (Vol. 5). New York: Basic Books.

Bowen, M. (Ed.) (1978). *Family therapy in clinical practice*. New York: Aronson.

Bowen, M., Dysinger, R. H., & Basamania, B. (1959). The role of the father in families with a schizophrenic patient. *American Journal of Psychiatry, 115*, 1017–1020.

Bowen, M., Dysinger, R. H., Brody, N. M., & Basamania, B. (1957, March). *Study and treatment of five hospitalized families each with a psychotic member*. Paper presented at the Annual Meeting of the American Orthopsychiatric Association, Chicago.

Broderick, C. B., & Schrader, S. S. (1981). The history of professional marriage and family therapy. In A. S. Gurman & P. J. Krishern (Eds.), *Handbook of family therapy*. New York: Brunner/Mazel.

CSWE Commission on Accreditation. (1984). *Handbook of accreditatin standards and procedures*. New York: Author.

Erickson, G. D., & Hogan, T. P. (1976). *Family therapy: An introduction to theory and technique*. New York: Aronson.

Guerin, P. J., Jr. (1976). Family therapy: The first twenty-five years. In P. J. Guerin, Jr. (Ed.), *Family therapy*. New York: Gardner.

Gurman, A. S., & Kniskern, D. P. (Eds.). (1981). *Handbook of family therapy*. New York: Brunner/Mazel.

Hansen, J. C., & L'Abate, L. (1982). *Approaches to family therapy*. New York: Macmillan.

Hoffman, L. (1981). *Foundations of family therapy*. New York: Basic Books.

Johnson, S. (1984). AAMFT profile: Growth and opportunity. *Family Therapy News, 15*(3), 20.

Kadushin, A. (1978). Social work and the American family then and now, 1920–1978. *Smith College Studies in Social Work, 49*(1), 3–24.

Meier, E. G. (1954). *A history of the New York School of Social Work*. New York: Columbia University Press.

Mitchell, C. B. (1960). The use of family sessions in diagnosis and treatment of disturbance in children. *Social Casework, 41*(6), 283–290.

Mitchell, C. A casework approach to disturbed families. (1961). In N. W. Ackerman, F. L. Beatman, & S. N. Sherman (Eds.), *Exploring the base for family therapy*. New York: Family Service Association of America.

Mitchell, C. Integrative therapy of the family unit. (1965). *Social Casework, 46*(2), 63–69.

Mitchell, C. Problems and principles in family therapy. (1967). In N. W. Ackerman, F. L. Beatman & S. N. Sherman (Eds.), *Expanding theory and practice in family therapy*. New York: Family Service Association of America.

Moggridge, M. W. (1882). *Method of almsgiving–handbook for helpers*. London: John Murray.

Nicols, M. (1984). *Family therapy: Concepts and methods*. New York: Gardner Press.

Okun, B. F., & Rappaport, L. J. (1980). *Working with families*. North Scituate, MA: Duxbury.

Olson, D. H., Sprenkle, D. H., & Russell, C. S. (1979). Circumplex model of marital and family systems: Cohesion and adaptability dimension, family types and clinical applications. *Family Process, 18*(1), 3–28.

Papp, P. (1976). Family choreography. In P. J. Guerin, Jr. (Ed.), *Family therapy*. New York: Gardner Press.

Papp, P. (1980). The Greek chorus and other techniques of family therapy. *Family Process, 19*(1), 45–58.

Quaranta, M. A. (1979). The family as the unit of attention in social work. *Smith College Studies in Social Work, 6*(1), 16–18.

Richmond, M. E. (1917). *Social diagnosis*. New York: Russell Sage.

Sanborn, F. B. (1890). Indoor and outdoor relief. In *Proceedings of the National Conference of Charities and Correction*. Boston: George H. Ellis.

Satir, V. (1964). *Conjoint family therapy*. Palo Alto, CA: Science and Behavior Books.

Saunders, B. E. (1980). *Social work with families. An analysis of domain issues*. Paper presented at the Annual Meeting of the Southeastern Council on Family Relations, Mobile, Alabama.

Scherz, F. H. (1962). Multiple-client interviewing: Treatment applications. *Social Casework, 43*(3), 111–113.

Scherz, F. Exploring the use of family interviews in diagnosis. (1964). *Social Casework, 45*(4), 209–215.

Siporin, M. (1980). Marriage and Family Therapy in Social Work. *Social Casework, 61*(1), 11–21.

Smith, Z. D. (1890). *Proceedings of the National Conference in Charities and Corrections.*

Tuckerman, J. (1832). An introduction. In B. Gerando (Ed.), *The visitor of the poor.* Boston: Hilliard, Gray, Little and Wilkins.

Wilson, G. (1976). From practice to theory: A personalized history. In R. W. Roberts & H. Northern (Eds.), *Theories of social work with groups.* New York: Columbia University Press.

SECTION FIVE

SPECIAL ISSUES

Introduction

As the field of family therapy has become more sophisticated, so has the training and supervision literature. Whereas the early literature tended to focus on generic training issues and program descriptions, the present decade has witnessed an expansion of this literature to include a wide variety of highly specialized issues in family therapy training and supervision. For example, special training formats now exist to teach specific family therapy techniques, such as circular questioning (Fleuridas, Nelson, & Rosenthal, 1986), and family therapy concepts, such as triads (Coppersmith, 1985) and family development (Liddle, 1988). The impact of training on broader issues such as gender (Caust, Libow, & Raskin, 1981; Hare-Mustin, 1987; Okun, 1983), feminism (Goldner, 1987; Hare-Mustin, 1981; Libow, 1985; Wheeler, Avis, Miller, & Chaney, 1985), culture (Falicov, Chapter 21, this volume), and ethics (Piercy & Sprenkle, 1983) has also been addressed. Therapists are now trained to work with special populations (e.g., stepfamilies, abusive families), special problems (e.g., drug abuse, bulimia), or family processes (e.g., divorce). The importance of evaluative research on family therapy training is being recognized (see Kniskern & Gurman, Chapter 23, this volume), as is the importance of trainees' responses to the training they receive (see Liddle, Davidson, & Barett, Chapter 25, this volume).

The integration of these special training issues into the philosophy of training programs is still a matter of debate. Academic programs may offer courses on special issues, and free-standing institutes sometimes devote some of their didactic seminars to these issues. Falicov (Chapter 21) notes that such compartmentalizing of special issues can convey a message to trainees that the issue is somewhat separate from other family or clinical issues. Falicov recommends that, if the issue is sufficiently central, it be integrated with other training objectives. Wheeler *et al.* (1985) have adopted a similar position with regard to feminism, and offer a set of training objectives that integrate a feminist perspective. A program with an interest in a particular issue may successfully integrate that issue without having to restructure the program, but when this is attempted with several issues, the additional emphases necessitate additional time, which eventually extends the length of training. Recently proposed changes in the AAMFT accrediting standards reflect this dilemma. As a field we are clearly struggling to articulate and accommodate the breadth of training required to produce a competent family therapist.

In Section Five we have also included chapters by two of the leaders in the field of family therapy and family therapy training. Jay Haley (Chapter 22) provides reflections on family therapy supervision, and Cloé Madanes (Chapter 24) takes a humorous metaperspective to the subject of training.

References

Caust, B., Libow, J., & Raskin, P. (1981). Challenges and promises of training women as family systems therapists. *Family Process, 20,* 439–448.

Coppersmith, E. I. (1985). Teaching trainees to think in triads. *Journal of Marital and Family Therapy, 11,* 61–66.

Fleuridas, C., Nelson, T., & Rosenthal, D. M. (1986). The evolution of circular questions: Training family therapists. *Journal of Marital and Family Therapy, 12*(2), 113–128.

Goldner, V. (1987). Instrumentalism, feminism, and the limits of family therapy. *Journal of Family Psychology, 1*(1), 109–116.

Hare-Mustin, R. (1981). A feminist approach to family therapy. *Family Process, 17,* 181–194.

Hare-Mustin, R. (1987). The problem of gender in family therapy theory. *Family Process, 26,* 15–27.

Libow, J. A. (1985). Training family therapists as feminists. In M. Ault-Riche (Ed.) *Women and family therapy.* Rockville, MD: Aspen.

Liddle, H. A. (1988). Integrating developmental thinking and the family life cycle paradigm into training. In C. Falicov (Ed.). *Family transitions: Continuity and change over the life cycle.* New York: Guilford Press.

Okun, B. F. (1983). Gender issues of family systems therapists. In B. Okun & S. T. Gladdings (Eds.), *Issues in training marriage and family therapists.* Ann Arbor, MI: ERIC/CAPS.

Piercy, F., & Sprenkle, D. (1983). Ethical, legal and professional issues in family therapy: A graduate level course. *Journal of Marital and Family Therapy, 9*(4), 393–401.

Wheeler, D., Avis, J. M., Miller, L. A., & Chaney, S. (1985). Rethinking family therapy education and supervision: A feminist model. *Journal of Psychotherapy and the Family, 1*(4), 53–72.

21

Learning to Think Culturally

CELIA JAES FALICOV
La Jolla Marital and Family Institute, La Jolla, California

> *Dr. Ackerman:* If I were in your spot, I'd feel exactly as you do.
>
> *Richard:* That you feel the same way? But if, you see . . . if you were in my spot it wouldn't *be* because you're white.
>
> *Dr. Ackerman:* Supposing I were black? That's right, I could only be in your spot if I were black.

The scene is from a simulated interview in the late 1960s. The actors are beginning therapists in a training setting. They are being interviewed by experienced family therapists (Carl Whitaker, Robert McGregor, Nathan Ackerman, and Thomas Brayboy) in a situation designed to examine the particular problems therapists encounter in their initial contacts with families of different ethnic and socioeconomic groups. This experience took place at the American Group Psychotherapy Association Conference in 1969 (and was documented in a book by Sager, Brayboy, and Waxenberg [1970]). After many simulations of middle-class white families interviewed by middle-class white therapists, an increased sociocultural awareness prompted the organizing group to challenge the consultants with the task of interviewing a simulated black ghetto family.

Over time, this and other pioneering efforts succeeded in raising consciousness about cultural differences. Much as in the dialogue above, a recognition of the different existential "spots" of families ensued. But then, as now, beyond each therapist's demonstration of her or his personal artistry in interviewing the family, there was a glaring absence of a framework with which to approach families in their cultural context. The search for such a framework continues today, often giving rise to conflicting positions (Falicov, 1983; McGill, 1983; McGoldrick, Pearce, & Giordano, 1982; Montalvo & Gutierrez, 1983). A growing number of family therapy training programs include ethnicity and other aspects of culture, each exploring avenues to introduce cultural issues.[1]

This chapter presents a framework for the integration of culture in family therapy training. A cultural framework is a way of thinking about families and family therapy. It is not a theory or a defined set of techniques that can be easily tried out, accepted, or discarded. Rather, it is a necessary posture that develops through awareness of the role that values play for families, for therapists, and for their encounter with each other.

The framework presented here selects areas and topics where culture is a relevant consideration and suggests ways to integrate a cultural perspective with other training objectives. The approach taken reflects a middle course between a "universal" position, wherein all families are considered to be alike regardless of their background, and a "particular" position, wherein each group is considered to have such culture-specific behaviors that the trainee is required to become an anthropological expert.

The trainer interested in cultural perspectives must find an answer to several interconnected questions: (1) What is the definition of culture to be used? (2) What are the objectives of "cultural training"? (3) Is it preferable to teach a special course on cultural issues, or to articulate them with the other training experiences? (4) What should the content and format of cultural training be? The answers depend, to some extent, on contextual considerations (setting, type of training program, type of trainee, and client population). The responses offered here generalize from experiences teaching family therapy at a free-standing postgraduate institute with a beginning-level group. The trainees are of various cultural backgrounds, but with a significant representation (one-third) of Mexican-American ancestry. The population of clients is ethnically varied and of middle-class, working-class, and poor socioeconomic levels.

WHAT IS MEANT BY CULTURE?

Most discussions of culture in family therapy have focused on ethnicity as an important determinant of family behavior (McGoldrick, Pearce, & Giordano, 1982; Papajohn & Spiegel, 1975). This chapter offers a more comprehensive definition of "culture." It is defined as those *sets of shared world views and adaptive behaviors derived from simultaneous membership in a variety of contexts*, such as ecological setting (rural, urban, suburban), religious background, nationality and ethnicity, social, class, gender-related experiences, minority status, occupation, political leanings, migratory patterns and stage of acculturation, or values derived from belonging to the same generation, partaking of single historical moment, or particular ideologies. Thus, cultural differences result from simultaneous contextual inclusion (that is, participation and identification) in different types of groups. Since families partake of and combine features of the many contexts to which they belong, it is necessary for therapists to be aware of the family's membership in all the relevant contexts simultaneously. Taken altogether, each family is unique precisely because of its specific ecological niche, which is that combination of the multiple settings in which it is embedded. Believing that culture, ethnicity, or social class have equal impact on all families ignores the complex of contexts that create variability.

WHAT ARE THE OBJECTIVES OF INTRODUCING CULTURAL THINKING INTO THE TRAINING SITUATION?

The first objective is an effort to prevent focusing exclusively on the interior of the family to understand its function and dysfunction. The investigation of family process without attention to the larger sociocultural contexts is often insufficient to explain and influence behavior.

The second objective is to differentiate among universal, transcultural, culture-specific, and idiosyncratic family behaviors. Universal or transcultural similarities are to be emphasized, while recognizing that all families have culture-specific and idiosyncratic behaviors.

The third is to discriminate between family situations where cultural issues may be of clinical relevance from those where cultural issues are tangential.

The fourth is to attain a culturally relativistic framework for assessment and intervention, and to recognize culturally bound concepts and behaviors that may lead to ethnocentric biases.

The fifth is to avoid the use of negative or positive stereotypes. They blur the specificity and simplify the complexity of influences on individuals and families, and may lead to errors of assessment that are often as serious as those that stem from ethnocentric views.

The sixth is to recognize that alternative value systems may be not only possible but valid, and that each set of cultural values has inherent strengths and weaknesses.

The last objective of thinking culturally is to develop an exploratory, sensitive, and respectful attitude toward the client's cultural identity that is integrated with skills in joining, defining a problem, and selecting interventions.

HOW SHOULD CULTURAL ISSUES BE TAUGHT?

Is it better to offer a separate course, or should cultural issues be integrated with other aspects of the training objectives? When is the best time to introduce cultural issues in the training situation?

A Separate Course

Trainers often entertain the possibility of offering a course on cultural issues, generally focused on ethnicity. However, such courses usually fail to generate sufficient trainee interest in the topic, and tend to have low attendance. After taking such a course trainees seldom show evidence of having integrated sociocultural factors in the cases they bring for supervision. This suggests difficulties in applying the learned concepts to the realities of the therapeutic encounter. Furthermore, the trainees tend to invoke cultural factors as a last resort when befuddled by behavior resistant to change, implying that culture is a less important and more static element than other considerations.

These outcomes may be linked to several messages implicit in the act of offering a separate course: (1) it conveys a separateness of cultural issues from other family issues; (2) it singles out cultural factors and labels them—"By the way, this is something you ought to know also"—rather than making them relevant, if not central, to the trainees' clinical experience; (3) it also marks everything else being offered in the training program as "not-cultural," when in fact the notion one wants to advance is that culture appears in myriad ways in family life and family therapy.

When culture is taken out of context, it is easy to forget how cultural abstractions are constructions that fit more or less with observation, but are not true realities. As constructions, they are sometimes helpful ways to organize experiences. In any given therapeutic context, however, they might be less than helpful. For example, the overly literal use of cultural data to create "terminal" hypotheses that invoke cultural traits as fixed, precludes change, and presents obvious difficulties (Falicov, 1985; see also Montalvo & Gutierrez, 1988).

Integration with Learning Objectives

Rather than teach a separate course, a more congruent, exciting, and economical approach is to incorporate cultural perspectives into the training objectives which guide many training programs (Cleghorn & Levin, 1973; Falicov, Constantine, & Breunlin, 1981; Tomm & Wright 1979). Training objectives usually include observational, conceptual, and therapeutic skills. Cultural thinking can be taught simply by making it a part of acquiring those skills, by regularly placing an ecological–cultural lens over all didactic and clinical training experiences. This integration helps to move from the description of ethnic norms to an understanding of each family's reality. Since the map is always different than the actual territory, this integration also encourages "deutero-learning" (Bateson, 1971), that is, learning to learn about cultural similarities and differences rather than only absorbing specific content. Thus, the student learns to ask relevant questions about culture, instead of stereotyping a family by misapplying a culturally normative pattern to a particular case.

WHAT TRAINING FORMAT AND CONTENT IS CONDUCIVE TO HELPING TRAINEES BECOME CULTURALLY ATTUNED?

Didactic Lectures

During the initial didactic lectures of the training program two main constructs may interweave cultural perspectives with the basic systems and family therapy concepts. The first is that cultural relativism can be grasped best through an *ecosystemic view* that constantly places the family in its social context. The second is the degree of *cultural consonance–dissonance* between the world views of the family and of the therapist. The latter is a corollary of another construct: that family therapy ideals, and the interventions that follow from them, are culturally relative. Widely used concepts, such as family organization and family development, are central, since many cultural variations are manifested in the way the family is organized or how it undergoes developmental transitions. It is in these areas that cultural dissonances between families and therapists most blatantly occur. A more detailed account of these concepts appears later in this chapter.

Readings

Since cultural contexts are patterned rather than amorphous or unpredictable, readings or lectures about the specific populations (socioeconomic, ethnic, religious) most often treated by the trainees have a helpful orienting function. It is difficult, however, to move from this academic information to the practical realities of perceiving and acting on cultural issues in the therapy situation. In fact, normative cultural descriptions may present a number of problems for the trainee who attempts to use them pragmatically. In the first place, these descriptions portray cultural ideals and typical—perhaps statistically average—styles and expectations, rather than the actual variations. When norms and ideals are confused with particular causes, complexities can be reduced to stereotypic, and hence invalid, simplifications. Furthermore, when the descriptions are based on inferences from clinical practice, a so-called normative view may be distorted by experience with clients seen in distress, seldom considering that dysfunctional families (by virtue of their rigidity or constraints), may be either more culture-bound, or more deviant from cultural norms, than functional families. Thus, the behavior of clients (distressed people seeking help) may be intermingled or confused with the norms of the cultural group (people at large not seeking help). In the absence of cross-cultural normative research data, it is very important, then, to ensure that trainees do not compare unstable and rigid ethnic families with stable dominant-society families, and conclude thereby that the differences observed are primarily cultural in nature.

Experiential Exercises

To make the academic information more relevant to the clinical situation, a series of exercises ties the conceptual to the practical. One way for trainees to learn to think culturally is for them to interview a nonclinical family of a distinct ethnic or socioeconomic group. Using the concepts from didactic sessions, the trainee develops an interview protocol that includes exploration of the family's ecological setting, level of acculturation, family development, and family organization. There are several reasons for this choice of learning format. The message about differentiating functional from dysfunctional behavior is more poignantly delivered if the rudiments of learning to think culturally begin by interviewing a nonclinical family.[2] The trainee also learns to rely on his or her own observations rather than presuppositions about a family's culture. Finally, the nonclinical situation has the advantage of allowing an exploration of cultural matters without the pressures of resolving a presenting problem.

THE CONCEPTUAL FRAMEWORK

Although culture is everywhere, not all clinical situations warrant the same degree of attention to cultural issues. The position taken here is that an ecosystemic view provides the best initial avenue to discover when and how cultural differences really make a difference to therapists.

An Ecosystemic View

An ecosystemic view is based on a notion of "ecological fit," or family–environment match. This view maintains that the behavior of individuals and families represents interactive adaptations to ecological requirements. A pronounced lack of fit between the family's behavior and the social environment is psychologically and socially stressful. A lack of fit often stems from the interaction of ethnic and socioeconomic minority factors with the dominant society's values and customs.

For the therapist-in-training it is helpful to have a model that locates the potentially stressful interactions between the family and the social context. Bronfenbrenner (1977) developed a model for an ecology of human development that can be adapted to the study of the family in context. The model (See Figure 21-1) is ecological because it is

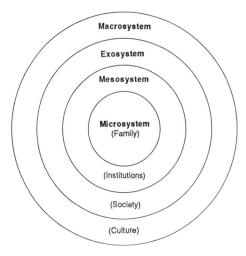

Figure 21-1. Ecosystems levels: Mutual accommodation between family and larger contexts.

concerned with the total field of a problem and deals with "layers of contexts" (individual, family, community, societal institutions, culture).

The definitions of Bronfenbrenner's terms are as follows. "Microsystem" is the complex of relationships within the family. "Mesosystem" refers to the interrelations among the major settings (extended family, workplace, school, peer group, neighborhood). "Exosystem" refers to the major institutions of the society, such as the mass media (and their image of minoritities). "Macrosystem" refers to the general prototypes or ideals of the culture or subculture that set the patterns for the interactions that occur at the concrete level. Events occurring at one level influence those at other levels. An ecosystemic model considers the joint effects of a family's exposure to more than one level, and analyzes interactions among levels (home and school; family and peer group; peer group, family, and school). In the therapy situation, intervention occurs at the micro- or mesosystemic level, but family problems often replicate tensions at other levels. It is important to have an appreciation of the family's ecological fit, as this will determine the therapist's position in the total ecology and will guide the choice of interventions.

Ecological Fit and Family Adaptation

Under stable living conditions, there is a reciprocity or "fit" between the family's functioning and the societal levels that has the properties of a system, with a stability and a "sense" of its own. The family's organizational and developmental norms, beliefs, and other crucial aspects of family (microlevel) life are, in fact, interactive adaptations that fit more or less well with other levels (macro-, exo-, and mesolevels). Although the "ecological fit" is never perfect, a pronounced lack of fit seriously impairs family functioning. To assess the fit, it is helpful for the therapist to have research-based knowledge of sociocultural normative patterns.

Cultural issues become most salient in situations of instability. These include cultural transitions caused by migration or relocation (from one country to another, or urban–rural and even local moves), acculturation stresses (such as language difficulties), and other forms of dislocation (such as unemployment). These situations disrupt the family's ecological balance by changing its equation or fit, and provoke cultural dissonance among family members, and between the family and the surrounding institutions. The interactions between the family and the various levels of the social context become points of cleavage rather than points of consonance.

Disruptions of ecological fit precipitated by culture change are illustrated in Figure 21-2, by comparing the ecological balance of Mexicans in their country of origin with the points of cleavage they face after migration to the United States, since the American culture is based on a totally different ecological balance. This figure shows that Mexicans moving to the United States are likely to experience cultural dissonances in a number of areas. It is probable that Mexican immigrants grew up in large families that value interdependence, and stress hierarchical and complementary interactions; individual needs may be secondary to family loyalties. Inclusiveness of others in the kinship network in the mesosystem, and a low reliance on the institutions of the exosystem, are more highly valued than among Anglo-Americans. When moving to the United States, Mexican people move to a society where families tend to live in smaller arrangements and have greater reliance on secondary institutions. Cultural ideals tend toward symmetry with others, and individual boundaries are clearly marked. Self-realization through achievement and active self-assertion are relatively more important than interpersonal proximity and conformity with authority figures. A corollary of these attitudes

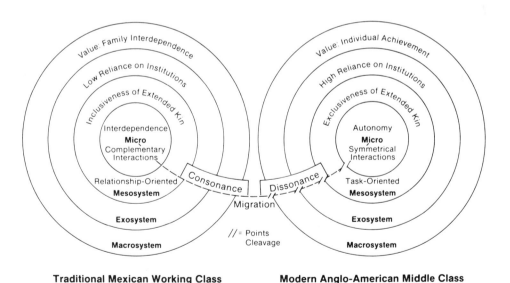

Traditional Mexican Working Class   **Modern Anglo-American Middle Class**

Figure 21-2. A comparison of Mexican and Anglo-American ecological fit, and points of cleavage.

for Americans is to favor a task orientation over the relatedness orientation preferred by Mexicans. These changes of rules during cultural transition create considerable confusion.

Two areas of questioning help the trainee assess the ecological fit.

INQUIRING ABOUT MIGRATION

If the family has recently relocated, and belongs to a small ethnic, religious, or other minority group, the trainee needs to be sensitive to the family's subjective sense of cultural fit with the newly encountered institutions, including the therapist's domain and expectations. Information about the previous ecological setting, the reasons for migration, the separations and reunions, the necessary adaptations, the reception encountered in the new community and the support networks, allows the therapist to evaluate the stage of the family's migratory process and to design the therapeutic interventions accordingly.[3]

INQUIRING ABOUT THE PRESENT ECOLOGICAL CONTEXT

By definition a family's culture is tied to its ecological settings. To inquire about ecological features of each family, the trainee explores the family's socioeconomic and living conditions (income, housing, safety), its employment conditions (occupation, job stability, satisfaction, schedules), the degree and and quality of insertion of the family in the extended family and friendship networks, and the cultural norms of the surrounding community. When children are involved, exploration of the school and parent–teacher relationships are in order. An assessment of the family's ecological situation can be facilitated by learning to draw an *eco-map* that portrays family–environment relationships, a useful method developed and illustrated by Hartman and Laird (1983). Meyerstein (1979) also provides a comprehensive outline of areas related to the family's ecological context.

ECOLOGICAL FIT AND ACCULTURATION

The concept of ecological fit need not be applied only to the family in culture shock after migration. The reverberations of culture change spread over time and alter the ecological fit over several generations.

Indicators of Ecological Stress over the Generations. There are certain regularities in the experiences of cultural transition for each succeeding generation of an immigrant family. The ecological fit of each generation can be associated with different degrees and types of ecological stress (Falicov, 1982a).

In Table 21-1 the adaptations and conflicts within the family, and between the family and the surrounding institutions, are summarized for the first, second, and third generations of an immigrant family. The dimensions on the left side of the table are assessed during the initial interview. The exploration of those variables provides an index of ecological stress and underlines situations where culture may be a relevant treatment issue.

Awareness about generational differences guides the therapist toward specificity and helps avoid overgeneralization, since families of the same ethnic group vary enormously depending on their level of acculturation. The table provides an estimate of the "pile up" and the location of stress at different levels of the enivornment for the various generations. These have many implications for therapeutic action. The therapist's role, biases of assessment, and effective therapeutic approaches vary when treating the different genera-

TABLE 21-1. Stresses of Cultural Transition

Ecosystem level	Dimensions	Acculturation stages		
		Immigrant family (first generation)	Immigrant/American family (second generation)	American family of immigrant descent (third generation)
Macro	*Value Systems*	Cultural Dissonance	Emergent Consonance	Biculturalism, Assimilation
Exo (Society)	*Immigrant Status*	Legal Alien, Undocumented	Undocumented, Citizen	Citizen
	Economic Status	Unemployment, underemployment	Underemployment, Employment	Stable
	Reception	Discrimination, Welcome	Equal or Less Discrimination	Less Discrimination
Meso (Institutions)	*Language*	Monolingual Native	Bilingual	Monolingual Adoptive
	Institutional Use	Very Limited or Excessive:	Greater Reliance	Widespread Use
	Social Network	Fear & Alienation Lack of Models Ethnic Community	Sense of Marginality Emergent Models, Emergent Participation	Sense of Belonging Demands Equality Peer Models
	Ethnic Identity	Split, Idealization, Denigration	Marginal, Mimetic, Duality	Ethnic, or American, Integrated
Micro (Family)	*Adaptation*	Culture Shock Situational Problems	Moderate Adaptation	High Adaptation
	Membership	Migratory Separations and Reunions	Stable	Stable
	Supports	Very Low to High	Moderate	Moderate
	Organization (Proximity, hierarchies)	In Flux to Cope, e.g., increased marital proximity; decreased extended proximity.	Transitional Patterns: e.g., intergenerational conflicts, incongruent hierarchies.	Patterns Rigidified or Restructured
	Developmental Norms	Original, or Shift in Dominant dyad	In Flux or Conflict	Integrated or Parallel

First generation: All family members are born in native country. *Second generation:* Some members born in country of origin; others in country of adoption. *Third generation:* All members born in country of adoption.

tions. Table 21-2 summarizes the therapeutic implications of the concept of ecological balance for three generations.

When pressing problems arise between the immigrant family and the new cultural institutions, the therapist has to assume a role of *social intermediary*. For the second-generation family, the therapist is more often placed in the position of *family intermediary*, helping to resolve intergenerational conflicts. A fuller discussion of these therapist's roles with clinical examples can be found in Falicov (1982b).

The two most common pitfalls in cross-cultural work are maintaining an ethnocentric position and thereby minimizing cultural differences, or maximizing the differences by using ethnic stereotypes to understand families (Falicov, 1983). Both pitfalls can occur with any of the three generations. Other therapeutic biases are related to the positions the therapist takes (Table 21-2). With immigrant families, the therapist may unwittingly set out to rescue the family from dissonance with the larger society when care should be taken instead to help empower them and encourage initiative. With the second generation, the therapist runs the risk of siding with one generation against the other when helping to resolve the intergenerational conflicts typical of this stage. With the third generation, the therapist may be inducted into either ignoring or paying exaggerated attention to cultural issues, when in fact culture may be a mask or a camouflage for other family processes.

Once an assessment of generational status has been made, many family therapy approaches can be used successfully, but some seem to fit better than others with the life circumstances of a particular generation. Those congruences are summarized in Table 21-2 under the heading "Helpful Approaches."

By beginning with an ecologically oriented approach, we launch a journey toward cultural awareness using the concept of consonance–dissonance. The status of cultural consonance is assessed at the interfaces between the individual, the family, and the surrounding institutions. The result is quite different from starting the journey by developing specific sensitivities to various cultural groups.

The ecosystemic approach regards all behaviors as interactive adaptations and includes a perspective on the values of the host culture, the reactions of the "natives" to the "foreigners," and the adaptations required from each over the generations. In the following sections two areas of great relevance to family therapists are discussed: family organization and family life cycle. Value differences between the therapist and the family in these areas may prevent the formation of a therapeutic alliance, misguide the choice of interventions, or create divergent therapeutic goals.

FAMILY ORGANIZATION

Most family therapy models include parameters relevant to issues of proximity or cohesion, and others relevant to issues of power and hierarchy. The labels may vary, but the concepts appear to be similar and are thought to be fundamental dimensions of family organization (Beavers, 1977; Epstein & Bishop, 1981; Kantor & Lehr, 1975; Minuchin, 1974; Olson, Sprenkle, & Russell, 1979; Wood & Talman, 1983).

As constructs, these dimensions have universal validity. Most models of family functioning, however, also carry implicit or explicit expectations about the normative

TABLE 21-2. Ecological Balance and Therapeutic Implications

	Immigrant family	Immigrant/American	Immigrant descent
Biases in assessment	Ethnocentrism Ethnic stereotyping Disregard: a. Cultural shock b. Situational constraints c. Impact of separations and reunions Rescuing the family	Ethnocentrism Ethnic stereotyping Disregard conflicts of: a. Cultural code b. Ethnic identity Siding, e.g., induction into generational split	Ethnocentrism Ethnic stereotyping Disregard or overemphasize ethnic issues (induction into cultural theme, camouflage family processes)
Therapeutic role and interventions	Social intermediary: Advocate Organizational consultant Network facilitator Educator Crisis intervention Catalyst Help restore ecological order	Family intermediary: Cultural philosopher Negotiator Balancer Help restore hierarchies Encourage differentiation Use cultural strategies (i.e., language as boundary) Values clarification	Activate system to change factors that impede adaptation: Reconnect Revive rituals Retribalize Derigidfy
Helpful approaches	Ecological Structural Networks	Structural Intergenerational Experiential Communication	Networks Existential Strategic

degree of cohesion or the type of hierarchy associated with health and deviance. Until recently, these norms were applied to all families, ignoring cultural differences in the expression of proximity or the types of hierarchies preferred.

Olson, Russell, and Sprenkle (1980) predict cultural variations along the dimensions of cohesion and adaptability of their circumplex model. They maintain that the American, white, middle-class culture attempts to balance family togetherness and individual autonomy, but the theme favoring autonomy prevails (see Figure 21-2). Families from various ethnic groups (Greek, Slovak, Mexican, Italian), families from religious groups (Amish, Mormon, born-again Christian), sectors of the working-class and poor families, all stress traditional values of family interdependence through physical and emotional proximity, loyalty, and interpersonal consensus. A culturally relativistic view recognizes that this cultural emphasis on family interdependence is functional unless it seriously interferes with social or individual adaptation.

Principles of Family Organization: The Cultural Code

To help train culturally attuned therapists, the models of family functioning taught must satisfy three criteria: (1) they must be free from culturally biased normative expectations; (2) they must take into account cultural–transactional styles; (3) they must differentiate those styles from dysfunctional traits. Principles of family organization are tied to culture; they are contained, as it were, in a cultural code that determines these and many other aspects of family life.

The Concept of the Dominant Dyad

A cultural lens on issues of family organization such as proximity and hierarchy can be introduced by utilizing the concept of "dominant dyad" (Falicov & Brudner-White, 1983; Hoffman, 1981; Hsu, 1971.) This concept is based on the assumption (derived from anthropological evidence) that cultures vary in the prominence they give to certain dyadic bonds over others in the total family configuration. In many cultures the husband–wife dyad is central, but in others the dominant dyad may be different. For example, in Chinese and Middle Eastern families the father–son dyad is the most central; in traditional Hindu society the dominant dyad is mother–son; in some African societies, it is brother–brother (Hsu, 1971).

The Cultural Code

Many principles of family organization vary depending on the dominant dyad. For example, depending on which dyad is central, differences exist in the continuity and discontinuity of the generations, the inclusion of others in family subsystems, and the rules about authority and leadership.

Section I of Table 21-3 summarizes the characteristic *cultural code* that gives prominence either to the intergenerational or to the marital dyad. Those differences have many implications for family therapy interventions, beginning with the initial communications between the family and the therapist. It is more likely that families organized on

TABLE 21-3. Differences in Cultural Code: The Nuclear and the Extended Family

	Nuclear family	Extended family
I. Cultural code	Dominant Dyad	
Principles of organization	Marital bond	Intergenerational bond
	Discontinuity	Continuity
	across generations	
	Exclusiveness	Inclusiveness of others
	Symmetry	Complementarity
II. The marital bond in each family type		
Boundaries	Clear and firm	Clear but permeable
	Equal proximity with children	Unequal proximity with children
Hierarchies	Egalitarian	Complementary
	Symmetry	Asymmetry
	Negotiation	Preguidelines
Values	Marital closeness	Intergenerational closeness
	Parental consensus	Respect for authority and tradition
	Balanced quid pro quo	
Ideal triad	Family of origin Family of origin Mother══════Father Child	Family of origin Family of origin Mother – – – – –Father Child
Coalition	Intergenerational	Same-generation
	threatens ideal values and hierarchies	

the extended family principles will prefer complementary types of interactions with the therapist-as-expert, compared to the nuclear family's tendency toward symmetry. Even more important are the implications of the concept of the "dominant dyad" for intervention in family triangles.

Family therapists agree on the central importance of the marital bond for family functioning; however, the possibility is seldom considered that the attributes of the marital bond depend on the cultural context. Indeed, there is ample anthropological and sociological evidence that the marital dyad functions differently internally and in relation to the kinship and friendship networks in families based on intergenerational bonds than in families that give prominence to the marital bond. These variations, listed in Section II of Table 21-3, need to be taken into account for correct assessment and intervention. To take one example, in situations involving family triangles, family therapists usually make a negative evaluation and proceed by applying a typical solution: to strengthen the marital bond. But some healthy families are more prone to "triangling" others than is considered ideal by middle-class nuclear family ideals. In fact, there are many families where a less sharply delineated boundary between the marital dyad and the extended family (or friends) is not only acceptable, but may even enhance the stability of the marriage (Bernard, 1985; Bott, 1957; Komarovsky, 1967).

Inclusiveness of kin, and even triangles involving the extended family and friends, are more readily tolerated by poor and working-class families, partly because they favor the intergenerational tie, but also because relatives serve many support functions. In this context, a phenomenon that family therapists consider to be a universal indicator of family pathology, the cross-generational coalition (Haley, 1967), may turn out to be culturally relative as long as it is not overly rigid.

The emergence of a cross-generational coalition, therefore, may have a different meaning and impact for dysfunction, depending on the cultural values (see Table 21-3). A cross-generational coalition is *incongruent* with the ideals of marital unity, parental equidistance from children, and egalitarian hierarchies that typify the nuclear middle-class American family—the model implicitly advocated by much of family therapy theory. The same coalitionary processes are not as threatening when families do not rely as much on clear boundaries around the marital dyad and where the leadership structure of the family is not solely dependent on parental consensus. On the other hand, in families where continuity over the generations, complementarity of functions, and hierarchical differences are important, same-generation coalitions (such as a husband–wife dyad or peer relationships that seriously diminish intergenerational influence) may be incongruent and therefore become associated with relationship problems.

Trainees must be taught that observed family coalitions should be screened through the corresponding cultural code to distinguish triangles generated by the cultural patterns from those that are dysfunctional triangles. This screening guards against the tendency to gravitate toward and intervene in those triangles that may indeed endanger the integrity of nuclear middle-class American families but are of different significance to families with different cultural codes. This topic has been developed in detail elsewhere (Falicov & Brudner-White, 1983).

Family Organization and Ecological Fit

The concept of the dominant dyad can also be used to conceptualize conflicts of cultural transition. Ethnic families often move from traditional settings, where there is stability of values and continuity of the generations, to rapidly changing settings in which the family is based primarily on the marital dyad. Families who migrate are often faced with the need to resolve the contradictory demands implicit in different dominant dyad priorities. This could also be counted as a source of stress.

When formulating therapeutic goals, trainees are taught to develop answers to the following questions. Do the couple's interactional rules need to change in the new setting to fit a new cultural code that supports the autonomy of the marital dyad? Or does the nuclear unit need to remain simultaneously congruent with the values of the extended family that surrounds them? Answers to questions like these provide valuable guidelines regarding which dyads in the system need reinforcement. Most families adapt success-fully, but some develop symptoms when attempting to blend two contradictory sets of rules. In these situations, the trainee needs to be guided to open and close doors selectively between the old and the new structures through approaches to be imple-mented in the supervisory situation.

Experiential Exercise

To assist trainees' ability to observe and experience the triadic configurations that occur in nuclear and extended families, several triangular interactions can be simulated by the training group. In each simulated triad the dominant dyad varies; special emphasis is given to a subsystems analysis that compares the marital, the parent–child, and the sibling dyads in various cultural contexts. Once the patterns are delineated and their organization understood, a discussion and simulation takes place that is centered on the types of appropriate interventions. Trainees thus see how interventions in triangles can create excessive or insufficient dislocations of the habitual patterns embedded in the cultural context.

FAMILY LIFE CYCLE

Family therapists use life cycle concepts to understand family and individual behavior, to recognize crisis points, and to formulate treatment goals (Carter & McGoldrick, 1980; Haley, 1973; Liddle, 1983; Solomon, 1973). In fact, it is common practice to associate a family crisis with transition points in the life cycle, usually marked by addition and losses of membership requiring a renegotiation of interactional rules. Furthermore, therapists often evaluate family dysfunction on the basis of age-appropriate behavior. Yet, transition points and perception of age-appropriateness are embedded in a cultural fabric.

The sequence of events in the family life cycle is probably universal, in that it is tied to biological events; mating, having offspring, raising and launching them, and growing old. But the timing of the stages and transitions, the themes, the rituals, and even the mechanisms by which the developmental changes take place are influenced by culture. Modal descriptions of the family life cycle have concentrated on the middle-class American individual and family (Haley, 1973; Schulz, 1976; Solomon, 1973). Little attention has been paid to cultural variations in the life cycle (Falicov, 1984; Falicov & Karrer, 1980; McGoldrick & Carter, 1982).

Training provides opportunities to learn about the life cycle of the population most often seen by the trainees. A rudimentary model of the life cycle is introduced, along with a discussion of universal dimensions and those where cultural variations can be expected. Cultural variations in sequence, timing, stages and transitions, rituals, age-appropriate behavior, and solutions to life cycle predicaments are discussed. An illustration may be given of a cultural variation from the Anglo-American family life cycle by describing the life cycle of the traditional Mexican family. (Falicov & Karrer, 1980). Examples of these differences are a longer state of interdependence between the mother and young children (often mistaken for overprotection), the absence of a launching period from the family of origin into an independent living situation for young adults, and the absence of an "empty nest" and a middle-age crisis. These differences appear to be associated with a lesser emphasis on individual pursuits in Mexico than in the United States. With acculturation, many developmental expectations gradually change to accommodate American norms, but some remain minimally changed over the generations.

Rather than judging families with the norms of their theories or their culture, trainees are taught to adopt an exploratory attitude about when and how a developmental task is dealt with in the family's original culture. The transition of launching children or leaving home provides an illustration. Most therapists are trained in the middle-class Anglo-American norms, which consider late adolescence and young adulthood to be the crucial times for the development of autonomy, self-sufficiency, and independence. Failure to disengage at an "appropriate time" has been linked to schizophrenia, drug addiction, and psychosomatic problems, and has given rise to the hypothesis that the deviant behavior stabilizes the family so that they do not have to face the threat of separation and change. But for many ethnic groups, and working-class or poor families, there is little threat during late adolescence, since actual leaving occurs later and usually through marriage. In many traditional families, individuation and personal identity—a universal expectation—are manifested in behaviors other than leaving home or achieving financial independence from the family. The test of successful disengagement may come later and be manifested in the establishment of a marriage free from paralyzing loyalty conflicts and excessive interference from the family of origin. Understanding the function that unity, loyalty, and communal behavior have for families of rural, traditional, or impoverished backgrounds may bring a different perspective on the issue of individuation and make it less essential for mental health than our middle-class, urban background prescribes. Awareness about life cycle differences helps to recognize crisis points, raises questions of whether certain types of transitional difficulties may be more common in some cultures than in others, and warns against culturally biased theories of psychopathology.

Rites and Rituals

Rites of passage and even rites of continuity are common features of life cycle events. Inquiring about the culture's rites of passage and the family's adherence to rituals over the generations may reveal the definition of the developmental moment for the particular family. Schwartzman (1983) suggests that there are two types of situations where the family's accepted cultural premises are highlighted and made obvious to the "clinician as ethnographer." These are *calendrical rites* (rituals celebrated at particular times during the year, such as birthdays, anniversaries, and civil and religious holidays) and *rites of passage* (rituals commemorating changes in the life cycle, such as weddings, graduations, and puberty rites). Through these rites the social organization of the family is acted out. Who attends and what role they play in the performance reveals important aspects of the social structure. In general, when compared with modern middle-class families, traditional ethnic families are characterized by more communal behavior and more family rituals. For a comprehensive description of cultural rituals and their ties to social organizations, see van der Hart (1983).

Family Development, Ecological Fit, and Family Organization

From an ecosystems framework, developmental transitions occur more smoothly when the family is operating with one shared set of cultural agreements backed by the various levels of the total ecological context. If the family relocates, it faces internal and external dissonances in developmental expectations. Sometimes family members try to reconcile the new and the old cultural codes. A young couple that migrates from a traditional rural setting may attempt to develop a more cohesive and egalitarian marital dyad to cope with the demands of early parenthood in a modern, urban context. But they may also attempt to maintain strong intergenerational alliances and the friendships that were adaptive in the native environment. Often there is asynchrony between husband and wife on the readiness to adopt one or the other culture code. Symptoms may develop through attempts to force and merge two contradictory sets of developmental codes.

An interface between family development and migration also occurs when there are migratory separations and reunions that result in changes of membership similar to the stressful additions and losses of developmental transitions. Difficulties in adaptation to the new culture may not become apparent until the time of a developmental transition, for example, in the transition from home to school, when the family comes in contact with the mesosystem or the exosystem (Falicov, 1982a; Falicov & Karrer, 1980; Montalvo, 1974; Montalvo & Gutierrez, 1983). Dissonances in developmental expectations among family members at different stages of acculturation has been associated with family dysfunction (Stanton, 1979; Szapocznick, Scopetta, & Tillman, 1978).

Experiential Exercise

To increase awareness about cultural variations in sequence, staging, and timing of developmental events, a sculpting technique is used (Duhl, Kantor, & Duhl, 1973). It consists of asking the trainees to form a simulated family and sculpt a longitudinal sequence of events from the time two young adults meet and decide to form a family until they die. Several changes in cultural context can be depicted that modify the family life cycle. The life cycle of the various generations of the immigrant family can also be determined.[4] At transition points, a "freeze" command is given to the moving group sculpture and a discussion takes place about the developmental tasks, the reorganizations, and the change of rules involved. The total exercise results in a comparative outlook and an exploratory attitude about life cycle issues in different cultures.

PRACTICAL APPLICATIONS

Application of Concepts to Nonclinical and Clinical Families

In the initial didactic lectures and experiential exercises of the program (four weeks), the trainee develops an outline for an interview format, with questions and observations that will tap the cultural information being sought. The interview covers four areas of family functioning: ecological context, acculturation, organization, and development.

The trainee then uses the outline to interview a nonclinical family selected from among friends, colleagues, or other volunteers. Two families are usually interviewed during the training sessions by a cotherapy team of trainees, while the rest of the training group observes. An alternative for those trainees who cannot secure a nonclinical family is to explore the culture of their own family of origin, via a written or audiotaped interview based on the same guidelines. It is not essential that this family belong to a minority ethnic group, given the definition of culture that includes majority and minority ethnic and social class issues, religion, and occupation. (Some of the most fascinating interviews, because of the complexity of cultural blends, are with second-generation families that have clearly identifiable ethnic roots.) This exercise encourages appreciation of cultural relativity and introduces appreciation of intragroup variability and generational differences.

PRECONCEPTIONS
Before conducting the interview, trainees are encouraged to write down all their *a priori* ideas about the cultural group they are about to interview, on the basis of very general information (for example, "an interracial middle-class family, father engineer, mother a social worker, two adolescent children," or "a working-class, second-generation Latino family with three school-age children"). Trainees are free to disclose their preconceptions or not, as they choose. This exercise helps prevent the possibility that the interviewers would only attempt to confirm their own stereotypes and thus preclude exploration of variability. Also, by including the observers and their own values and ideas as part of the observation, an interactional lens is introduced that highlights the mutual preconceptions between the therapist and the family (Sluzki, 1982).[5]

FAMILY AND THERAPIST CONSONANCE-DISSONANCE
Videotaped segments of the interviews are then reviewed by the training group to discover areas of consonance and dissonance. Special attention is paid to the family's and the therapist's styles of communication, the therapist's questions or comments that join or transgress the family's style, and the statements that open up or preclude new alternative behaviors for the family. The trainee's subjective impression, level of comfort, empathy, and degree of understanding are also discussed.

From this material a "Family Map" and a "Therapist Map" (Figure 21-3) are drawn. These maps serve a dual purpose. First, they summarize the specific dimensions of assessment within the major areas of family functioning, and thus serve as an interview guide. Second, by overlapping the maps, the trainee examines and compares his or her own maps about healthy family behavior with the maps of those families being interviewed. The overlaps of these two maps in the four areas of family functioning result in a qualitative estimate of *cultural distance* between the family and the therapist. A concept of *social distance* has been used by Yamamoto (1967), Lefley (1982), and Jenkins and Morrison (1978) to tap individual or institutional racism. In our training context this concept is used to summarize issues of consonance–dissonance, and as a device to detect prejudice.

A moderate degree of cultural distance is optimal. If there is too much cultural distance, the therapist may become too cautious and superficial, or too confused and judgmental. Too much cultural distance can cause the family to drop out of treatment. But there are also advantages to cultural distance, since the therapist may introduce alternative world views precisely by belonging to a different culture. Too little cultural distance can block the therapists' change orientation, and organize their behavior to become part of the family system. A moderate range of consonance–dissonance allows for a perception of difference between what is cultural and what is dysfunctional, and increases the range of alternative behaviors for the therapist–family system.

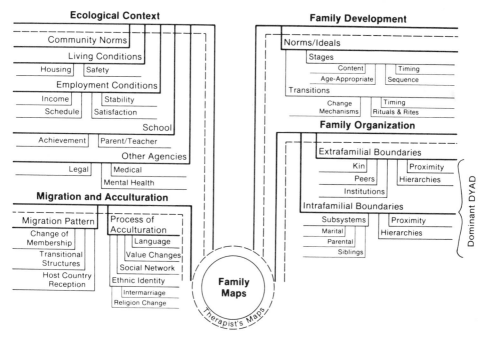

Figure 21-3. Family maps and therapist's maps.

Implications for the Therapeutic Process

The total exercise outlined above serves as a laboratory for learning to perceive or to think culturally. The exercise takes up about four two-hour sessions that follow the didactic lectures, and are concentrated at the beginning of the program. The payoffs far outweigh the amount of time involved.

The byproducts of this experience will be manifested later in the process of joining, defining a problem, and selecting culturally attuned interventions. First, mutual accommodation and recognition of cultural consonances and dissonances between therapists and family are good starting points for the process of joining and forming a therapeutic alliance. Once a trainee becomes aware that families have cultural preferences—for example, in complementary or symmetrical attitudes toward family members or toward outsiders—then the approach selected for building an alliance is readily and effectively adjusted. Cultural considerations tend to slow down this phase of therapy, but a slower pace often turns out to be an advantage. The trainee also learns the need to pursue a cultural theme with a "balance of risk and respect" and with constant "reading of the family's verbal and non-verbal feedback" to the therapist's comments, which in turn should increase the family's trust and comfort with the therapist (Lappin, 1983).

Second, in the area of assessment and defining the problem, the trainee's clinical judgment is sharpened through the experience of deciding when and how cultural issues are of relevance to a presenting problem. Adopting a perspective that takes into account the effects of multiple contexts appears to open up more systemic avenues for intervening in the family's total situation. Another eventual by-product of this way of thinking may be to stimulate the development of more complex models of family functioning. The process of selecting a focus of therapeutic work then becomes more comprehensive and more closely targeted.

Third, the delineation of therapeutic goals takes into account the family's perception about fundamental aspects of family life. The challenge to trainee and trainer is to devise means of producing change without excessive pattern and value dislocation; only then does therapy not become a form of involuntary acculturation to the therapist's values.

Fourth, the definition of the therapist's role and the interventions that accompany it becomes sharply delineated. Whether the interventions take place within the family or between the family and other institutions, a number of specific culturally-attuned strategies are possible.

As experience grows, more refined and strategic uses of cultural issues as tools for change are possible (Falicov, 1985; Falicov & Karrer, 1984), which go beyond the rudiments of learning to think culturally and are best put into practice with trainees who have mastered the essentials of family therapy theory and technique.

SUMMARY

This chapter presents a framework for the integration of cultural perspectives in family therapy training. Culture is defined as those shared sets of world views and adaptive behaviors derived from membership in various contexts simultaneously. The articulation of "cultural training" with other training objectives is accomplished through the introduction of two basic positions. The first is an ecosystemic view that constantly places the family in its social context. This view is based on the notion of "ecological fit," or family–environment match. A model has been presented that helps trainees to locate potentially stressful interactions and the social context for the immigrant family and subsequent generations. This model guides the trainees to discover when and how cultural differences make a difference through exploring a number of variables that render an index of ecological stress. This index, in turn, guides the trainee toward choosing appropriate therapeutic goals and interventions.

The second position focuses on the degree of cultural consonance–dissonance between the world view of the family and that of the therapist. Concepts and interventions related to family development and family organization in various cultures are paid particular attention, since many cultural dissonances between therapist and families occur in those areas. A format that involves a series of experiential exercises enables trainer and trainee to move from normative cultural descriptions to the practical realities of perceiving and acting "culturally" in the therapy situation. Practicing a cultural way of thinking takes place initially through the experience of interviewing, observing, and evaluating cultural aspects of nonclinical families. A rationale for beginning cultural training by differentiating between functional and dysfunctional families is also offered. In sum, this chapter addresses questions about appropriate format, content, and timing of cultural training in the context of other family therapy training objectives.

Notes

1. Among the training programs that include cultural perspectives on the family are John Spiegel's group at Brandeis University in Massachusetts, which was actually the first program on ethnicity training; David McGill's at the Smith School of Social Work; Monica McGoldrick's group at the Community Mental Health Center of Rutgers Medical School in New Jersey; Joel Feiner and Fred Takemoto's at the Psychiatric Residency, Einstein's Bronx Psychiatric Center; Francesca Farr's at the Family Practice Residency Program, San Francisco General Hospital; Guillermo Bernal's in the Department of Psychiatry at the University of California at San Francisco, and the Family Systems Program at the Institute for Juvenile Research in Chicago.

Several programs have developed very interesting cross-cultural training methodologies for individual therapists. Notable among them are Paul Pedersen at Syracuse University and Harriet Lefley at the Department of Psychiatry, University of Miami.

2. I am indebted for this idea to Dr. Bertha Melgoza. For a description of expectable or normal behavior in ethnic families, see M. McGoldrick (Walsh, 1982), and for a description of myths about normality in American culture, see Walsh (1983).

3. In a pioneering article, Sluzki (1979) presents a useful and parsimonious model of the conflicts regularly encountered by families at different phases of migration and acculturation.

4. Landau's (1982) use of dual sculpting in cases of cultural transition is a related and very useful technique.

5. Sluzki (1982) is one of the few theorists who considers macrolevel systemic perceptions and behaviors between individuals of different cultures. In this article he also underscores the self-fulfilling prophecies inherent in stereotypes.

References

Bateson, G. (1972). *Steps to an ecology of the mind.* New York: Ballantine.

Beavers, W. (1977). *Psychotherapy and growth: A family systems perspective.* New York: Brunner/Mazel.

Bernard, J. (1985). The marital bond vis-à-vis the male bond and the female bond. *American Family Therapy Association Newsletter, 19,* 15–22.

Bott, E. (1957). *Family and social network: Roles, norms, and external relationships in ordinary urban families.* New York: Free Press.

Bronfenbrenner, U. (1977). Toward an experimental ecology of human development. *American Psychologist, 45,* 513–530.

Carter, E., & McGoldrick, M. (Eds.). (1980). *The family life cycle: A framework for family therapy.* New York: Gardner Press.

Cleghorn, J., & Levin, S. (1973). Training family therapists by setting learning objectives. *American Journal of Orthopsychiatry, 43,* 439–446.

Duhl, F. J., Kantor, D., and Duhl, B. S. (1973). Learning, space and action in family therapy: A primer of sculpture. In D. A. Block (Ed.), *Techniques of family psychotherapy: A primer.* New York: Grune & Stratton.

Epstein, N., Bishop, D. (1981). Problem-centered systems therapy of the family. In A. Gurman & D. Kniskern (Eds.), *Handbook of family therapy.* New York: Brunner/Mazel.

Falicov, C. J. (1982a). *An ecosystemic framework for the study of families in cultural transition.* Paper read at Conference on the Effects of Migration Over the Generations, sponsored by the University of California at San Francisco, San Francisco, California.

Falicov, C. J. (1982b). Mexican-American families. In M. McGoldrick, J. Pearce, & J. Giordano (Eds.), *Ethnicity and family therapy.* New York: Guilford Press.

Falicov, C. J. (Ed.). (1983). Introduction. *Cultural perspectives in family therapy.* Rockville: Aspen Systems.

Falicov, C. J. (1984). Focus on stages: Commentary to C. L. Proudfit's developmental analysis of V. Wolff's novel *To the lighthouse. Family Process, 23*(3), 329–334.

Falicov, C. J. (1985). Cross-cultural marriages. In N. Jacobson & A. Gurman (Eds.), *Handbook of marital therapy.* New York: Guilford Press.

Falicov, C. J. (Ed.). (1988). *Family transitions: Continuity and change over the life cycle.* New York: Guilford Press.

Falicov, C. J., & Brudner-White, L. (1983). The shifting family triangle: The issue of cultural and contextual relativity. In C. J. Falicov (Ed.), *Cultural perspectives in family therapy*. Rockville, MD: Aspen.

Falicov, C. J., Constantine, J., & Breunlin, D. (1981). Teaching family therapy: a program based on training objectives. *Journal of Marital and Family Therapy, 3*, 497–506.

Falicov, C. J., & Karrer, B. (1984). Therapeutic strategies for Mexican-American families. *International Journal of Family Therapy, 6*(1), 16–30.

Falicov, C. J. & Karrer, B. (1980). Cultural variations in the family life cycle: The Mexican-American family. In Carter, E. & McGoldrick, M. (Eds.). *The family life cycle: A framework for family therapy*. New York: Gardner Press.

Haley, J. (1967). Toward a theory of pathological systems. In G. Zuk & I. Boszormenyi-Nagy (Eds.), *Family therapy and disturbed families*. Palo Alto, CA: Science and Behavior Books.

Haley, J. (1973). *Uncommon therapy: The psychiatric techniques of Milton Erickson, MD*. New York: Ballantine Books.

Hartman, A., & Laird, J. (1983). *Family-centered social work practice*. New York: Free Press.

Hoffman, L. (1981). *Foundations of family therapy*. New York: Basic Books.

Hsu, F. (Ed.). (1971). *Kinship and culture*. Chicago: Aldine.

Jenkins, S., & Morrison, B. (1978). Ethnicity and service delivery. *American Journal of Orthopsychiatry, 48*(1), 160–165.

Kantor, D., & Lehr, W. (1975). *Inside the family*. San Francisco: Jossey-Bass.

Komarovsky, M. (1967). *Blue-collar marriage*. New York: Vintage Books.

Landau, J. (1982). Therapy with families in cultural transition. In M. McGoldrick, J. K. Pearce, & J. Giordano (Eds.), *Ethnicity and family therapy*. New York: Guilford Press.

Lappin, J. (1983). On becoming a culturally conscious family therapist. In C. J. Falicov (Ed.), *Cultural perspectives in family therapy*. Rockville, MD: Aspen.

Lefley, H. P. (1982). Final report on cross-cultural training for mental health personnel. Coral Gables, FL: University of Miami School of Medicine. Department of Psychiatry.

Liddle, H. (1983). *Clinical implications of the family life cycle*. Rockville, MD: Aspen.

McGill, D. (1983). Cultural concepts for family therapy. In C. J. Falicov (Ed.), *Cultural perspectives in family therapy*. Rockville, MD: Aspen.

McGoldrick, M. & Carter, E. (1982). The family life cycle. In F. Walsh (Ed.), *Normal family processes*. New York: Guilford Press.

McGoldrick, M., Pearce, J. K., & Giordano, J. (Eds.). (1982). *Ethnicity and family therapy*. New York: Guilford Press.

Meyerstein, I. (1979). The family behavioral snapshot: a tool for teaching family assessment. *American Journal of Family Therapy, 7*(1), 48–56.

Minuchin, S. (1974). *Families and family therapy*. Cambridge, MA: Harvard University Press.

Montalvo, B. (1974). Home–school conflict and the Puerto Rican child. *Social Casework, 55*(2), 100–110.

Montalvo, B., & Gutierrez, M. (1983). A perspective for the use of the cultural dimension in family therapy. In C. J. Falicov (Ed.), *Cultural perspectives in family therapy*. Rockville, MD: Aspen.

Montalvo, B., & Gutierrez, M. (1988). The emphasis on cultural identity: A developmental ecological constraint. In C. J. Falicov. (Ed.,), *Family transitions: Continuity and change over the life cycle*. New York: Guilford Press.

Olson, D. H., Russell, C. S., & Sprenkle, D. H. (1980). Circumplex model of marital and family systems: II. Empirical studies and clinical intervention. *Advances in Family Intervention, Assessment and Theory, 1*, 129–179.

Olson, D. H., Sprenkle, D. H., & Russell, C. (1979). Circumplex model of marital and family systems: I. Cohesion and adaptability dimensions, family types and clinical applications. *Family Process, 18* (1), 3–28.

Papajohn, J., & Spiegel, J. (1975). *Transactions in families: A modern approach to resolving cultural and generational conflict*. San Francisco: Jossey-Bass.

Sager, C., Brayboy, T., & Waxenberg, B. (1970). *Black ghetto family in therapy: A laboratory experience*. New York: Grove Press.

Schulz, D. (1976). *The changing family: Its function and future*. Englewood Cliffs, NJ: Prentice-Hall.

Schwartzman, J. (1983). Family ethnography: A tool for clinicians. In C. J. Falicov (Ed.), *Cultural perspectives in family therapy*. Rockville, MD: Aspen.

Sluzki, C. (1979). Migration and family conflict. *Family Process, 18*(4), 379–390.

Sluzki, C. (1982). The Latin lover revisited. In M. McGoldrick, J. K. Pearce, & J. Giordano (Eds.), *Ethnicity and family therapy*. New York: Guilford Press.

Solomon, M. A. (1973). A developmental, conceptual premise for family therapy. *Family Process, (12)*, 179–188.

Stanton, M. D. (1979). Family treatment approaches to drug abuse problems: A review. *Family Process, 18*(3), 251–280.

Szapocznik, J., Scopetta, M. A., & Tillman, W. (1978). What changes, what stays the same and what affects acculturative change? In J. Szapocznik & M. C. Jerrers (Eds.), *Cuban Americans: Acculturation, adjustment and the family*. Washington, DC: COSSMHO, The National Coalition of Hispanic Mental Health and Human Services Organizations.

Tomm, K. M. & Wright, L. M. (1979). Training in family therapy: Perceptual, conceptual and executive skills. *Family Process, 18*, 227–250.

van der Hart, O. (1983). *Rituals in psychotherapy: Transition and continuity*. New York: Irvington Publishers.

Walsh, F. (1983). Normal family ideologies: Myths and realities. In C. J. Falicov (Ed.), *Cultural perspectives in family therapy*. Rockville, MD: Aspen.

Wood, B. & Talmon, M. (1983). Family boundaries in transition: A search for alternatives. *Family Process, 22*(3) 347–357.

Yamamoto, J. (1967). Racial factors in patient selection. *American Journal of Psychiatry, 124*, 630–639.

22

Reflections on Supervision

JAY HALEY
The Family Therapy Institute of Washington, D.C., Rockville, Maryland

In the therapy field there is no consensus on the nature of clinical supervision or how to teach a trainee to do therapy. Presumably the task of a teaching supervisor is to supervise in such a way that a trainee is successful with the particular case being supervised, and learns from that experience how to be successful with others. Yet, because there is no agreement about the nature of therapy or how to do it, there is confusion about what a supervisor should do.

PARALLELS BETWEEN THERAPY AND TRAINING

At one time there was more consistency between clinical practice and training therapists. A clinician interviewed an individual client and offered insight into emotional problems, exploring past experiences and childhood. Change was expected to occur spontaneously as a result of self-understanding. Similarly, training was done by putting the therapist-in-training in therapy and offering insight into emotional problems, exploring childhood and past experiences. Competence in doing therapy was expected to occur spontaneously as a result of insight into problems. Just as the individual client was never observed in action with intimates, but only reported about them, a therapist-in-training was never observed dealing with patients, but only reported on them. Therapy and supervision were consistent. The ideas used behind the one-way mirror for trainees were formally the same as those in front of the mirror for clients.

When we turn to the new developments in therapy, particularly in the family therapies, the situation is different. There no longer seems to be the same kind of parallel between therapy and training. Family therapy was born when individuals were observed in action with their intimates. Because of what was seen, and the influence of cybernetic theory, a revolutionary set of premises about psychological problems appeared. Symptoms were no longer viewed as a response to childhood experiences, but were seen as a reaction to the current social situation. Rather than being maladaptive and irrational misperceptions of reality, symptoms were viewed as appropriate and adaptive to the person's system of intimates. The therapeutic task was to change a current system involving several people, not to explore the past of one of them.

LACK OF PROGRESS

Given these new ideas about human beings and the new focus of change, how should a supervisor train a family therapist? The most obvious first step is for the supervisor to see the therapist in action with clients, just as he or she would first see the individual client in action with family members, and not depend on self-report. The logic of this view led to training with the one-way mirror and live supervision. Just as observing the client in his or her social context changed ideas about psychology, so did observing a therapist actually at work change ideas about the nature of therapy and how to teach it. Yet have the premises of family therapy been accepted in the training of family therapists? I do not think so. There has been slow progress in changes in training procedures. On the basis of travels about the country, I think the vast majority of therapy supervision—and this includes family therapy training—is still being done without the supervisor ever seeing the trainee do therapy, and with an emphasis on the individual nature of the therapist.

I think that therapy today is more effective than it has ever been, and that supervision techniques have improved steadily over the years. With therapists and teachers more skillful, there are some difficult human problems that can be resolved rapidly today. Yet I think such progress has occurred only with a minority in the field. The most common focus of supervision still seems to be on the personality of therapists, and there is a reluctance to teach directive skills by live supervision. For half a century the entire teaching ideology did not include instructing a therapist in interview skills or teaching directive therapy techniques, so the change to including these skills and techniques requires innovation in therapy training programs.

THREE AREAS OF FOCUS

There are no sound research data on which to base our ideas about how to supervise therapists. We can only speculate on how it should be done. As I look around at supervision approaches, there seem to me to be three major areas of focus when teaching therapy.

The Problem Situation

There is a long tradition of teaching a trainee to do therapy by describing the client's situation. The etiology of the neurosis, and the dynamics of intrapsychic life, occupied much of the training in individual therapy. To teach expertise in the meaning of dreams was considered teaching therapy. As family therapy developed, many supervisors continued that tradition, teaching therapists the nature of families and their problems. Family dynamics, family structure, and circular systems are discussed at length in such training programs. If a client has an eating disorder, the training focuses on what kind of family presumably produces such a disorder. Issues of how to raise chidren, the role of women in families, and how to bring out information by skillful questioning are all taught. What is not taught is how to change anyone.

The merit of the problem situation approach is that the supervisor does not have to teach in a setting where therapy is being done. Clients need not even be available, and so the individual and family problems can be discussed at length in universities, using texts on different types of abnormal psychology. The problem approach can also be used in clinics at staff conferences. Traditionally the staff conference has been a diagnostic conference, not a conference to select the kind of therapeutic intervention to use in a case. The results of intelligence and psychological tests and discussions of pathology can all be presented without the issue of actual therapy coming up. I recall a young woman who had the responsibility of curing a young child who started fires. She waited for testing, for the interviews, and finally for the staff conference, expecting to be advised how to cure the child. At the staff meeting, there was a one-hour discussion of the dynamics of fire setting and the testing results, but not a single suggestion for stopping the child from starting fires. The staff was pleased with the conference, feeling they had covered the case as thoroughly as they should. The young woman, however, wept because her supervisor and the staff had no suggestion to give her about what to do.

The Therapist's Personality

Another supervisory focus that has been common is the assumption that training in therapy is accomplished by resolving the emotional problems of the trainee. Individual therapy for the trainee is usually compulsory in this approach, and the supervisory sessions deal with the trainee and his or her life. It is assumed that the therapy will be successful if the trainee is cleared of his or her problems. As one supervisor in family therapy put it, "As soon as I saw the trainee talking with a family, I knew his problem was with his own family. When he realized that, everything would be solved." In such training programs, the obligation of the supervisor becomes how to help the trainee with personal problems, not teach how to do therapy. For example, if a supervisor notes that a trainee has difficulty interviewing adolescents, the focus is on his or her emotional response to these youths. Therapy is recommended for the trainee, or the trainee simulates his or her personal family with special emphasis on the adolescent period. It would be assumed that if he or she worked through feelings about young people, he or she would be able to deal therapeutically with any adolescent who walked in the door without needing to be taught how to deal with them. From this viewpoint, psychological problems are said to prevent the therapist from making appropriate therapeutic interventions. Further, it is assumed that if the trainee becomes aware of what is behind the psychological problem in his or her personal life, he or she will be an effective therapist with any client. When this emphasis on the trainee's personality is used in the supervision of family therapists, different procedures are included; besides requiring individual or family therapy of the trainee, the entire group of trainees takes turns simulating their families of origin. Trainees also do genograms of their family trees, and are sent off to visit their relatives. The basic premise of self-exploration appears to have been adopted from psychoanalysis without considering that family therapy offers new opportunities for training. Sometimes such training never includes actually seeing a client family.

The merit of this approach is that the supervisor does not have to know how to change anyone. Any teaching problem that arises can be dealt with by suggesting the trainee has emotional problems. This approach also encourages all trainees to have therapy, often with the staff of the training program, so there is more business for everyone. It was estimated that over 40% of the people in psychoanalysis were professionals, not the public.

Some training programs not only require the trainee to undergo personal therapy, but also require the trainee to bring in spouse and children and have family therapy. A special problem arises from this compulsory family therapy: family members must have therapy even if they do not need it, and they must reveal their family life in public if the trainee is to get an academic degree. Such a requirement is probably illegal, but teachers in the psychoanalytic tradition require it without thinking the matter through.

It is remarkable that, apparently, there has not been a research study demonstrating that a therapist who has had personal therapy, family or otherwise, has a better outcome with clients than one who has not. One would think that an idea that has existed for almost half a century, and involves millions of dollars in training money, would have led to hundreds of such studies. My own experience has been that the more personal therapy trainees have had, the more difficult they are to teach. They become so preoccupied with themselves that clients have trouble getting their attention.

Skill Supervision

A third type of supervision focuses on teaching the trainee skills in doing therapy interviews. It is assumed that therapy is like any other operational skill, such as playing the piano, and must be taught under observation. The emphasis is not on the personal life or on the psychological problems of the trainee. If the trainee has difficulty dealing with adolescents, it is assumed that the supervisor's responsibility is to teach him how to deal with adolescents in a therapeutic way. The maturity and self-confidence of a trainee is assumed to come from gaining competence in his or her work, not from exploring personal emotional problems.

Skill supervision goes back to the last century, when clinical hypnosis was taught with live observation: a trainee observed the teacher doing hypnosis with a patient, and then the teacher observed and guided the trainee with a patient. That kind of supervision disappeared from the field with Freud's emphasis on confidentiality and the abandonment of hypnosis. With the appearance of the one-way mirror in the 1950s, a focus on skill in interview technique again became an issue.

Skill supervisors tend to work with one-way mirrors or recordings because they must know what actually happens in therapy. While the personality supervisor makes personal therapy compulsory, the skill supervisor makes therapy under observation compulsory.

When the supervisor does live supervision behind the mirror, the ideology of the training group mirrors the ideology in the family therapy room; the therapy, and the training, are directive and not insightful. The training group is not allowed to interpret each other's personal problems, but must focus on positive suggestions for what is to be done. Just as each client and family is treated with a different plan, each trainee is taught with a concern about his or her particular needs. The behavior in front of the mirror and behind it is consistent. That is, the concern of the supervisor in this situation is not the family in therapy, or the trainee, but the trainee–family unit.

The task of the supervisor is to devise a plan that will change the particular family but can be implemented by this particular trainee. Different trainees have different limitations and assets, and the supervisor must design an intervention that is appropriate to that person, just as a plan for the family must be appropriate for that particular family.

Since the behavior behind and in front of the mirror is parallel, the supervisor will use directive techniques with the trainee to teach how to use directive techniques. The supervisor will attempt to enlarge the range of skills of the trainee, while the trainee will try to enlarge the opportunities in a family. If straightforward insistence that the trainee try a procedure would be effective, the supervisor will use a straightforward directive. If a trainee is shy and nervous, on the other hand, the supervisor might encourage that behavior, thereby using a paradoxical technique. The emphasis on respecting hierarchy required in the therapy will be followed in the training program, as will the use of humor and metaphor. The supervisor needs a theory and practice in training that allows a range of interventions with trainees who are various in their natures, just as the trainee must learn a range of interventions with the various kinds of families who appear at the door.

CONSEQUENCES OF A TRAINING FOCUS

One might add other kinds of supervision besides those discussed above, but if we examine these three from the point of view of the parallels between supervision and therapy, the consequences of a training approach become evident. Let me outline some supervision premises.

1. A supervisor who uses a single method of teaching for all trainees will produce therapists who follow a method with all clients and do not adapt therapy to each one.

2. If a supervisor requires all trainee therapists to explore their families with genograms and visits to relatives, no matter what the trainee's problem in doing therapy, the therapist will require the family to do genograms and visit relatives, no matter what their presenting problem.

3. If a supervisor spends training time largely talking about a family's structure and problems, in contrast to talking about how to change them, the trainee will spend his or her time talking to the clients about their nature and problems; the issue of change is not likely to come up explicitly.

4. If a supervisor implies that a therapist's personal problems are interfering with the progress of a case, the therapist will suggest, directly or indirectly, to the client that his or her deep emotional problems are interfering with the progress of the therapy.

5. The supervisor who focuses on the dynamics of the situation tends not to take responsibility for the success or failure of the case. Trained in that way, the therapist is not likely to take responsibility for failure of the therapy. Each will blame someone else: the supervisor is likely to blame the trainee for emotional problems, and the therapist will blame the family for being resistant or untreatable because of their emotional problems.

6. A supervisor who discourages experimentation by a trainee and emphasizes orthodoxy, indicating that inaction and reflection are best, will have trainees who do not encourage clients or families to experiment with new ways of living.

7. A supervisor who has not thought through a clear position on how to do therapy, but is eclectic, will typically have trainees who cannot decide how to do therapy and who try different approaches, aborting them before they are successful.

8. A supervisor who teaches a trainee that he or she has repressed ideas and inner emotional problems, which he or she might project on the client, is teaching that trainee self-distrust; one cannot trust one's impulses if taught to doubt oneself. In skill therapy, it is assumed that a therapist must trust himself or herself, and follow inner ideas and impulses to be able to deal immediately with the complexities of therapy interviews.

9. A supervisor who teaches by giving trainees insight into their problems will produce trainees who feel like cads if they do not give insight to their clients. People who are given insight by a therapist tend to get revenge on the therapist, usually by not changing. Trainees also do not appreciate supervisors interpreting their behavior or thoughts to them insightfully, and they will tend to take it out on other trainees, creating a group with low morale and bad feelings.

10. If a supervisor believes he or she should be a pal and not an authority figure with a trainee, the therapist will be a pal to the family and not be authoritative, even when necessary. For example, if there is a violent youth in a family, the parents need to get the youth under control. If the therapist is not firm with the parents, they will not be firm with the youth. However, if the supervisor is not firm with the therapist, he or she will not be firm with the parents. When the therapy hierarchy is in confusion, the police may have to come and be firm. The hierarchy on one side of the mirror reflects the hierarchy on the other side. This applies even when there is no mirror.

11. The supervisor who wishes to give trainees full autonomy and never directs them will have trainees who never direct clients but instead listen to their dilemmas and commiserate about their misery.

12. The supervisor who emphasizes analysis of the situation, rather than how to change it, will think he or she is teaching therapy by interviewing a family at a public demonstration. Actually, in that situation, he or she is not teaching trainees how to do therapy but only how to interview at a public demonstration a family they will never see again.

Sometimes these demonstrations take place with simulated families. The supervisor who focuses on the situation, and not on actual therapy, does not mind that. I recall a colleague asked to attend a national meeting and simulate supervision of a person simulating a therapist with a family being simulated by colleagues. All was fantasy.

Although the list could be extended, these axioms about supervision indicate that teaching and therapy have close parallels. To illustrate the issue, let me cite some problems. For example, suppose a couple comes to therapy where the husband is beating the wife. A supervisor who is focused on the problem situation will dwell at length on wife abuse and its cause and nature, relating it to childhood abuse experiences, and so on. The personality supervisor will emphasize the therapist's own problems about marriage and abuse. The skill supervisor would teach the therapist ways to stop the abuse, and would focus on how to do that with this particular couple.

As another example, suppose an anorexic adolescent comes in, who weighs 70 pounds and is wasting away. Half a dozen hospitalizations have had no effect. The problem situation supervisor would discuss the families of anorexics and explore the causes of the misperceptions of the client and the dynamics and structure of the family. The personality supervisor would consider the weight and diet of the therapist relevant to the problem, particularly if the therapist was over- or underweight. In contrast, the skill supervisor would teach the therapist how to organize the family to make the girl eat and gain weight, beginning in the first session.

As another illustration, I can cite a milder and more routine case. I was supervising a therapist who was dealing with a young married couple. The wife had become interested in another man and was uncertain whether to go with him or stay with her husband. The husband wanted his wife to stay with him and was both angry about the other man and trying to please and placate the wife.

The therapist was having difficulty helping them resolve this issue. A supervisory problem was the fact that the therapist seemed to be siding with the wife against the husband. Ostensibly he was being evenhanded with the couple, but covertly he and the wife were implying that the husband was not quite up to what he should be. This coalition seemed to be incapacitating the husband. That is, the therapist had involuntarily triangulated on the side of the wife in such a way that change was being prevented.

The wife couldn't make up her mind, the husband was angry at the therapist and wife and was making only halfhearted efforts to keep his wife, the therapist was under pressure from me to resolve the problem, and he hesitated to act because he did not know what I wanted. I had not come up with anything to help the therapist. Everyone was stuck.

A supervisor focused on the problem situation would discuss with the trainee the nature of marriage, the issue of involvements with other men or women, the stages of marriage, and so on. There would be an emphasis on gathering more information. The question of how to change this situation would not come up.

A supervisor focused on the personality of the therapist would point out that the therapist was siding with the wife against the husband. Personal therapy would be recommended, or the supervisor would talk to the therapist about his own marriage (assuming there was indecision about someone leaving that marriage, or else there would not be a problem in therapy). Perhaps the supervisor would have the trainee simulate his marriage, or his parents' marriage, to work through his dilemma in dealing with this couple.

A skill supervisor would assume that this situation often happens and that any therapist might at some time get into an involuntary coalition with one spouse against the other. It is a consequence of doing marital therapy. In fact, even prominent therapists can get into such coalitions.

With a trainee in this situation, the skill supervisor would assume it is his or her task to help the therapist disengage from this unhelpful involvement. Whether the therapist has a problem in his own marriage would not be considered relevant, or allowed as an excuse. Emotional problems should not be allowed to interfere with one's work. A skill supervisor would also assume that the therapist does not need insight into the fact that he is in coalition with the wife. He already knows that. The problem is to do something about it. A skill supervisor would also assume that if the coalition was insightfully interpreted to the therapist as his problem, it could cause harm. The therapist would be likely to withdraw from the wife and try to side with the husband in order to please the supervisor. The wife would be bewildered and wonder what she had done wrong. The husband would be likely to feel the therapist was joining him in an artificial and phony way. Thus, insightful interpretations could make the situation worse for everyone, in therapy or in supervision.

Behind the mirror with a group of trainees, I watched the therapist and the wife rather patronizingly talking to the husband about how he was trying to please his wife but was not quite capable. I was looking for some way to change the balance of the couple in relation to the therapist; the husband was in a weak position, while the wife was in a strong position because of the therapist's support of her. The therapist needed to put the wife down and lift the husband up to get a change in his relationship with them, but not in a way that would offend or reject the wife. I was assuming the couple could not change in relation to each other unless the therapist changed in relation to them. The therapist was not likely to change in relation to them unless I changed in relation to *him*.

As I searched for a directive, a therapist behind the mirror mentioned that the wife was not very feminine, wearing jeans and a man's shirt. Perhaps she was trying to look less attractive because she wanted more distance from her husband. I found that observation helpful, and I telephoned the therapist. I suggested that he say to the husband that he would know when he was more successful in pleasing his wife because she would respond to him in a more feminine way.

The therapist said that to the couple, and the wife immediately said she did not agree with that. Coming to life for the first time in the interview, the husband looked pleased and said he understood that. The wife protested defensively that if her husband wanted a more feminine woman, he would have to look elsewhere. The therapist said he just thought he'd mention that in passing, and he went on to other things. After that simple intervention, the wife and husband behaved toward each other more as equals, and the therapist was no longer in coalition with the wife against the husband. At the next interview the husband insisted she make her choice of men, and she did so.

THE ROLE OF INSIGHT IN TRAINING

A supervision question is raised by this example. The therapist followed the directive of the supervisor and found himself free of the handicapping coalition without knowing why that had happened. In this therapy approach, the clients would not be told why the change had taken place with an explanation of the therapeutic intervention. Should the trainee be told? Is noninsight therapy logically and clearly taught by noninsight training? Many therapists are now comfortable with the idea that they can change a family without the family being aware of how the change was carried out. It should logically follow that a supervisor could change the problem of a trainee by manipulating him or her outside the trainee's awareness.

Whether awareness should be offered can be determined by the goal of the therapist or the supervisor. The goal of a therapist is to change the problem that the family wishes changed; awareness of how that is done should not be shared with the family if it would interfere with the change. That is, there is nothing wrong with making a family aware of what the therapist is doing unless that awareness will prevent a change. When awareness may interfere, the obligation of the therapist is not to share that awareness. The machinery of therapy is the therapist's business, not the family's.

When the supervisor is teaching a trainee, the machinery of the therapy is what he or she is teaching. Therefore, the supervisor should explain to the trainee what he or she did, and why he or she did it. The task of the supervisor is not only to have the trainee change the family, but also to teach the trainee to change other families in the future when the supervisor will not be present. To achieve that goal, some conceptualization of the trainee's involvement with a family is necessary. However, one should note that many expert therapists are not conceptualizers. As a researcher watching therapists at work, I saw many competent therapists who knew what to do, but who, when asked why, could only invent reasons. The action in the therapy room can be so complex that conscious conceptualization as one works is improbable.

In the example cited above, I explained to the therapist why I had suggested he make that comment to the wife and why I thought it helped him disengage from his coalition with her: he corrected the imbalance without offending her, and the husband became more equal to her in relation to the therapist. I am not sure that explanation was necessary for him to solve a similar situation in the future. The action itself could have been sufficient.

It would seem to be best for the supervisor to have the freedom to influence trainees outside their awareness, particularly if making them aware of an intervention would oversimplify it or interfere with their learning to do it. The principle is the same when conducting therapy. The difference is that a therapist-in-training must learn to influence many kinds of people in many situations, and so needs education as a people changer. The family just needs to know how to live together without a certain problem.

It is different if the trainee is to become a teacher and supervisor. In that case he or she must learn the conceptualizations in order to pass them on, and so the process of how to teach is itself a learning situation.

CHANGING THE TRAINEE'S SOCIAL CONTEXT

All supervisors presumably have the goal of training therapists in such a way that the particular case in training is successful, and the therapist learns from that experience to be successful with other clients. If we take family theory seriously, whether trainees do well or fail should be explained in terms of their social situation. According to this premise, the reason the intimates of a patient are involved in therapy is because the family finds it convenient to adapt to the abnormal behavior; the failing of a person has some function in the family situation. Granting some physiological limitations, changing a person requires changing his or her social situation so that new behavior occurs. If we apply the same logic to training, it follows that the incompetence or inappropriate behavior of a trainee is an adaptation to the teaching situation. Within certain physiological limitations, such as the trainee being stupid, the explanation of a trainee's difficulties should be found in his or her social context, not psychological nature or childhood experiences. The question is what to include in the definition of that social context. Certainly the training context, including the conflicts about therapy among different authorities and supervisors in the trainee's life, should be considered. The particular family in therapy is also part of the context of the therapist-in-training. Should the context also be broadened to include the personal marriage of the therapist, or his or her family of origin? Rather than use a method of teaching that starts by exploring every trainee's past and present emotional problems, which teaches him or her to be uncertain, it seems more reasonable to begin teaching by focusing on the work as a craft. If, after being taught the basic skills, the trainee is deemed incompetent, his or her IQ and family situation might then be explored.

If one accepts the influence of the social context, as we do in family-oriented therapy, it follows that supervisors have a responsibility toward the workplaces as well as the training places. When the individual was the focus of therapy, it was argued that insight was needed to avoid a relapse. That idea changed as a result of the relapses after insight therapy, but also because of the logic of family theory. It was argued by family therapists that change persists for an individual because his or her social system is changed; the new behavior is an adaptation to the new situation, and an individual cannot relapse if such behavior is inappropriate in the new situation. The same argument can be applied to therapists-in-training.

We often see trainees who learn a particular family approach, but in a year or two are doing therapy as they did before they went through a training program. We can explain this "relapse" in terms of the individual, or as an adaptive response to a social situation. Whether therapists work in the way they were trained can have more to do with where they work than with what they were taught. For example, many work in social agencies where they must spend their time diagnosing and cannot see whole families. Others work in inpatient institutions where the training in therapy they received cannot be done. Some teach therapy, but in settings where they cannot observe a trainee, and so cannot focus on skill as they were taught.

The potential of a client, or a therapist-in-training, cannot be developed in a setting that prevents development. Therapists who have learned new ways do not necessarily need insight to persist in, and develop, their new skills. They need places to work that welcome more effective therapy. All of us who teach have a responsibility to train competent therapists and improve training programs. We also need to improve the workplaces in the therapy field where our trainees will function.

23

Research

DAVID P. KNISKERN
University of Cincinnati College of Medicine

ALAN S. GURMAN
University of Wisconsin Medical School

THE EMPIRICAL BASE FOR FAMILY THERAPY TRAINING

In a recent publication we reviewed the history of research in the field of family therapy (Gurman, Kniskern, & Pinsof, 1985). We summarized the gradual process by which outcome and process research, important in the initial phase of family therapy development (the 1950s), became separated from the field as a whole and diminished in both visibility and importance. Research continued to be done, but was generally of such poor quality and so scarce that few conclusions could be drawn. It was during this period, from the late 1950s to the mid-1970s, that family therapy grew explosively, growth that was almost wholly unguided by empirical examination.

Our review (Gurman & Kniskern, 1978) of over 200 outcome studies may have signaled that research was again to have a place in the family therapy field. While it is immodest to describe one's own work as a turning point in a field, it seems that since 1978 research has had an increasingly significant place in the family therapy field.

In the past few years, family therapy research has begun to be taken so seriously that there has been controversy among researchers about the "proper" conduct of research on systemic psychotherapy (Gurman, 1983; Keeney, 1983; Kniskern, 1983; Manicas & Secord, 1983; Schwartz & Breunlin, 1983; Tomm, 1983). These debates between advocates of what has become known as the "new epistemology" and the "old epistemology" seem to have spurred even greater interest in the domain of family therapy research.

Family therapy researchers seemed initially to focus on the naive question "does it work?" As interest in research has increased, researchers in the field have become increasingly sophisticated in the questions they are asking. Some researchers have even begun investigating the efficacy of training.

Almost from its beginning as a field, family therapy has been concerned with the transmission of knowledge, understanding, and technique to clinical students and other professionals. In fact, almost without exception, the grandfathers and grandmothers of the field have worked in settings where training was a primary, if not *the* primary, goal of the organization. Despite the importance and magnitude of these training endeavors (Bloch & Weiss, 1981), until recently the empirical evaluation of family therapy training has seldom been viewed as important enough to undertake.

In our earlier summary and evaluation of the existing research on training in marriage and family therapy (Kniskern & Gurman, 1979), we found little that could be considered as evidence of training effectiveness. Research on training in family therapy had not yet reached the point where it could be an important part of the family therapy landscape. In this chapter, we will review the progress that has been made in training research, and suggest directions that the field could fruitfully explore.

We consider the evaluation of any training program to be a five step process. The first step is the *identification and specification of training goals*. The second is the *development of a training model*. The third is the *development of measures that can evaluate training-induced change*. The fourth is the *demonstration of the expected change in trainees* who participate in the program. The final step is the *demonstration that trainees who have shown expected change on the measures are better able to help families in therapy*.

Before discussing these steps in detail, it is worth noting that at the time of our 1979 paper the training literature consisted almost exclusively of articles that described programs and discussed training and supervision goals (e.g., Ferber, Mendelsohn, & Napier, 1972; Flomenhaft & Carter, 1974; Garrigan & Bambrick, 1977; Lange & Zeegers, 1978; Liddle & Halpin, 1978). The only measures of change used were anecdotal reports of trainees and trainers, or gross estimates of amount of family therapy done by trainees before and after their involvement in a particular training experience. In the last six years the field has progressed to the point where there have now been several measures published that assess change resulting from training. Several studies have even evaluated training programs and offered evidence that trainees have changed in ways expected by program developers. However, we are still unaware of any study that links training with therapeutic outcome.

THE PROCESS OF EVALUATING FAMILY THERAPY TRAINING PROGRAMS

Identification of Training Goals

Most published accounts of training programs have described their goals as achieving an increase in trainees' conceptual, perceptual, and technical or executive skills. This way of describing learning objectives (e.g., Falicov, Constantine, & Breunlin, 1981; Tomm & Wright, 1979) follows the proposal of Cleghorn and Levin (1973). Conceptual skills are those that relate to the therapist's ability to formulate problems systemically, and to understand the way rules govern family behavior and make family interaction predictable. Perceptual skills are those skills that relate to a therapist's ability to evaluate a particular family within his or her conceptual framework. Conceptual skills can be evaluated by purely paper-and-pencil methods. To evaluate perceptual skills, however, the therapist must be presented with family behavior, whether live or recorded. It should be obvious that gains in conceptual and perceptual skills seldom occur independently of each other. More discriminating perceptions allow for better conceptualization, and better conceptual skill allows for better perceptual acuity.

The third type of skill has been called executive or technical, and refers to the therapist's ability to act in family sessions in ways that are consistent with the goals of the training program. These skills are obviously the ultimate goal of training, even if the more immediate goal is to increase conceptual or perceptual skills. The first step in the evaluation of family therapy training is to specify learning objectives in terms that allow for empirical evaluation of their acquisition.

Despite the limited data on the ability of training to help trainees acquire or apply conceptual, perceptual, or technical skills, and the total lack of data about the consequent effects on therapeutic outcome, an increasing body of data does exist about therapist factors that influence the outcome of family therapy. We cite family therapists' experience level, therapy structuring skills, and relational skills as factors that influence the outcome of family therapy (Gurman & Kniskern, 1978). Of these three factors, the latter two are potentially teachable. Experience cannot be taught, but since high levels of experience have been correlated with positive therapeutic outcome, the behavior of experienced therapists can be an indirect criterion for training success. For example, Pinsof (1981) found that advanced therapists used a wide range of interventions and were significantly more active than beginners. Later, Tucker and Pinsof (1984) provided preliminary evidence that trainees became more active and used a wider range of interventions over the course of training. These reports together suggest that trainees became more like experienced, and arguably more successful, therapists during the course of training.

The other two therapist factors associated with positive outcome have been investigated by several researchers: structuring skills (Alexander, Barton, Schiavo, & Parsons, 1976; Sigal, Guttman, Chagoya, & Lasry, 1973; Sigal, Rakoff, & Epstein, 1967) and relationship skills (Alexander et al., 1976; Beck & Jones, 1973; Burton & Kaplan, 1968; Mezyold, Wauck, & Foley, 1978; Thomlinson, 1973). Structuring skills include directiveness, clarity, self-confidence, information-gathering, and stimulating interaction. Relationship skills include warmth, humor, and affect–behavior integration. Both of these skills appear to be related to positive outcome, regardless of therapeutic orientation.

Specification of a Training Model

After objectives for training are determined, the next logical step in an evaluation project is to describe specifically the means by which these objectives are to be met. The progress of therapy outcome research has in the past been impeded by the frequent lack of specificity about change procedures (Gurman & Kniskern, 1978). Without a clear articulation of the training package (or treatment package in outcome research), no understandable conclusions or experimental replication can be accomplished.

As we have described elsewhere (Gurman & Kniskern, 1978), objectives for training are typically based on specific beliefs about important family therapy skills held by various schools of therapy, or empirical research about the behavior of effective therapists of recognized experts. Training procedures cannot initially be derived empirically or even by utilizing logical necessity as a criterion. Some family therapists have suggested that training procedures should be isomorphic with the behavior or attitude to be learned by trainees (Liddle & Halpin, 1978), but there is no evidence that this should be the case. That is, there is no evidence to date that training methods that parallel the stance and technique used in the school's therapeutic endeavors are more effective than methods that are different or perhaps even antithetical to the therapeutic methods.

With our current knowledge base, we are unable to offer guidelines about the kind of training procedures trainees might use. We can only ask that training programs evaluate those methods that they believe are most effective in reaching their objectives, and that they describe these methods adequately in their publications and presentations.

So little has been done to date in evaluating training effectiveness that, in contrast to research evidence on the outcome of family therapy (Gurman *et al.*, 1985), it is not possible to cite a particular school as having more empirically validated training methods. It seems apparent, however, that trainees representing the more technique-oriented family therapies are working more actively in evaluating their training methods.

Development of Measures of Change

The third step in our five-step evaluation process is the development of measures or instruments that evaluate the hoped-for changes in trainees. As previously stated, goals of different types require the use of different types of change measures. Some of the effects of family therapy training can be evaluated by simple paper-and-pencil examinations, not unlike a college final exam. The evaluation of perceptual and technical skills, however, require that the trainees be confronted with clinical or simulated clinical material.

Since the ultimate goal of family therapy training is to increase the effectiveness of trainees in actual therapy, the closer one gets to the evaluation of real therapy behavior, the more powerful the measure of this effectiveness. Anyone who has conducted therapy research knows the practical problems that arise with the use of dysfunctional families in research (e.g., lack of standardization, no-shows, confidentiality).

Because of the difficulties in the use of "real" families in actual sessions, family researchers have used written descriptions of family behavior (Byles, Bishop, & Horn, 1983), live simulated families (Tucker & Pinsof, 1984), or taped simulated families (Breunlin, Schwartz, Krause, & Selby, 1983; Mohammed & Piercy, 1983).

In addition to the problem of the development of a standard stimulus for evaluation, there is also the problem of developing a rating scale that evaluates the trainee/therapist's response to the stimulus.

Several excellent descriptions of the development and validation of therapist rating scales have been published within the last few years (Breunlin *et al.*, 1983; Piercy, Laird, & Mohammed, 1983; Tucker & Pinsof, 1981). Each of these papers details a different approach to the problem of scale development. Piercy and colleagues (1983) began with a pool of 375 items that were believed to reflect family therapy skills from all theoretical orientations. Experienced family therapists repeatedly reduced the pool until it became 10 items in each of five skill categories. Tucker and Pinsof (1981) utilized a scale (the Family Therapist Coding System) that was developed to allow for the description of all therapist behavior, whereas Breunlin and colleagues (1983) began with a list intuitively derived and then refined it empirically. To the degree that we know which therapist behaviors lead to positive outcomes, we can indirectly evaluate the success of training programs by measuring the degree to which these behaviors increase during training. The field of family therapy has increased its knowledge about these "change-inducing" behaviors since our earlier review of training research (Kniskern & Gurman, 1979), but there is still a remarkable empirical ignorance of what types of activity or styles of intervention should be fostered in trainees.

One study that offers promise in the area of the development of change measures is that of Breunlin and colleagues (1983). This study, along with Tucker and Pinsof's (1984), represent, we think, the current high water marks in the empirical evaluation of family therapy training.

THE STUDY BY BREUNLIN AND COLLEAGUES (1983)

The goal of this project was to develop an instrument (the Family Therapy Assessment Exercise, or FTAE) that would assess whether trainees in their structural–strategic training program benefited from the training. The process by which this instrument was constructed is worth describing in detail because it demonstrates the level of sophistication in the area of training research that is possible, and provides a model for the development of future research instruments.

A videotaped first session with a family was selected which the research group felt demonstrated with fidelity the knowledge and technique of structural–strategic therapy. A script was transcribed, edited, and added to until it was judged that the session adequately depicted family dynamics of modern complexity, and therapist behaviors that were both "correct" and "incorrect" from a systems perspective. Actors then played the script to develop a final videotape.

A test was then constructed that measured how well trainees could apply the observational, conceptual, and therapeutic skills that a consensus of four experienced family therapists judged were portrayed by the tape. The authors note, however, that the test measures only how similar the trainee's thinking is to what the test developers believe are correct answers. It does not measure clinical skill directly. The test developed was piloted by administering it before and after several training programs. Breunlin and his group report on three versions of the FTAE. The first version (T_1) used open-ended questions. The second version (T_2) converted the open-ended questions to a multiple choice format, and the third version (T_3) was constructed by analysis of the results of T_2 and adding new questions and deleting some questions with the goal of improving the content and predictive validity.

Breunlin and Schwartz (1986) report that they have refined the instrument well beyond the level reported in the 1983 article. Based on the feedback from the T_3 and the newer T_4 versions, they have developed a T_5. With T_5, while Breunlin and Schwartz report continued difficulties with the observational scale, there is accumulating evidence that both the conceptual and therapeutic scales of T_5 discriminate well, as does the total score.

Two dissertations have studied the FTAE. In one study, Hernandez (1985) classified 75 subjects as either novice, mid-range, or experienced in family therapy. Subjects were drawn from 7 family therapy training programs in Illinois and Indiana and ranged from first-year graduate students to AAMFT-certified supervisors. Three and 6-week test–retest reliabilities were .76 and .62, respectively. Hernandez found that the FTAE total score, conceptual score, and therapeutic score all discriminated well between novice and experienced therapists. She concluded that this instrument, with the exception of the observational dimension, genuinely measures trainee acquisition of constructs specific to structural–strategic family therapy.

In another study, Pulleyblank and Shapiro (1986) used the FTAE to evaluate a structural family therapy training program and found that all the scores of the FTAE differentiated between trainees in a structural family therapy training program and a comparison group. The generalizability of her study is limited, however, by small sample size.

Demonstration of Change in Trainees

After measures of change are developed that adequately tap the dimensions thought to be important for effective family therapy, the next step is to demonstrate that the training program produces change in the expected direction. In our previous training paper we stated, "There now exists no research evidence that training experiences in marital–family therapy in fact increase the effectiveness of clinicians" (Kniskern & Gurman, 1979). Happily, we are no longer able to say that unequivocally. Tucker and Pinsof (1984) offer evidence that training does effect change in trainees at least on some important dimensions.

THE TUCKER AND PINSOF PROJECT (1984)

Recognizing that it will be years before "reliable and valid information exists about what skills are associated with good outcome," Tucker and Pinsof (1984) set as their goal evaluating "to what extent psychotherapy training programs achieve their skills training goals." In so doing, they tackled the same methodological problems as did the Breunlin group (1983), that is, the development of a standard stimulus and a battery of instruments for evaluating trainee change.

This study, evaluating change in the first year of study at the Center for Family Studies/Family Institute of Chicago (CFS/FIC), is the first comprehensive empirical evaluation of any family therapy training program. The study investigated change in the three attributes in which the training faculty at CFS/FIC expected change to be demonstrated: (1) clinical cognition, (2) techniques, and (3) self-actualization. Clinical conceptualization was measured with the Family Concept Assessment (FCA) (Tucker & Pinsof, 1981), in-therapy technique with the Family Therapist Coding System (FTCS) (Pinsof, 1981), and self-actualization with the Personal Orientation Inventory (POI) (Shostrom, 1974).

The in-therapy behavior of trainees was evaluated by rating the trainee's response to a "live family simulation." Four professional actors were trained to represent a family referred to therapy because the son had committed a petty crime. The training of the actors "was designed to enable them to improvise in response to each therapist, while maintaining the prescribed and consistent mode of family interaction" (Tucker & Pinsof, 1984, p. 441). Two different but similar families were used for pretraining test and posttraining test. Empirical evidence demonstrated that the simulated families were equivalent in interactional patterns for trainees in both pre- and posttraining situations.

The results reported by Tucker and Pinsof (1984) suggest that trainees did change significantly on several dimensions in the direction desired by the training staff. The pre–post scores showed a significant increase on one of the three subscales of the FCA. This change indicated that trainees thought more in terms of circular rather than linear causality at the posttraining test than at the pretraining test. In-therapy verbal behavior, as measured by the FTCS, was expected to change in 25 code categories. Of these, 3 were found to have changed significantly in the expected direction, while 1 changed significantly in the unexpected direction. The POI showed no increase in self-actualization during the year of training, but also suggested that most trainees began the program highly actualized.

Tucker and Pinsof's findings support the belief that family therapy training can have clinically meaningful effects on trainees. Training had its intended impact of increased systemic thinking, increased activity level, and increased range and specificity of interactions. Obviously, many directional hypotheses were not confirmed, which could indicate that the training had a more limited effect than many experts would have assumed or predicted, and that only longer periods of training, or training of a different type, will produce effects on those other dimensions.

Perhaps more important than the specific results of the Breunlin and colleagues and Tucker and Pinsof studies is the fact that these studies were done at all. They both break methodological ground and provide models for future investigators. Taken together, these studies suggest that the empirical study of family therapy training is possible. The results they have reported also confirm that research may be a useful guide for tailoring family therapy training programs to maximize impact and effectiveness.

Linkage of Change to Positive Outcome

The final step in the evaluation of a training program is the empirical linking of trainee change to positive outcome in treated families. In the accomplishment of this step, the domains of training research and family therapy outcome literature converge. We must reiterate at this point that there is no empirical study of which we are aware that has attempted to evaluate the effects of training in this most direct manner.

It should be obvious that the problems of evaluating change in trainees are many, but are not insurmountable. Still, to integrate the problems of outcome research with those of training research compounds the difficulties of conducting research. Fortunately, many of the methodological problems of outcome and process research on family therapy have been solved, or are close to being solved (Gurman et al., 1985). This is not to say that there is not a great deal of empirical work left to accomplish. As we emphasize (Gurman et al., 1985), few of the major schools of family therapy have ever begun to investigate either the process or outcomes of their methods of therapy. Moreover, the schools that have developed some empirical base have not investigated many of their most cherished theoretical tenets.

Methodologies are now in place for a comprehensive evaluation of family therapy training programs. Such a project will have to be a long-term enterprise that will focus on the type of training experiences that are potent in producing effective therapists *within a particular model of therapy*. Researchers investigating training programs should avoid the overly generalized question "Does family therapy training work?" Investigation of the analogous question "Does family therapy work?" by family therapy researchers has wasted a good deal of time and effort, with only a moderate return in knowledge and understanding.

CONCLUSION

Our five-step approach to the evaluation process emphasizes the delineation of specific goals and objectives for trainee learning. Most of these goals and objectives by definition have to be stated in school-specific terms, and must be tied to parts of the training program.

All training programs in family therapy utilize three primary methods for training: didactic, supervisory, and experiential. Each training program uses these three methods in varying ways, to varying degrees, and at different points in the training process. Programs also differ in that some focus on the work of a single theorist, while others present a variety of orientations of the trainee. At this time, all training programs have developed their format of training intuitively, or based on imitation of other programs; none have been empirically derived. We have delineated (Kniskern & Gurman, 1979) a long list of important and researchable questions which could be answered about training in a particular setting. Since few, if any, of the questions have even been initially addressed, we repeat them here as a framework for the future of training research. Each of these questions could usefully be asked of any training program that emphasizes a particular approach to treatment:

Selection:

- What type(s) of previous training best prepares a trainee for training?
- Are there any types of previous training that inhibit training?
- Does the developmental stage of the trainee (for instance, never married versus married) influence the trainee's learning?
- Can success be predicted without a personal interview? Based on what criteria?
- Does a sample of therapy behavior improve selection?

Didactic methods:

- Does reading about families help the trainee learn therapy?
- Should reading be done before, after, or during the bulk of therapy training practice?
- Does the live observation of "experts" help or hinder development of skills?

Supervision:

- When are audio- or videotapes most helpful? When are they harmful?
- What are the demonstrable advantages and disadvantages of cotherapy supervision and of live observation supervision?
- What are the measurable strengths and weaknesses of problem-oriented supervision and of therapist-oriented supervision?
- Should all cases be supervised?
- What differences do different forms of supervision make for different trainees?

Experiential methods:

- What specific changes are produced by different types of personal therapy?
- What are the positive and negative effects of personal therapy when it is required?

- At what point in one's training in family therapy are personal therapy experiences most beneficial, and when may they be harmful?
- Does working with one's own family via family genograms facilitate cognitive (conceptual) change more than it facilitates personal emotional change?
- Are role-playing experiential methods more effective in producing technical skill than in reducing neophyte family therapists' anxieties about their competence?

We predict that, just as family therapists will be most attracted to and influenced by outcome research that speaks directly to the approaches to which they are conceptually committed (Gurman *et al.*, 1985), family therapy trainees will be most affected by training research that addresses their preferred models. At the same time, we would encourage research that evaluates the impact of factors that may not be specific to any given "school," but which may be potent variables in the learning and skill enhancement process in various schools, on trainee learning and clinical skill. Thus, for example, one might ask the following sorts of illustrative nondenominational questions: (1) Are trainees' clinical skills enhanced more by supervisory processes that foster their own therapeutic problem-solving than by those that emphasize following directives from observing supervisors? If such enhancement is found, is it especially marked at the more advanced, rather than the beginning, stages of supervision? (2) Are there relatively enduring personality factors (e.g., psychological-mindedness, tendency toward convergent rather than divergent thinking) that predict trainees' success regardless of the "school" of training? (3) Does conceptual exposure to multiple points of view about family therapy enhance or diminish specific types of learning within a given model of therapy? (4) Does experiential training (e.g., use of family genograms, personal couples or family therapy) enhance or diminish learning, and do such experiences have different effects at different stages of training?

Despite the lack of empirical guidelines, family therapy training continues to increase in importance within the entire field of mental health. Just as many patients were drawn to marital–family approaches not because of empirical validation but because of the logic and intuitive appeal of treating a natural system, therapists have been drawn to family therapy training. It is intuitively reasonable that training increases effectiveness. While this assumption needs to be empirically validated, of more importance is the development of particular training procedures that maximize the learning that takes place and most efficiently leads to increasing a therapist's effectiveness with families. Research that addresses training issues that are specific to given schools of therapy, and also relevant across various schools, offers a basis for enhancing the effectiveness of neophyte family therapists.

REFERENCES

Alexander, J., Barton, C., Schiavo, R., & Parsons, B. (1976). Systems–behavioral intervention with families of delinquents: Therapist characteristics, family behavior, and outcome. *Journal of Consulting and Clinical Psychology, 44*, 656–664.

Beck, D., & Jones, M. (1973). *Progress on family problems: A nation-wide study of clients' and counselors' views on family agency services.* New York: Family Service Association of America.

Bloch, D., & Weiss, H. (1981). Training facilities in marital and family therapy. *Family Process, 20*, 133–146.

Breunlin, D., & Schwartz, R. (1986). Personal communication.

Breunlin, D., Schwartz, R., Krause, M., & Selby, L. (1983). Evaluating family therapy training: The development of an instrument. *Journal of Marital and Family Therapy, 9,* 37–47.

Burton, G., & Kaplan, H. (1968). Group counseling in conflicted marriages where alcoholism is present: Clients' evaluation of effectiveness. *Journal of Marriage and the Family, 30,* 74–79.

Byles, J., Bishop, D., & Horn, D. (1983). Evaluation of a family therapy training program. *Journal of Marital and Family Therapy, 9,* 299–304.

Cleghorn, J., & Levin, S.. (1973). Training family therapists by setting learning objectives. *American Journal of Orthopsychiatry, 43,* 439–446.

Falicov, C., Constantine, J., & Breunlin, D. (1981). Teaching family therapy: A program based on training objectives. *Journal of Marital and Family Therapy, 7,* 497–504.

Ferber, A., Mendelsohn, M., & Napier, A. (1972). *The book of family therapy.* New York: Jason Aronson.

Flomenhaft, K., & Carter, R. (1974). Family therapy training: A statewide program for mental health centers. *Hospital and Community Psychiatry, 25,* 789–791.

Garrigan, J., & Bambrick, A. (1977). Introducing novice therapists to "Go-between" techniques of Family Therapy. *Family Process, 16,* 211–218.

Gurman, A. S. (1983). Family therapy research and the "new epistemology." *Journal of Marital and Family Therapy, 9,* 227–234.

Gurman, A. S., & Kniskern, D. P. (1978). Research on marital and family therapy: Progress, perspective, and prospect. In S. Garfield & A. Bergin (Eds.), *Handbook of psychotherapy and behavior change* (2nd ed.). New York: Wiley.

Gurman, A. S., Kniskern, D. P., & Pinsof, W. M. (1985). Research on the process and outcome of marital and family therapy. In S. Garfield & A. Bergin (Eds.), *Handbook of psychotherapy and behavior change* (3rd ed.). New York: Wiley.

Hernandez, K. (1985). Validational studies on two instruments that measure therapists' level of systemic thinking. *Dissertation Abstracts International, 46,* 46107B.

Keeney, B. P. (1983). *Aesthetics of change.* New York: Guilford Press.

Kniskern, D. P. (1983). The new wave is all wet. *The Family Therapy Networker, 7,* 38, 60, 62.

Kniskern, D. P., & Gurman, A. S. (1979). Research on training in marriage and family therapy: Status, issues and direction. *Journal of Marital and Family Therapy, 5,* 83–94.

Lange, A., & Zeegers, W. (1978). Structured training for behavioral family therapy: Methods and evaluation. *Behavior Analysis and Modification, 2,* 211–225.

Liddle, H., & Halpin, R. (1978). Family therapy training and supervision literature: A comparative review. *Journal of Marriage and Family Counseling, 4,* 79–98.

Manicas, P., & Secord, P. (1983). Implications for psychology of the new philosophy of science. *American Psychologist, 38,* 399–413.

Mezyold, L., Wauck, L., & Foley, J. (1978). The clergy as marriage counselors: A service revisited. *Journal of Religion and Health, 22,* 278–288.

Mohammed, Z., & Piercy, F. (1983). The effects of two methods of training and sequencing on structuring and relationship skills of family therapists. *American Journal of Family Therapy, 11,* 64–71.

Piercy, F., Laird, R., & Mohammed, Z. (1983). A family therapist rating scale. *Journal of Marital and Family Therapy, 9,* 49–59.

Pinsof, W. M. (1981). *The family therapist coding manual.* Chicago: Center for Family Studies/The Family Institute of Chicago.

Pulleyblank, E., & Shapiro, R. (1986). Evaluation of family therapy trainees' acquisition of cognitive and therapeutic behavior skills. *Family Process, 25,* 591–598.

Schwartz, R. C., & Breunlin, D. L. (1983). Research: Why clinicians should bother with it. *The Family Therapy Networker, 7,* 23–27, 57–59.

Shostrom, E. (1974). *The Personal Orientation Inventory* (2nd ed.). San Diego: Educational Industrial Testing Service.

Sigal, J., Guttman, H., Chagoya, L., & Lasry, J. (1973). Predictability of family therapists' behavior. *Canadian Psychiatric Association Journal, 18,* 199–202.

Sigal, J., Rakoff, V., & Epstein, N. (1967). Indications of therapeutic outcome in conjoint family therapy. *Family Process, 6,* 215–216.

Thomlinson, R. (1973). A behavioral model for social work intervention with the marital dyad. *Dissertation Abstracts International, 34,* 1288b.

Tomm, K. (1983). The old hat doesn't fit. *The Family Therapy Networker, 7,* 39–41.

Tomm, K., & Wright, L. (1979). Training in family therapy: Perceptual, conceptual and executive skills. *Family Process, 18,* 227–250.

Tucker, S., & Pinsof, W. M. (1981). *The family concept assessment (FCA) task and rating system manual.* Chicago: Center for Family Studies/The Family Institute of Chicago.

Tucker, S., & Pinsof, W. M. (1984). The empirical evaluation of family therapy training. *Family Process, 23,* 437–456.

24

Family Therapy Training—
It's Entertainment

CLOÉ MADANES
The Family Therapy Institute of Washington, D.C., Rockville, Maryland

Family therapy training coordinates the traditional transmission of knowledge and skills with the modern technology and culture of entertainment. The word "entertainment" is defined here as imaginative presentations that make money. Entertainment is a specialized form of popular art that is not subject to the aesthetic and political scrutiny reserved for "real art." In this sense television, Hollywood movies, and wrestling and other popular sports are all entertainment, even though the argument that they are art has been offered, mainly by French authors such as Roland Barthes and Jean Luc Godard (Barthes, 1966).

In contrast, traditional education communicates information through lectures and readings, as well as apprenticeships where a disciple learns a trade from a master. Entertainment relies heavily on metaphorical communication and often plays with confusion and misunderstandings. Education involves information and the transmission of skills, and here the confusion and misunderstandings of symbolic communication have no place. The exception might be the teaching of therapy—when the subject to be taught is how to solve the problems of living. When posed a question, the Zen master may offer a metaphor. When asked about a problem in therapy, Milton Erickson would tell the story of another patient. In this sense the teaching of therapy is metaphorical.

Much has been said about whether therapy is a science or an art. Political implications have been addressed, and the importance of aesthetics has become an issue. But if therapy is an art, who is the audience? If there is an audience, it is a very limited group. There are no exhibits, no auctions, no performances for the general public. Compared to the audience for the mass media, this audience is limited in numbers, even though recently it has expanded to include large numbers of people at conferences and workshops who expect to be instructed in entertaining ways. These people are interested in acquiring a practical education with the least possible effort, so it could be said that if therapy is an art, it is a form of entertainment to be assimilated as effortlessly as possible.

This is not to say that therapy is not also a science. We understand the stages of life, the organization of the family, hierarchy, power, the function of a symptom, institutionalization. We know how to change sequences, reverse hierarchies, use paradox, change metaphors. When we try to teach these skills, however, we can only do so through metaphor. Generalizations and rules are difficult if not impossible to make. The respect for the uniqueness of each individual and each family that characterizes a systems view makes classification, the basis of science, anathema to the approach. As teachers, we vacillate: Should we attempt to be scientific, should we teach as the Zen master does, or should we offer an entertaining performance?

To make the dilemma even more peculiar, there are critics from within and from outside the field. Some critics say that all attempts to intervene in a system are futile or detrimental; others see therapists as agents of social control; some evaluate therapy on the basis of whether it is aesthetic; and the whole field is said to have deliberately or unwittingly collaborated in the oppression of women, homosexuals, and social deviants. Even the very idea that there should be a profession that attempts to solve the problems of living has been questioned. Some of the criticisms are similar to the attacks on television, "where owners of thousand-dollar sets think nothing of calling them 'idiot boxes,' and where a well pronounced distaste for TV has become a prerequisite for claims of intellectual and even of ethical legitimacy" (Marc, 1984). There have even been serious proposals for the elimination of television. But television, like psychotherapy, is part of the mind industry. It is beside the point to think that either could be arrested or abolished.

These dilemmas about art, entertainment, science, political oppression, and whether therapy should exist as a field at all are the context in which we have to teach. And all this while we try to do something about the concrete problems of real people, and while we attempt to teach some skills to real students. I know of no other field dealing with practical issues that is so consistently self-critical.

The effect this criticism has on teachers is that we teach what we know while simultaneously attempting to justify (1) the fact that we are teaching, (2) the content of what we teach, and (3) the idea that there is anything to teach at all. And this is where entertainment comes in. When teaching must take place at many levels, a teacher must rely on metaphors, symbols, and narratives that will influence the audience directly and indirectly. Drama becomes essential. But how can we produce this drama without violating the privacy of the therapist's office? How can we create the theater in which the student will be the audience, a sensitive and understanding witness to the human dilemmas that will become his or her area of expertise. Here technology enters: the one-way mirror and the video camera. With this technology a family therapy training institute begins to share more and more the elements of the world of entertainment that we are all familiar with as we sit in the family room watching television.

The students sit behind the one-way mirror watching the drama unfold on the other side of the glass. Sometimes they watch the action on a television screen that reproduces with close-ups and at different angles the view from behind the mirror. They take turns being the therapist, the observer, and the observed. The supervisor is the drama's director, organizing the action on both sides of the screen and arranging simultaneously the solution to the client's problems and the education and entertainment of the students— whose attention span seems to become shorter every year as new generations raised in front of the television set expect fast-paced action, and who engage in the learning process while simultaneously eating and conversing. Some sit, mesmerized and spaced out. Others rise to the occasion—to consciousness—and are able to preserve their integrity and autonomy by analyzing and comparing what they see on the screen or on the other side of the mirror with other therapies of the past or of the present. Similarly, television's most interesting moments occur, as David Marc (1984) points out in his article "Understanding Television," when new series are compared to old reruns. "Miami Vice" and "Hill Street Blues" make "Starsky and Hutch" obsolete, while "Dragnet" and "The Mod Squad" have lost all credibility as police mysteries and have become comedies of obsolescence.

It is important to distinguish between taking television on one's own terms and taking it the way it presents itself. The television viewer who watches a rerun or a soap opera with an understanding that emerges out of the culture of television itself is protected from the homogenizing, authoritarian influence that is claimed by television's pessimistic critics. Similarly, the student of therapy can save himself or herself from the monolithic, authoritarian teacher through the autonomy of his or her imagination, and through a knowledge of the culture of therapy.

Some of today's therapy students, accustomed to the world of the sitcom, where months become weeks and years become months, are bored with long-term therapy. In the television soap opera each episode ends with uncertainty as to the possible rescue of characters from danger, torture, or even apparently hopeless anxiety, which device is used to entice the viewer to watch the next episode in the series. In the sitcom, in contrast, the central tensions are almost always alleviated before the end of each episode—each episode resembles a short self-contained play. Modern therapy has incorporated these aspects of modern television mostly through the use of the directive as the main therapeutic tool. The use of the directive creates suspense within the session as it addresses the family drama: What directive will the supervisor come up with? Will the student be able to deliver it? How will the family respond? There is drama beyond the confines of the interview, however: Will the directive solve the problem? Will the clients return to the next session transformed? Will they return at all? These are the elements that create tension between sessions and entice the students to return to the next day of training.

The teacher must entertain. Boredom must be avoided, and the directive is the main tool to create drama and excitement in the limited context of therapy. The movie screen and the television set have limitless possibilities for thrilling the audience: the viewers can be flooded with hordes of characters, transported out of this world, and made to suffer innumerable illusions. The possibilities of the theater, in contrast, are limited to what can transpire on a stage, where there are obvious physical constraints, and where editing to create distortions is impossible. The ideal play, in terms of the expense of production, is one with three actors and one set. Modern playwrights, limited by this constraint, struggle to produce thrills, action, and drama within these limitations. The supervisor in modern therapy suffers from similar restrictions. The set of characters is limited. Even though relatives and friends of the family in therapy are invited, they often do not come to the sessions. There is usually only one therapist. The set is always the same. The possibilities of what action and interaction can actually take place in the therapy room are limited by the code of ethics of the various professions; in most therapies, sex, violence, nudism, and anything but restricted physical contact is discouraged. Furthermore, in general terms, the plot is always the same. A family or a couple comes in, distressed by what appears to be an insurmountble problem, estranged from each other, unhappy. The therapist questions, prods, sets up a different scenario. The problem is solved, and the family ties are strengthened. The ending must be happy, or the therapy has failed. If it is impossible to arrange a happy ending, it is essential to bring out in the therapy all the qualities of a warm human drama. There is almost as much satisfaction for therapists in revealing the unsolvable dilemmas and the tragedies of life as there is in finding the best possible solutions. Just as in theater, where the audience can be entertained by the tragedy of Hamlet even though they know what the outcome will be, so the audience of therapists can be fascinated by how a family came to be as they are, irrespective of the outcome of therapy or of any effort to influence them.

What are the possibilities for the supervisor as playwright, who assumes the task of entertaining by writing, for each family and therapist, a script that will produce a happy ending, or reveal a warm human drama, within a very limited context? One possibility is intelligent questioning that will reveal unsuspected elements and uncover carefully concealed secrets, thereby unraveling right in front of the eyes of the students glued to the one-way mirror the fabric of the mystery of why the family has come to be the way it is. Among strategic therapists, the Milan group excels at this skill, although we all can claim a certain proficiency in this area. It is the basis for the drama that will subsequently unfold.

Another possiblity is enactment. The family can be asked to reproduce their conflicts and difficulties in the therapy room. In this way some action is introduced; the clients may stand up and move around the room. The most famous playwright of enactment is probably Minuchin, who has reproduced in the therapy room the struggle of the fathers of anorectics to feed their daughters during his now classic lunch sessions.

As in a play or a novel, once the characters and the conflict have been introduced, the obstacles to the resolution of the conflict must be presented. These obstacles must be serious enough to create tension, yet they cannot be insurmountable, since the ending has to be happy. Reframing is one way to present such obstacles. The therapist explains to the family that the origin of the problem, the motivations of the characters, and the nature of the conflict are not as they appear. That is, the family comes to the therapy with one view of what the obstacles are that they find overwhelming. The therapist transforms these obstacles into new difficulties that can be solved. The members of the Mental Research Institute are probably the most famous reframers, having proposed that the obstacle is the attempted solution to the conflict. Virginia Satir, however, has probably made the most memorable contribution in her famous reframing of a murderous husband who, she said, had been running after his wife with an axe because he was trying to reach out to her. With reframing, magic is introduced: hatred becomes love, avoidance protection, and rebellion submission.

Vargas Llosa has said that fiction was created to appease man's appetite for a life different from the one he leads. The truth of the novel does not depend on facts. It is written and read to provide people with lives they are unresigned to not having (Vargas Llosa, 1985). Similarly, reframing introduces to the family meaning, drama, and the possibility of being someone else, of relating and living in ways that had gone unsuspected. The truth of the reframing depends on its own persuasive powers, on the skill of its magic. Every good therapy tells the truth and every bad therapy lies. Truth in therapy is to make the client experience an illusion; manipulation and lies mean to be unable to accomplish that trickery. Therapy has its own ethic, one in which truth and falsehood are secondary concepts.

Reframing involves taking what is presented by the clients and throwing a new light on it. A different approach is to introduce totally new obstacles. Milton Erickson was probably the best known master of this. In his therapies, the obstacle would often become climbing Squaw Peak, enduring the desert sun, approaching a stranger. This was a therapy of adventure, where the main action occurred outside of the therapy room. There was no video or live supervision in Erickson's day, and he entertained his disciples with stories of his own feats and of those of his patients. The adventures he proposed involved overcoming not only physical obstacles but also intellectual and spiritual ones, and his characters changed as they struggled to solve a puzzle, understand a difficult subject, and improve themselves in various ways.

Once the obstacle has been redefined, or a new obstacle has been created, it must be overcome. Here is where directives and metaphors are the main tools of the supervisor. Directives may be simple or complex, straightforward or paradoxical, to be carried out in or out of the session. They may be an ordeal to be performed as a punishment if the problem occurs, or they can be a pleasurable experience. Erickson was the originator of directive therapy, and Jay Haley has probably been the most thoughtful presenter and theorist of the approach. It is in the directive that the greatest possibilities for entertainment exist, and where the future may bring the most spectacular developments. It is also where therapy may become comedy or slapstick, when clients are asked to do what appears absurd or ridiculous. Here is also where it is possible to develop the play within the play. I have asked families to pretend to have other problems than those they offered, and to pretend to solve these imaginary problems in make-believe ways (Madanes, 1981, 1984).

Sometimes, instead of directives, metaphors are used. Erickson used to tell stories to his patients in which fictional characters solved problems that were similar to the clients' problems. I have developed this approach into what I call "prescribing the metaphor." The clients are given the ingredients of a fictional situation that resembles their own conflict and asked to resolve it in the form of an essay, story, movie script, or play. This is another type of play within a play, where the clients create their own metaphors and are influenced by the metaphorical solutions that they themselves create. As they solve the problems of their fictional characters, they extend the solution to their own situation, which the fiction represents.

It is currently in the realm of directives that the most creative work is being done, as well as the most interesting theorizing about interpersonal influence. The directives and the theories can become so sophisticated that supervisors are protected from noticing that their efforts are often focused on banality and trivia, such as the problem of a 12-year-old who refuses to take out the garbage, or of a couple who quarrel over who will do the dishes. Therapists and teachers in the past dealt with mental illness and with emotional problems. In the present, perhaps because of our attempts to get away from the medical model, perhaps because of a need to drum up business for ourselves, we find that we are working more and more with banalities. Just as popular sitcoms deal with trivia—little everyday problems that are cheerfully resolved by the characters in shows such as "Three's Company," "Family Ties," and "The Cosby Show"—so also therapists deal with the normal difficulties of living related to the stages of development of family life.

What is normal is important for television. A program is successful if it portrays what is currently normal in the culture. Similarly, a teacher of therapy is concerned with normality and must be constantly in tune with what is normal in the culture so that student therapists can adjust to that "normality" and can in turn help their clients to do the same. Cultural norms come to us through the mass media, so that culture determines what television will portray as normal and television tells us what we should tell our families is normal, except for the problem of censorship.

Hollywood used to produce only musical comedies, romances, or police dramas because there was an implicit rule that the mass media should not discuss certain ideas or make certain issues explicit. Apart from constraints on the subject matter, there were also constraints as to what moral could be derived from a story. For example, it used to be that nobody could be portrayed stealing and not go to jail. Gradually, other unhappy endings became possible, and script writers were able to arrange imaginatively for the thief to die in an accident, or become maimed for life, or lose the woman he loved.

Censorship both in entertainment and in therapy is primarily self-imposed. Explicit rules and regulations are not necessary, but a healthy fear of financial ruin is useful. A television show might be taken off the air; a therapist might be sued for malpractice. Our freedom to decide what should be done in a therapy is sometimes determined more by the apprehensiveness of a therapist concerned about malpractice suits than by the particular needs of a client.

Family therapy has its own shows and its own microcosmos of mass media. Just as the sitcom presents its own abbreviated version of life, so we edit our videotapes and present our own abbreviated, censored version of therapy to the large crowds that come to our workshops for training. Those of us who provide training for large groups of students must often create training materials in the form of videotapes that have to be as entertaining as television shows, lest we lose the attention of our students. Errors, hesitations, and instructions from the supervisor are edited out, and students admire the smoothness and intelligence of therapists who are becoming performers as they grow accustomed to carrying out instructions from behind the one-way mirror. Just like the director and the actor, supervisor and therapist are lost without each other. The supervisor's instuctions can make a timid therapist appear bold or a boring therapist hilarious, and the final edit of the videotape can make a rambling therapist look intelligent and precise.

The interest of the audience determines the success of the show, and there is no question that family therapy is quite a show. More than seven thousand people attended the "Evolution of Psychotherapy" conference sponsored by the Erickson Foundation in 1985. I know of no other field or scientific endeavor that attracts an audience turnout worthy of a rock concert or a political rally. This is a unique phenomenon of therapy in our times.

In the old days, music and therapy were live and could only be enjoyed on stage or through audio recordings. Today, with clever marketing, the endless technological improvements carried out behind the closed doors of the studio result in pop videos available for rent or for purchase. A whole new market has opened.

With the "Live Aid" benefit concert, rock and roll became a major political force, bridging the lack of communication between nations and making us all one big family.

Just as rock music has broadened its audience, so have we. Virginia Satir has said in a recent interview that she is now admitting the general public to her workshops, since they also deserve to be enlightened. Perhaps this is what the future holds. We are truly entering the world of real entertainment.

Acknowledgment

This paper was read at the Twenty-fifth Anniversary Meeting of the Mental Research Institute, Palo Alto, California, August 1985.

References

Barthes, R. (1966). *Critique et vérité*, Paris: Ed. du Seuil
Madanes, C. (1981). *Strategic family therapy*, San Francisco: Jossey-Bass.
Madanes, C. (1984). *Behind the one-way mirror*, San Francisco: Jossey-Bass.
Marc, D. (1984, August). "Understanding Television." *The Atlantic, 254*(2).
Vargas Llosa, M. (1985, June). "Is Fiction the Art of Lying?" *The Writer.*

25

Outcomes of Live Supervision: Trainee Perspectives

HOWARD A. LIDDLE
University of California, San Francisco

GAIL S. DAVIDSON
Seton Hall University, South Orange, New Jersey

MARY JO BARRETT
Midwest Family Resources Associates, Chicago

Studies have increasingly begun to evaluate systematically various aspects of family therapy training (Allred & Kersey, 1977; Byles, Bishop, & Horn, 1983; Churven, 1977; Churven & McKinnon, 1982; Crane, Griffin, & Hill, 1986; Doehrman, 1976; Dowling, Cade, Breunlin, Frude, & Seligman, 1979; Fenell, Hovestadt, & Samuel, 1986; Garfield & Lord, 1982; Green & Kolevzon, 1982; Henry, Sprenkle, & Sheehan, 1986; Kolevzon & Green, 1983a; Mead & Crane, 1978; Mohammed & Piercy, 1983; Pulleyblank & Shapiro, 1986; Reilly & Bayles, 1981; Sutton, 1985; Tomm & Leahey, 1980; West, Hosie, & Zarki, 1985; Zaken-Greenberg & Neimeyer, 1986).[1] Progress has been made in the development of instrumentation suitable for evaluating training (Breunlin, Schwartz, Krause, & Selby, 1983; Kolevzon & Green, 1983b; Piercy, Laird, & Mohammed, 1983; Pinsof, 1979; Tucker & Pinsof, 1984), and in the theoretical and conceptual domains of training and supervision (Grunebaum & Chasin, 1982; Liddle & Saba, 1983, 1984, in press; McDaniel, Weber, & McKeever, 1983; Piercy & Sprenkle, 1985). Still, several papers have called for continued investigation of these and other aspects of training (Kniskern & Gurman, Chapter 23, this volume), most notably of live supervision (Berger & Dammann, 1982; Liddle & Schwartz, 1983). Research has recently addressed such specific issues as the impact of live supervision on a therapist's conceptual development and therapeutic functioning (Draper, 1982; Forman, 1984; Gershenson & Cohen, 1978; Kaslow & Gilman, 1983; Lowenstein, Reder, & Clark, 1982; O'Hare, Henrich, Kirschner, Oberstone, & Ritz, 1975; Stedman & Gaines, 1978). These anecdotal descriptions or small-sample studies are useful preliminary guides to the process and consequences of live supervision.

Between 1977 and 1985 we investigated trainee reactions to live supervision. Eighty-five trainees from a broad variety of training sites participated in the study.[2] No trainees refused to be interviewed, and a wide range of trainee experience level was represented in the study. The amount of experience as a therapist (pre- and postdegree) was 2.1 years, and the average age of respondents was 26.4 years. Of the 85 respondents, 46 (54%) were female and 39 (46%) were male. Thirty-five respondents (41%) had completed a terminal degree (master's or doctoral program) and were seeking specialized advanced training in family therapy, while 50 respondents (59%) were enrolled in degree-granting programs at the time they were interviewed for the study, their live supervision experience being obtained as part of their regular graduate program. Study participants were interviewed by a family therapy trainer other than their supervisor. Interviews averaged 45 minutes in length and were audio or video tape-recorded. The data of the study were obtained through a theme and content analysis of the interview tapes. Finally, when appropriate, the findings will be presented separately for less experienced and more experienced trainees.

Five categories of training experiences were explored in the interview:

1. Initial expectations of live supervision
2. General opinions about training and live supervision
3. Experience with and evaluation of the particulars of live supervision
   a. Phone-ins
   b. During-session consultations
   c. The observing group, or in some cases the observing and participating therapy team[3]
   d. Supervisor–supervisee relationship
4. Observations of the interrelationship between therapy and training
5. Advice to future trainees

INITIAL EXPECTATIONS OF LIVE SUPERVISION

In the majority of cases, trainees reported that they applied to the training program because of its live supervision component. Thus these trainees were positively inclined toward what they perceived to be the promise of close attention to and feedback about one's clinical work. Despite this positive bias, live supervision still aroused predictable responses of anxiety. The less experienced trainees worried about being judged incompetent and unlikable. Some of these beginning trainees experienced more fear prior to the actual start of live supervision, whereas others felt their trepidations peak just as their program began. Additionally, the less experienced trainees were initially quite accepting of the hierarchically organized live supervision context. They appeared to have little difficulty in, as many of them described, "placing myself in the role of a learner." The more experienced therapists, however, were less concerned with being viewed as incompetent, and instead were apprehensive about potential power and control struggles with their supervisor-to-be. This group hoped that their supervisor would acknowledge, and in some cases approve of, their previous training and experience. However, they were cautious about the hierarchy of live supervision, and often adopted a wait-and-see stance toward the assumption of supervisor competence. In general, these therapists did not have an *a priori* assumption of trainer competence. They were more likely to accept the hierarchical nature of the relationship once the supervisor, in the words of many trainees, "had proven himself or herself." In sum, regardless of experience level, trainees were ambivalent about live supervision. Overall, however, they were committed to learning the family therapy model being taught and willing to tolerate some discomfort in the process.

GENERAL OPINIONS ABOUT TRAINING AND LIVE SUPERVISION

Issues of Competency and Performance Anxiety

Less experienced trainees reported a rapid, but not complete, reduction of their preoccupation with being evaluated and appearing inept once they began to conduct interviews. The more experienced clinicians found that their skeptical, show-me attitude diminished when *they* felt respected by the trainer. Beginning therapists' apprehensions and awkwardness were greatly reduced when the contract and rules (i.e., the mutual expectations) of the live supervision context were clearly defined, understood, and accepted. Additionally, they believed they were better able both to follow supervisory directives and to understand the context of the directive or suggestion when they felt personally supported by the supervisor. This support was most frequently defined as having a supervisor who commented positively on some aspect of the interview or the trainee's therapeutic style. Their anxiety also lessened as a result of their involvement in an ongoing didactic seminar with assigned readings and supervisor presentations. Trainees not working in a context with such seminars reported they were similarly helped through assigned readings structured by the supervisor.

Trainees in degree-granting programs, expectably, often explained that their concerns about competency were compounded by their fears about grades and the overall evaluative aspects of the program. These trainees often believed that they would learn more about the difficult art of family therapy, or at least feel more at ease, in a private or institute setting where they could receive specialized therapy training without the same type of evaluation pressure.

Issues of Trainee Dependence and Independence[4]

Trainees in degree-granting programs were frequently receiving supervision on other cases from a variety of theoretical orientations simultaneously. In these situations, many trainees felt the depth of their experience in any one of these therapeutic models (e.g., family therapy, behavior therapy) was lacking. They believed they assumed less responsibility for the planning and outcome of the cases in the training program than they normally did with their usual caseload (i.e., with families seen in their agency position or private practice). These trainees often reported feeling, especially initially, that the case was not "theirs" in the usual sense, and that they were mere extensions of the supervisor.

Interestingly, during the beginning phase of training, trainees were not particularly bothered by their lack of control. As trainees learned the therapeutic model through didactic input, observation of others, and supervision, their confidence increased; concomitantly, they wanted to have more input into the creation of therapeutic strategy and intervention. Moreover, these therapists believed that it was very difficult for them to contribute successfully to the treatment planning session, for instance, if their supervisor failed to acknowledge their progress and degree of skill development. They felt that a supervisor should work actively to decrease trainee dependence. Fewer and different kinds of supervisory interventions (e.g., during-session *consultations* of a more collaborative nature rather than unidirectional *commands*), and the supervisor's capacity to minimize his or her control of both the trainee and the case, were the most frequently cited suggestions from trainees in this regard.

From the beginning the more experienced trainees struggled with issues of autonomy. These trainees disliked supervisory behavior that, in their view, fostered dependence. In particular, they were disturbed by "too many" in-session phone-ins from their supervisor. Furthermore they believed that, at a certain stage of trainee development, supervisors should routinely solicit trainee ideas about how to proceed with a case; that at these later stages of training, supervisor and trainee should have a distinctively collaborative relationship. Many trainees believed that it was possible to have a collaborative supervisory partnership within a hierarchically organized relationship.

Trainee as Performer and Supervisory Instrument

At the outset, beginning trainees in particular were bothered by the performance and the demand characteristics of the live supervision context. They frequently were more preoccupied with performing well for the supervisor and observers than with learning complex clinical skills. Additionally, early in the training, therapists often felt as if they were mere instruments of their supervisors, "with no mind of my own." At the end of their training, however, a majority of trainees endorsed the belief that live supervision does not ultimately hinder development of independent thinking on the therapist's part. Trainees generally attributed their change in perception about live supervision to changes in the supervisor's behavior over time (i.e., from more to less intrusive, and less to more solicitous of therapist viewpoint), as well as to their own increased clinical competence.

The more experienced therapists were inclined, especially at the start of training, to want a rationale for supervisory suggestions. They wanted, as many phrased it, "the big picture or context in which any given intervention fits." As these trainees were increasingly able to integrate the therapy model with their personal identities as therapists, the previously foreign methods of that model felt less like techniques and more like the logical and personal extension of the approach and oneself. In this sense, what we could call the "self-as-performer" and "self-as-supervisory-instrument" problems dramatically subsided as the gulf between the person of the therapist and the therapeutic model was bridged.

EXPERIENCES WITH AND EVALUATION OF LIVE SUPERVISION

Phone-ins

Beginning therapists believed that if the calls were skillfully executed, they could then integrate them without difficulty. Most trainees, however, initially interpreted phone-ins as reprimands: "the supervisor is calling because I've made a mistake." Gradually their interpretation became more benign: trainees began to see the phone-ins as guides to the conduct of a session ('It's like the rudder on a boat, keeping things on course"), and in this sense they reported that eventually they relied on and actually welcomed the phone-ins. Trainees generally appreciated phone-ins that were well timed and that caught a diversion and refocused the session. During the middle and later phases of training, supervisees wanted time to implement or complete an intervention on their own, or to be given the opportunity for independent, unprompted action in a session ("to find my own way in the room with the family") without supervisory interruption. This point was strongly expressed by many trainees and was seen as a crucial variable in decreasing the dependency aspects of live supervision.

As stated previously, trainees worried about the frequency of phone-ins, especially with respect to how the calls might contribute to the family's negative evaluation of the therapist, as well as possible adverse effects on the family and the therapy. Many therapists also stated that although they frequently were concerned about the disruptive effects of the phone-ins, afterward they often appreciated and realized that the calls facilitated the therapeutic process. Trainees had mixed opinions on the impact of live supervision on the case. Many indicated that their clients commented positively about the extra attention they received, whereas other families accepted live supervision as a necessary, but nonetheless sometimes problematic, aspect of therapy.

Trainees tend to find brief, directive phone-ins useful at the beginning of live supervision. In this regard, they spoke of the necessity for exposure to the theoretical aspects of family therapy, and instruction and discussion that links theory to their practice experiences in live supervision. Later in their training, therapists reported that it was easier to remember and use more complex phone-ins. There were many instances in which trainees preferred behind-the-mirror consultations: (1) when the phone-in was complex or lengthy, or if trainees believed the suggestions needed further refinement or discussion; (2) when they felt self-conscious listening to the supervisor's directive in front of the family (this was expressed by beginning-level trainees); and (3) in cotherapy sessions.

In their final analyses of live supervision, therapists of all experience levels reported that the immediacy of phone-ins and during-session consultations was a distinct advantage. As one trainee said; "The phone calls and consultation breaks are the absolute beauty and bonus of live supervision; it's there with you at the moment." Many therapists credited phone-ins with exerting an undeniably positive effect on the therapy. The respondents frequently reported that in comparison to their experience with other supervisory formats, live supervision, over time, facilitated more in-session focus, provided clearer direction for future sessions, and increased their feelings of appropriate and nonauthoritarian personal power.

Consultations

Often framed as "thought breaks," the respondents viewed during-session consultations with the supervisor very favorably. During the early and middle phases of training, the during-session consultations were most frequently initiated by the supervisor. Beginning therapists, again, tended to be concerned with the family's reaction to any break or interruption during a session. But, as with a similar worry about the phone-ins, this concern dissipated fairly quickly (especially in light of most families' low degree of reactivity to the components of live supervision). As trainees became more comfortable with live supervision, they wanted fewer supervisor-initiated and more self-prompted consultations. At later points of their training, trainees defined the consultations as a special time in which they could participate in designing and conceptualizing new in-session directions. More than phone-ins, consultations provided an opportunity for a collaborative and interactive supervisory context.

Significantly, this finding held across all levels of experience. This preference for active participation in the formulation of therapeutic plans, although more pronounced with trainees who saw themselves as having an active learning style, was expressed by the vast majority of interviewees. More advanced therapists, especially, wanted to generate alternatives with a supervisor and observing group or be permitted to choose indepen-dently a direction among several alternatives, rather than simply being directed what to do. Trainees at all experience levels agreed that consultations were an opportune time to discuss complex supervisory suggestions or ideas that were not yet fully or sufficiently formulated. Many trainees observed that it would be difficult, or at least less useful, to conduct live supervision only with phone-ins. Both consultations and phone-ins were thus perceived as valuable and complementary supervisory tools.

Although we did not specifically ask about videotape supervision, many therapists volunteered such information. They often characterized its advantages (e.g., a reflective emphasis) in relation to the disadvantages of live supervision (e.g., pressure to change in the moment). Therapists most frequently mentioned videotape supervision's capacity to help formulate and change elements of one's therapeutic or personal style.

The Training Group

The vast majority of respondents liked being trained in a group context. They saw the personal support, generation of ideas, and feedback about one's clinical style as benefi-cial. The opportunity to have others with whom to share the difficulties of exposing one's clinical work and feelings of self-doubt was perceived as quite important to most trainees. As time progressed, the observing groups often developed into a therapeutic team, even in contexts where this was not considered part of the therapeutic approach. Trainees often saw the use of the team in delivering or framing interventions as a means by which they could have more leverage in relation to the case.

Trainees often commented that an added benefit of a group training setting was the opportunity to observe other therapists directly. They believed that they learned a great deal from observing the supervision of other therapists (e.g., "It was as if I were actually having the opportunity to see several cases at the same time during the training"), and as time progressed, they felt committed to helping one another. A few trainees, however, mentioned that feelings of competition with other group members proved to be a handicapping factor in their learning, and others wished more time had been spent in processing group-related issues (e.g., competition, giving and receiving feedback).

Perceived Supervisor Characteristics and the Supervisor–Supervisee Relationship

The majority of family therapy trainees had clear opinions about effective and ineffec-tive supervisory behavior. The trainees in this study wanted their supervisors to be experts. They believed their trust in a supervisor, which was perceived as a crucial determinant of a productive supervisor–supervisee relationship and to effective outcome of training, was tied to this perception of the supervisor as a highly trained and experienced family therapist. The trainees perceived the relationship with their supervisors as a key element in the training process and in their evaluation of training. Trainees who reported difficulties in the supervisor–supervisee relationship were likely to have a more equivocal assessment of live supervision and the overall training experience than those who believed they experienced few relational problems.

TRAINEES' PERCEPTIONS OF SUPERVISOR COMPETENCE

The following list gives the most frequently cited criteria trainees used in evaluating their supervisor's competence. When a trainee judged these supervisory qualities to be present, there was a low likelihood that he or she would report supervisory relationship problems.

1. Supervisor's relationship skills:
   a. *Humor.* Helps trainees use their natural sense of humor in therapy, and also uses own sense of humor in the supervisory relationship.
   b. *Sensitivity.* Is aware of trainees' struggles to learn a new approach.
   c. *Communication.* Communicates clearly and directly about the supervisory situation and also about therapy matters.
   d. *Respect.* Shows respect for trainee's past professional and personal experience.
   e. *Challenge.* Confronts the trainee about unhelpful aspects of his or her therapeutic style.
   f. *Support.* Expresses understanding of the trainee's learning difficulties.
   g. *Enthusiasm.* Shows an enthusiasm about therapy and teaching.
2. Supervisory feedback. Regularly provides direct and clear feedback to trainee on in-session behaviors, responses to supervision, interpersonal style, and conceptual abilities.
3. Supervisor's conceptualization ability. Conceptualizes the case in a suitably complex, but clear and concrete way. Can communicate this thinking to the trainee in a variety of teaching contexts (e.g., verbally in case consultation, during video- or audiotape review, in individual and group supervision contexts), and actively teach the conceptualization ability to the trainee.
4. Supervisor as role model. Functions as a professional role model to trainees. This includes the professional socialization of therapists into the family therapy field, modeling task- and problem-focused behavior, group leadership, and organization skill.
5. Supervisor can provide:
   a. Guidance to a session *and* allow trainees to find their own way in an interview.
   b. Structure in training and supervision (e.g., tasks given to trainees such as directed readings and tape analyses).
   c. Help in making the model become concrete and personally replicable.
   d. A context where one's personal style of conducting therapy according to a model is shaped and refined.
   e. A flexible model of supervision that can adjust to the trainee's level of experience and skill.

    f. Direct teaching about the skills of the supervisor's model, provide ongoing feedback about trainee's progress and development as a therapist.

    g. Guidance in trainee's assessment of his or her own strengths and limitations.

    h. Support through availability to consult on cases outside of the training program's hours.

    i. A model of training that prescribes supervisory flexibility and change over time—supervisors have a clear sense of the trainee's developmental stage and what might be required at that phase (e.g., promoting more independence through greater trainee involvement in planning and decision making as supervision progresses).

OBSERVATIONS OF THE INTERRELATIONSHIP BETWEEN THERAPY AND TRAINING

Advanced trainees were particularly adept at recognizing the interconnectedness and mutually influencing processes of all levels of the training system (i.e., family, therapist, supervisor, training group, training program). At the beginning of training, mid-level and beginning trainees either did not recognize the isomorphism principle or only perceived its operation in select subsystems (e.g., as operational only in the family). During later phases of training, however, all trainees had a clear sense of the key features of this principle. The respondents often stated that an appreciation of the consistency between the principles of therapy and training was quite helpful in providing a rich understanding of the therapeutic approach they learned. This statement seems to reflect Bateson's (1979) ideas about the advantages of binocular versus monocular vision (i.e., the capacity to move from a two-dimensional to a three-dimensional experience).

    The specific dimensions of corespondence between the training and therapy subsystems most often identified by trainees were:

1. Action-oriented, present-focused treatment and training; emphasis on enactment (family member and family member/therapist and family).

2. Creation of workable realities and exploration of alternatives; emphasis on developing new frames or ways of seeing people and problems (i.e., creating a new reality of problem with a family member begins with the creation of that reality with oneself).

3. Stages of treatment and training; everything cannot change or be learned at once.

4. Expansion of self and others beyond usual limits; appreciation of the role that stress and crisis induction play in change.

5. Use of self as an instrument of change: pacing, language, timing, recalibration of interventions.

6. Appreciation of the importance of the relationship dimension in therapy and training.

7. Interconnectedness and interrelatedness of subsystems in families, training systems, and work systems.

8. Appreciation of the reverberations of change in all domains of life (personal, professional, workplace).
9. Perception of the relevance and application of the systemic view at many diverse levels, including cultural and societal.

ADVICE TO FUTURE TRAINEES

Finally, respondents were asked what recommendations they would offer other therapists about to engage in a training experience that has a live supervision component. Trainees reported that it is particularly important to accept the role of a learner: to accept the hierarchical nature of the supervisory relationship, and to maintain an open attitude toward learning. When supervisory input is given, it is not useful to conceive of oneself as an inept therapist or person. It might be helpful, instead, to remember that in a training setting, feelings of incompetence are normal aspects of being in new territory. Trainees stressed that time is precious, and it can be wasted by an overly defensive demeanor. Respondents also mentioned that practicing the new model in one's work setting, apart from the training context, is a primary, proactive means of integrating and making more accessible the unfamiliar skills.

They suggested that future trainees take an active learning stance in which they ask questions and demand satisfactory explanations. Further, they mentioned that thinking about and sharpening one's learning goals before, during, and after training will facilitate this stance. Next, they recommended that trainees use the training group, and the entire training context, as a source of encouragement, camaraderie, and intellectual stimulation. Finally, they suggest that trainees need to be ready for a certain lack of understanding or support for their family therapy viewpoint in their agency or clinic, and should be realistic about attempting to change their work sites.

SUMMARY AND CONCLUSIONS

This study assessed, through a structured interview format, 85 trainees from a variety of training contexts in which live supervision was a key component. The results provide an initial picture of the variables that might warrant further description and experimental inquiry. The study gives an in-depth portrait of the training experience, as characterized by the trainees themselves. Therapists stressed the need for supervisors to be flexible and change over the course of training and to provide in the process increasing opportunities for trainee independence. Respect also emerged as a key variable. Trainees very much wanted respect from their supervisors, and conversely wanted to respect their supervisors and perceive them as experts. Personal involvement in the learning process was seen as crucial to trainee success in supervision; passive learning styles were viewed as less beneficial than active ones.

Many issues remain inadequately addressed at this stage of our research.[5] To what degree are our findings an artifact of the therapy model that was taught? Given the isomorphism principle, it is likely that these results are, to a very large degree, a function of the structural–strategic therapy model (Liddle, 1985). Our generalizability will therefore be limited to this theoretical model, at least to some unverifiable degree. Although there were no findings in the present study that were gender-specific, this general topic is an unanswered question in the supervision field. Several contributions have been made that clearly detail some of the gender-related issues supervision research might explore (see Chapter 1, this volume). Another issue concerns the fit or interdependence of the live supervision format in relation to other supervisory modes. The precise ways of coordinating the use of videotape, case consultation, and live supervision are at an early stage of development. As more attempts at comprehensive training models are made, this issue of the orchestration of training components merits serious thought and planning.

An interesting and unanticipated finding, which has implications beyond the confines of therapy, concerned the degree to which trainees, at or beyond the later stages of training, thought about the applicability of the systems view to a number of domains of their lives. For example, trainees reported reading the newspapers and watching the evening news differently. They often remarked at how contemporary culture, as reflected in these media, rarely portrayed reality along systemic lines, preferring the more simple and simplistic Cartesian, unicausal, mechanistic epistemology. Various sources are useful in helping trainees articulate the manner in which society finds it difficult to construct a nonreductionistic vision of our world (Bellah, Madsen, Sullivan, Swidler, & Tipton, 1985; Berman, 1981; Capra, 1982).

Trainees also reported changes in the way in which they viewed their own personal relationships after training in family therapy. Trainees, like many of our clinical families after therapy, often reported having a more interdependent, or what from one perspective might be termed a more "responsible" (i.e., understanding of one's participation), view of their own relationships. This finding is especially interesting in light of the orientation of the programs in which the study's respondents were drawn; none had an orientation that included family-of-origin work as relevant to the training enterprise. As training programs become more sophisticated in evaluating their results, this area of outcome—effects on trainee world view and personal relationships—should be explored more fully.

Finally, supervisors can learn a great deal about the supervision they do by simply asking their trainees about it. The process of interviewing our therapists and listening to their comments on the supervisory process has been an enormously enriching one. For supervisors who accept the fact that not all trainee comments will be platitudinous, and that trainees' responses can even be enlightening, the experience of enlisting therapists' posttraining reactions is one we wholeheartedly recommend to our fellow supervisors.

Acknowledgment

Acknowledgment is gratefully given to Allan Tannenbaum, PhD, and Christopher Maloy, PhD, who served as interviewers at the early stage of this study. In addition, we wish to thank the therapists interviewed for this project, particularly those from the Temple University and Institute for Juvenile Research programs.

Notes

1. Family therapy's development in this area of research still lags behind training and supervision evaluation in counseling and clinical psychology, where there is a more firmly established research tradition.

2. These include: Temple University (Philadelphia); the Eastern Pennsylvania Psychiatric Institute (Philadelphia); Institute for Juvenile Research (Chicago); Midwest Family Resource Associates (Chicago); the University of California, San Francisco; and the Mental Research Institute (Palo Alto).

3. Programs at the different sites at which the study has been conducted sometimes defined the role of the observing group along more active, participatory lines. Most of the time, however, a traditional model of live supervision was used (Haley, 1976; Montalvo, 1973) in which the role of the observing group remained *mainly* as observers, and the supervision occurred between the supervisor and therapist/trainee.

4. We are again faced with the ways in which language orients and organizes conceptualization. In writing about "problems with trainees" in the supervisor–supervisee relationship domain, special care was taken to qualify the partial truths that our semantic structures convey (Liddle & Schwartz, 1983). The present usage also requires qualification. Trainee dependence and independence are, of course, relative terms arrived at via an arbitrary punctuation: they capture only a portion of the trainer–trainee interactional context in a unidirectional, attribute-providing manner. Trainee "dependence" and "independence" are, of course, only partial constructions of the picture. These behaviors exist and are elicited in context. They also serve as stimuli, as well as response behaviors on the part of others (trainees and supervisors). These qualifications serve as reminders of the partial, constructivistic nature of our daily observations, often treated as declarations of ultimate, empirical truth.

5. Those interested in family therapy supervision research would do well to carefully examine some of the aforementioned research in the clinical and counseling psychology supervision literature. Several studies have moved beyond extrapolating desirable and undesirable qualities or characteristics of trainees and trainers and determinants of effective supervision. On this front, the exact nature of supervisor-supervisee interaction is being examined as an essential correlate of good training outcome. The Epilogue to this volume covers some of this literature, as does Liddle (in press).

References

Allred, G., & Kersey, F. (1977). The AIAC, a design for systematically analyzing marriage and family counselors: A progress report. *Journal of Marriage and Family Counseling, 11*, 9–17.

Bateson, G. (1979). *Mind and nature.* New York: Dutton.

Bellah, R. N., Madsen, R., Sullivan, W. M., Swidler, A., & Tipton, S. (1985). *Habits of the heart: Individualism and commitment in American life.* Berkeley: University of California Press.

Berger, M., & Dammann, C. (1982). Live supervision as context, treatment, and training. *Family Process, 21,* 337–344.

Berman, M. (1981). *The reenchantment of the world.* Ithaca, NY: Cornell University Press.

Breunlin, D. C., Schwartz, R. C., Krause, M. S., & Selby, L. (1983). Evaluating family therapy training: The development of an instrument. *Journal of Marital and Family Therapy, 9,* 37–47.

Byles, J., Bishop, D., & Horn, D. (1983). Evaluation of a family therapy training program. *Journal of Marital and Family Therapy, 9,* 299–304.

Capra, F. (1982). *The turning point.* New York: Simon and Schuster.

Churven, P. (1977). Role playing, derolling, and reality in family therapy training. *Australian Social Work, 30,* 23–27.

Churven, P., & McKinnon, T. (1982). Family therapy training: An evaluation of a workshop. *Family Process, 21,* 345–352.

Crane, R., Griffin, W., & Hill, R. D. (1986). Influence of therapist skills on client perceptions of marriage and family therapy outcome: Implications for supervision. *Journal of Marriage and Family Therapy, 2,* 91–96.

Doehrman, M. J. G. (1976). Parallel processes in supervision and psychotherapy. *Bulletin of the Menninger Clinic, 40,* 3–10.

Dowling, E., Cade, B., Breunlin, D. C., Frude, N., & Seligman, P. (1979). A retrospective survey of students' view on a family therapy training program. In S. Walrond-Skinner (Ed.), *Family and marital psychotherapy.* London: Routledge & Kegan Paul.

Draper, R. (1982). From trainee to trainer. In R. Whiffen & J. Byng-Hall (Eds.), *Family therapy supervision: Recent developments in practice.* New York: Grune & Stratton.

Fenell, D. L., Hovestadt, A. J., & Samuel, J. H. (1986). A comparison of delayed feedback and live supervision models of marriage and family therapist clinical training. *Journal of Marriage and Family Therapy, 2,* 181–186.

Fisher, B., & Embree, T. (1981). *Supervision of beginning and advanced marital and family therapists: A comparative study.* Paper presented at the annual meeting of the American Association for Marriage and Family Therapy, San Diego, California.

Forman, B. (1984). Family of origin work in systemic/strategic therapy. *The Clinical Supervisor, 2,* 81–85.

Garfield, R., & Lord, G. (1982). The Hahnemann master's of family therapy program: A design and its results. *American Journal of Family Therapy, 10,* 75–78.

Gershenson, J., & Cohen, M. (1978). Through the looking glass: The experiences of two family therapy trainees with live supervision. *Family Process, 27,* 225–230.

Green, R., & Kolevzon, M. (1982). Three approaches to family therapy: A study of convergence and divergence. *Journal of Marital and Family Therapy, 8,* 39–50.

Grunebaum, H., & Chasin, R. (1982). Thinking like a family therapist: A model for integrating the theories and methods of family therapy. *Journal of Marital and Family Therapy, 8,* 403–416.

Haley, J. (1976). *Problem-solving therapy.* San Francisco: Jossey-Bass.

Henry, P. W., Sprenkle, D. H., & Sheehan, R. (1986). Family therapy training: Student and faculty perceptions. *Journal of Marital and Family Therapy, 12,* 249–258.

Kaslow, N. J., & Gilman, S. R. (1983). Trainee perspectives on family therapy supervision. *American Journal of Family Therapy, 11,* 70–74.

Kolevzon, M. S., & Green, R. G. (1983a). An experientially based inductive approach to learning about family therapy. *American Journal of Family Therapy, 11,* 35–42.

Kolevzon, M. S., & Green, R. G. (1983b). Practice and training in family therapy: A known group study. *Family Process, 22,* 179–190.

Liddle, H. A. (1985). Five factors of failure in structural–strategic family therapy. In S. Coleman (Ed.), *Failures in family therapy.* New York: Guilford Press.

Liddle, H. A. (in press). Family therapy training and supervision: A critical review and analysis. In A. Gurman & D. Kniskern (Eds.), *Handbook of family therapy* (2nd ed.). New York: Guilford Press.

Liddle, H. A., & Saba, G. (1983). On context replication: The isomorphic relationship of training and therapy. *Journal of Strategic and Systemic Therapies, 2,* 3–11.

Liddle, H. A., & Saba, G. (1984). The isomorphic nature of training and therapy: Epistemologic foundations for a structural–strategic family therapy. In J. Schwartzman (Ed.), *Families and other systems.* New York: Guilford Press.

Liddle, H. A., & Schwartz, R. C. (1983). Live supervision & consultation: Conceptual and pragmatic guidelines for family therapy training. *Family process, 22,* 477–490.

Lowenstein, S., Reder, P., & Clark, A. (1982). The consumer's response: Trainee's discussion of the experience of live supervision: In R. Whiffen & J. Byng-Hall (Eds.), *Family therapy supervision: Recent developments in practice.* New York: Grune & Stratton.

McDaniel, S., Weber, T., & McKeever, J. (1983). Multiple theoretical approaches to supervision: Choices in family therapy training. *Family Process, 22,* 491–500.

Mead, E., & Crane, D. (1978). An empirical approach to supervision and training of relationship therapists. *Journal of Marriage and Family Counseling, 4,* 67–76.

Mohammed, Z., & Piercy, F. (1983). The effects of two methods of training and sequencing on structuring and relationship skills of family therapists. *American Journal of Family Therapy, 11,* 64–71.

Montalvo, B. (1973). Aspects of live supervision. *Family Process, 12,* 343–359.

O'Hare, C., Heinrich, A., Kirschner, N., Oberstone, A., & Ritz, M. (1975). Group training in family therapy: The student's perspective. *Journal of Marriage and Family Counseling, 1,* 157–162.

Piercy, F. P., Laird, R., & Mohammed, Z. (1983). A family therapist rating scale. *Journal of Marital and Family Therapy, 9,* 49–59.

Piercy, F. P., & Sprenkle, D. H. (1985). Family therapy theory building: An integrative training approach. *Journal of Psychotherapy and the Family, 1,* 5–14.

Pinsof, W. (1979). The family therapist behavior scale (FTBS): Development and evaluation of a coding systems. *Family Process, 18,* 451–462.

Pulleyblank, E., & Shapiro, R. J. (1986). Evaluation of family therapy trainees: Acquisition of cognitive and therapeutic behavior skills. *Family Process, 25*, 591–598.

Reilly, I., & Bayles, T. (1981). Family therapy training—Give the customer what they want. *Journal of Family Therapy, 3*(2), 167–176.

Stedman, J. M., & Gaines, T. (1978). Trainee response to family therapy training. *Family Process, 5*, 1–12.

Sutton, P. M. (1985). An insider's comparison of a major family therapy doctoral program and a leading nondegree family therapy training center. *Journal of Psychotherapy and the Family, 1*(4), 41–50.

Tomm, K., & Leahey, M. (1980). Training in family assessment: A comparison of three teaching methods. *Journal of Marital and Family Therapy, 6*, 453–458.

Tucker, S., & Pinsof, W. (1984). The empirical evaluation of family therapy training. *Family Process, 23*, 437–456.

West, J. D., Hosie, T. W., & Zarki, J. J. (1985). Simulation in training family therapists: Process and outcome. *International Journal of Family Therapy, 7*, 50–58.

Zaken-Greenberg, F., & Neimeyer, G. J. (1986). The impact of structural family therapy training on conceptual and executive therapy skills. *Family Process, 25*, 599–608.

The Future of Family Therapy

One intention of this book has been to orient the reader to the range of training practices and assumptions in family therapy, and to the issues faced by trainers in different contexts or in using different techniques. A larger intention, however, has been to advance the field of family therapy itself by providing those who will have the most direct influence on its future—the trainers—with a sense of identity, an overview perspective, and some practical guidelines. We believe that the field will evolve no further than its trainers permit.

Family therapy has evolved from a movement sustained by free-standing institutes to a popular and respected mental health service taught in graduate programs of the major disciplines, and in newly formed degree-granting programs in marriage and family therapy. Family therapy is here to stay, but no one can accurately predict its future. Family therapy's development has been marked by tremendous creativity and the burgeoning of its body of knowledge. Today there is increasing awareness that family therapy should be rigorously examined (Schwartz & Perrotta, 1985) and made accountable for its claims (Cross, 1985). Which approaches to or aspspects of family therapy will survive is unknown. At the level of practice, family therapy may become more accountable through the establishment of criteria to determine competence and credentialing to legitimate practice. At the present time family therapy is unregulated, so virtually anyone can do it. The AAMFT has established criteria for clinical membership and is designated by the U.S. government Department of Education to regulate family therapy, but licensing occurs at the state level and currently only 11 states license marriage and family therapy.

Whether family therapy remains a field, emerges as a legitimate profession, or exists as some combination of the two will also shape its future. As a field, family therapy would remain accessible to all of the disciplines. The interaction of family therapy with these disciplines would affect and expand family therapy's body of knowledge. Some argue that the result would be a dilution of family therapy; others believe such interactions could enrich family therapy and rid it of its blind spots. For some, the fear remains that the disciplines would co-opt family therapy by shaping its identity to fit their needs.

In some quarters family therapy is already defined as a profession. It has become so by simply declaring itself so. The issues surrounding family therapy as a profession are complex. One major dilemma centers on the definition and regulation of family therapy's area of expertise. In the beginning, family therapy could be practiced by all disciplines because none could claim it exclusively, as, for instance, psychologists have claimed psychological testing. But if family therapy becomes a profession, will it desire or have the political power to lay claim to its area of expertise and, through credentialing, to limit its practice to members of that profession? The economics of professions suggest this possibility, just as obstetricians seek to prevent midwives from delivering babies. In this scenario family therapy would be regulated and accountable, but many would question the price paid for this change, especially in terms of the field's vitality.

The consequences to other training settings must also be questioned. If credentialing requires a degree, what becomes of the free-standing institutes? What sort of involvement can the graduate programs in the disciplines have with family therapy? Is there a danger that family therapy will end up competing against rather than collaborating with these disciplines? These thorny questions draw no easy answers, but these and versions of them will inevitably be asked in the future.

The fortunes of family therapy as a profession may be decided more in the marketplace than in the classroom. Currently only 11 states license marriage and family therapists. Barred from collecting insurance, family therapy as a profession will remain economically less desirable than psychiatry or psychology. This problem, however, may disappear in the long run if, as predicted, third-party payment schemes give way to a system of health care based on preferred providers and corporate conglomerates.

Family therapy training, as a body of knowledge and set of skills, will significantly affect this future. The way that the issues raised in this book are addressed and resolved will shape the future of family therapy training.

References

Cross, D. G. (1985). The age of accountability: The next phase for family therapy. *Australian and New Zealand Journal of Family Therapy, 6*(3), 129–135.

Schwartz, R. C., & Perrotta, P. (1985). Let us sell no intervention before its time. *The Family Therapy Networker, 9*(4), 18–25.

APPENDIX

The Family Therapy Training and Supervision Literature

Compiled by Howard A. Liddle and Douglas C. Breunlin

CONTENTS

1. BOOKS ON TRAINING

Duhl, B. (1983). *From the inside out and other metaphors: Creative and integrative approaches to training in systems thinking.* New York: Brunner/Mazel.

Flomenhaft, K., & Christ, A. (Eds.). (1980). *The challenge of family therapy: A dialogue for child psychiatry educators.* New York and London: Plenum Press.

Liddle, H. A., Breunlin, D. C., & Schwartz, R. C. (Eds.). (1988). *Handbook of family therapy training and supervision.* New York: Guilford Press.

Liddle, H. A., & Saba, G. (in press). *Training family therapists: Creating contexts of competence.* Orlando, FL: Grune & Stratton.

Schulman, G. (1982). *Family therapy: Teaching, learning, doing.* Washington, DC: University Press of America.
Whiffen, R., & Byng-Hall, J. (Eds.). (1982). *Family therapy supervision: Recent developments in practice.* New York: Grune & Stratton.

2. SPECIAL ISSUES OF JOURNALS ON TRAINING AND SUPERVISION

Journal of Marital and Family Therapy. (1979), 5(3), 3–106 (W. Nichols, Ed.).
Journal of Strategic and Systemic Therapies. (1983), 2(2), 1–78 (H. Liddle, Ed.).
The Clinical Supervisor. (1984), 2(2), 1–86 (Family of origin applications in clinical supervision). Also published as a book with Haworth Press.
The Clinical Supervisor. (1986), 2(2). (Supervision and training: Models, dilemmas, and challenges), (F. Kaslow, Ed.). Also published as a book with Haworth Press.
Journal of Psychotherapy and the Family. (1985), 1(4). (Family therapy education and supervision), (F. Piercy, Ed.). Also published as a book with Haworth Press.
Family Therapy Networker, (1983), 7(2).

3. OVERVIEWS OF TRAINING AND SUPERVISION

Ackerman, N. (1973). Some considerations for training in family therapy. In Career Directions (Vol. 2). East Hanover, NJ: Sandoz Pharmaceuticals, D.J.
Beal, E. (1976). Current trends in the training of family therapists. *American Journal of Psychiatry, 133,* 137–141.
Beavers, W. R. (1985). Family therapy supervision: An introduction and consumer's guide. *Journal of Psychotherapy and the Family, 1*(4), 15–24.
Bodin, A. M. (1969). Family therapy training literature: A brief guide. *Family Process, 8,* 272–279.
Bodin, A. M. (1971). Training in conjoint family therapy. In *Project summaries of experiments in mental health training.* Chevy Chase, MD: National Institutes of Mental Health, U.S. Department of Health, Education and Welfare.
Everett, C. A. (1975). *Clinical supervision of individual, marital and family psychotherapy; An annotated bibliography of articles and books published 1933–1975.* Unpublished manuscript.
Everett, C.A. (1980). Supervision of marriage and family therapy. In A. Hess (Ed.), *Psychotherapy and supervision* (pp. 367–380). New York: Wiley-Interscience.
Everett, C. A., & Koerpel, B. J. (1986). Family therapy supervision: A review and critique of the literature. *Contemporary Family Therapy, 8*(1), 62–74.
Fenell, D. L., & Hovestadt, A. J. (1985). Family therapy as a profession or professional speciality: Implications for training. *Journal of Psychotherapy and the Family, 1*(4) 25–39.
Ferber, A., & Mendelsohn, M. (1969). Training for family therapy. *Family Process, 8,* 25–32.
Ganahl, G., Ferguson, L. R., & L'Abate, L. (1985). Training in family therapy. In L. L'Abate (Ed.). *The handbook of family psychology and therapy.* Homewood, IL: Dorsey Press.
Glick, I. D., & Kessler, V. R. (1980). Training for the family therapist. In I. D. Glick & V. R. Kessler (Eds.), *Marital and family therapy.* New York: Grune & Stratton.
Haley, J. (1988). Reflections on supervision. In H. Liddle, D. C. Breunlin, & R. C. Schwartz (Eds.), *Handbook of family therapy training and supervision.* New York: Guilford Press.
Henley, R., & Weber, K. (1983). Training in marriage and family therapy. In B. Wolman & G. Stricker (Eds.). *Handbook for family and marital therapy.* New York: Plenum Press.
Kaslow, F. (1977). Training marriage and family therapists. In F. Kaslow (Ed.), *Supervision, consultation, and staff training in the helping professions* (pp. 199–234). San Francisco: Jossey-Bass.
Liddle, H. A. (1982). Family therapy training and supervision: Current issues, future trends. *International Journal of Family Therapy, 4,* 81–97.
Liddle, H. A. (1985). Redefining the mission of family therapy training. *Journal of Psychotherapy and the Family.* 1(4), 109–124.

Liddle, H. A. (in press). Family therapy training and supervision: A comparative review and critique. In A. Gurman & D. Kniskern (Eds.). *Handbook of family therapy* (2nd ed.). New York: Guilford Press.

Liddle, H. A., Breunlin, D. C., & Schwartz, R. C. (1988). Family therapy training and supervision: An introduction. In H. A. Liddle, D. C. Breunlin, & R. C. Schwartz (Eds.), *Handbook of family therapy training and supervision*. New York: Guilford Press.

Liddle, H. A., & Halpin, R. (1978). Family therapy training and supervision literature: A comparative review. *Journal of Marriage and Family Counseling, 4*, 77–98.

Nichols, W. C. (1973). The field of marriage counseling: A brief overview. *Family Coordinator, 22*, 3–13.

Nichols, W. C. (1975). *Training and supervision*. (Audiotape #123). Upland, CA: American Association for Marriage and Family Therapy.

Nichols, W. C. (1979). Education of marriage and family therapists: Some trends and implications. *Journal of Marital and Family Therapy, 5*, 19–28.

Parsons, B. V. (1972). *Family therapy training manual*. Unpublished manuscript, University of Utah.

Piercy, F., & Sprenkle, D. (1984). The process of family therapy education. *Journal of Marital and Family Therapy, 10*(4), 399–407.

Piercy, F. P., & Sprenkle, D. H. (1986) Supervision and Training. In *Family Therapy Sourcebook* (pp. 288–321). New York: Guilford Press.

Rosenbaum, I. S. (1978). *A review of the literature on training in family therapy, 1969–1978*. Unpublished manuscript.

4. GENERAL PAPERS ON TRAINING AND SUPERVISION

Knox, D. (1970). Supervision in marriage counseling. *Journal of Family Counseling, 4*, 24–26.

Madanes, C. (1988). Family therapy training—It's entertainment. In H. A. Liddle, D. C. Breunlin & R. C. Schwartz (Eds.). *Handbook of family therapy training and supervision*. New York: Guilford Press.

McKenzie, P., Atkinson, B., Quinn, W., & Heath, A. (1986). Training and supervision in marriage and family therapy. *American Journal of Family Therapy, 14*, 293–303.

Munson, C. E. (1980). Supervising the family therapist. *Social Casework, 61*, 131–137.

Novak, E. W., & Busko, B. P. (1974). Teaching old dogs new tricks: Issues in the training of family therapists. *The Psychiatric Forum, 14*(2), 14–20.

Rickert, V. C., & Turner, J. E. (1978). Through the looking glass: Supervision in family therapy. *Social Casework, 59*(3), 131–137.

Rubinstein, D. (1964). Family therapy. In H. Hoffman (Ed.). *Teaching of Psychotherapy: International Psychiatry Clinics* (Vol. 1). Boston: Little Brown.

Simon, R. (1982). Behind the one-way mirror: An interview with Jay Haley, Part I. *Family Therapy Networker, 26*(5), 19–25, 28–29, 58–59.

Simon, R., & Brewster, F. (1983). What is training? *Family Therapy Networker, 7*(2), 24–29, 66.

Sluzki, C. E. (1974). *Treatment, training and research in family therapy*. Paper presented at the Nathan W. Ackerman Memorial Conference, Cumana, Venezuela.

Stier, S., & Goldenberg, I. (1975). Training issues in family therapy. *Journal of Marriage and Family Counseling, 1*, 63–68.

5. ARTICLES ON CONCEPTUAL AND THEORETICAL FRAMEWORKS

Bateson, G. (1972). Experiments in thinking about observed ethnological materials. In *Steps toward an ecology of mind* (pp. 73–87). New York: Ballantine Books.

Bateson, G. (1972). Social planning and the concept of deutero-learning. In *Steps toward an ecology of mind*. New York: Ballantine Books.

Doehrman, M. J. G. (1976). Parallel processes in supervision and psychotherapy. *Bulletin of the Menninger Clinic, 40*(1), 3–10.

Grunebaum, H., & Chasin, R. (1982). Thinking like a family therapist: A model for integrating the theories and methods of family therapy. *Journal of Marital and Family Therapy, 8*, 403–416.

Liddle, H. A. (1988). Conceptual overlays and pragmatic guidelines for systemic supervision. In H. A. Liddle, D. C. Breunlin, & R. C. Schwartz (Eds.), *Handbook of family therapy training and supervision*. New York: Guilford Press.

Liddle, H. A. (1982). On the problems of eclectism: A call for epistemologic clarification and human scale theories. *Family Process, 4,* 81–97.

Liddle, H. A., & Saba, G. (1983). On context replication: The isomorphic relationship of training and therapy. *Journal of Strategic and Systemic Therapies, 2,* 3–11.

Liddle, H. A., & Saba, G. (1984). The isomorphic nature of training and therapy: Epistemologic foundations for a structural–strategic family therapy. In J. Schwartzman (Ed.), *Families and other systems*. New York: Guilford Press.

McDaniel, S., Weber, T., & McKeever, J. (1983). Multiple theoretical approaches to supervision: Choices in family therapy training. *Family Process, 22,* 491–500.

Piercy, F. P., & Sprenkle, D. H. (1985). Family therapy theory building: An integrative training approach. *Journal of Psychotherapy and the Family, 1*(4), 5–14.

6. TRAINING PROGRAMS

Betof, N. (1977). *The effects of a forty-week family training program on the organization and trainees.* Unpublished manuscript, Temple University.

Constantine, L. (1976). Designed experience: A multiple, goal directed training program in family therapy. *Family Process, 15,* 373–396.

Flomenhaft, K., & Carter, R. (1977). Family therapy training: Program and outcome. *Family Process, 16,* 211–218.

Kaslow, F. (1985). An intensive training experience: A six day post-graduate institute model. *Journal of Psychotherapy and the Family, 1*(4) 73–82.

Mendelsohn, M., & Ferber, A. (1972). Training program. In A Ferber, M. Mendelsohn, & A. Napier (Eds.), *The book of family therapy*. New York: Science House.

7. TRAINING MODELS

Andolfi, M., & Menghi, P. (1980). A model for training in family therapy. In M. Adolfi & I. Zwerling (Eds.), *Dimensions of family therapy*. New York: Guilford Press.

Ard, D. (1973). Providing clinical supervision for marriage counselors: A model for supervisor and supervisee. *Family Coordinator, 22,* 91–98.

Cohen, M., Gross, S., & Turner, M. (1976). A note on a developmental model for training family therapists through group supervision. *Journal Marriage and Family Counseling, 2,* 48–76.

Cromwell, R. E. (1979). Diagnosing marital and family systems: A training model. *Family Coordinator, 28*(1), 101–108.

Duhl, F., & Duhl, B. (1979). Structured spontaneity: The thoughtful art of integrative family therapy at BFI. *Journal of Marital and Family Therapy, 5,* 59–76.

Duncan, B. L., & Fraser, S. J. (1987). Buckley's scheme of schemes as a foundation for teaching family systems theory. *Journal of Marriage and Family Therapy, 13*(3), 299–305.

Ferguson, L. R. (1979). The family life cycle: Orientation for interdisciplinary training. *Professional Psychology, 10,* 863–867.

Keller, J. F., & Protinsky, H. (1984). A self-management model for supervision. *Journal of Marital and Family Therapy, 109*(3), 281–288.

Keller, J. F., & Protinsky, H. (1985). Family therapy supervision: An integrative model. *Journal of Psychotherapy and the Family, 1*(4), 83–90.

Kolevzon, M. S., & Green, R. G. (1983). An experientially based inductive approach to learning about family therapy. *American Journal of Family Therapy, 11*(3), 35–42.

L'Abate, L., & O'Callaghan, J. B. (1977). Implications of the enrichment model for research and training. *Family Coordinator, 26*(1), 61–64.

Liddle, H. A., & Saba, G. (1982). Teaching family therapy at the introductory level: A model emphasizing a pattern which connects training and therapy. *Journal of Marital and Family Therapy, 8*, 63–72.

Mead, E., & Crane, D. R. (1978). An emprical approach to supervision and training of relationship therapists. *Journal of Marriage and Family Counseling, 4*(4), 67–75.

Piercy, F., Hovestadt, A., Fenell, D., Franklin, G., & McKeon, D. (1982). A Comprehensive training model for family therapists serving rural populations. *Family Therapy, 9*, 239–249.

Protinsky, H., & Keller, J. F. (1984). Supervision of marriage and family therapy: A family of origin approach. *The Clinical Supervisor, 2*(2), 75–80.

Skynner, A., & Skynner, P. (1979). An open-system approach to teaching family therapy. *Journal of Marital and Family Therapy, 5*(4), 5–16.

Storm, C. L., & Heath, A. W. (1985). Models of supervision: Using therapy theory as a guide. *The Clinical Supervisor, 3*(1), 87–96.

Tucker, B., Hart, G., & Liddle, H. (1976). Supervision in family therapy: A developmental perspective. *Journal of Marriage and Family Counseling, 2*, 269–276.

Wendorf, D. J. (1984). A model for training practicing professionals in family therapy. *Journal of Marital and Family Therapy, 10*, 31–42.

TRAINING/SUPERVISION METHODS

A. Live Supervision

Berger, M., & Dammann, C. (1982). Live supervision as context, treatment, and training. *Family Process, 21*, 337–344.

Birchler, G. (1975). Live supervision and instant feedback in marriage and family therapy. *Journal of Marriage and Family Counseling, 1*, 331–342.

Bullock, D., & Kobayashi, K. (1978). The use of live consultation in family therapy. *Family Process, 5*(3), 245–250.

Gershenon, J., & Cohen, M. (1978). Through the looking glass: The experience of two family therapy trainees with live supervision. *Family Process, 17*, 225–230.

Hare-Mustin, R. (1976). Live supervision in psychotherapy. *Voices, 12*, 21–24.

Kempster, S. W., & Savitsky, E. (1967). Training family therapists through live supervision. In N. Ackerman, F. Beatman, & S. Sherman (Eds.). *Expanding theory and practice in family therapy.* New York: Family Service Association of America.

Kingston, P., & Smith D. (1983). Preparation for live consultation and live supervision when working with a one-way screen. *Journal of Family Therapy, 5*(3), 219–234.

Liddle, H. A., & Schwartz, R. C. (1983). Live supervision/consultation: Conceptual and pragmatic guidelines for family therapy training. *Family Process, 22*, 477–490.

Lowenstein, S., Reder, P., & Clark, A. (1982). The consumer's response: Trainee's discussion of the experience of live supervision. In R. Whiffen & J. Byng-Hall (Eds.), *Family therapy supervision: Recent developments in practice.* New York: Grune & Stratton.

McGoldrick, M. (1982). Through the looking glass. In R. Whiffen & J. Byng-Hall (Eds.). *Family therapy supervision: Recent developments in practice.* New York: Grune & Stratton.

Montalvo, B. (1973). Aspects of live supervision. *Family Process, 12*, 343–359.

Rickerts, V., & Turner, J. (1978). Through the looking glass: Supervision in family therapy. *Social Casework, 59*, 131–137.

Roberts, J. (1981). The development of a team approach in live supervision. *Journal of Strategic and Systemic Therapies, 1*, 24–35.

Roberts, J. (1983). The third tier: The overlooked dimension in family therapy training. *Family Therapy Networker, 7*(2), 30, 60–61.

Roberts, J. (1983). Two models of live supervision: Collaborative team and supervisor guided. *Journal of Strategic and Systemic Therapies, 2*(2), 68–83.

Schwartz, R. C., Liddle, H. A., & Breunlin, D. C. (1988). Muddles of live supervision. In H. A. Liddle, D. C.

Breunlin, & R. C. Schwartz (Eds.), *Handbook of family therapy training and supervision*. New York: Guilford Press.

Smith, D., & Kingston, P. (1980). Live supervision without a one-way screen. *Journal of Family Therapy, 2,* 379–387.

Whitaker, C. (1976). Comment: Live supervision in psychotherapy. *Voices, 12,* 24–25.

Wright, L. (1986). An analysis of live supervision "phone-ins" in family therapy. *Journal of Marriage and Family Therapy, 12,* 187–190.

B. Videotape Supervision

Berger, M. (Ed.). (1970). *Videotape techniques in psychiatric training and treatment*. New York: Brunner/Mazel.

Bodin, A. (1969). Video-tape applications in training family therapists. *Journal of Nervous and Mental Disease, 143,* 251–261.

Bodin, A. (1972). The use of video tapes. In A. Ferber, M. Mendelsohn, & A. Napier (Eds.), *The book of family therapy*. Boston: Houghton Mifflin.

Breunlin, D. C., Karrer, B., McGuire, D., & Cimmarusti, R. (1988). Cybernetics of videotape supervision. In H. A. Liddle, D. C. Breunlin, & R. C. Schwartz (Eds.), *Handbook of family therapy training and supervision*. New York: Guilford Press.

Fine, M., & McIntosh, D. N. (1986). The use of interactive videos to demonstrate differential approaches to marital and family therapy. *Journal of Marriage and Family Therapy, 11,* 85–90.

Kramer, T., & Reitz, M. (1980). Using video playback to train family therapists. *Family Process, 19*(2), 145–150.

Perlmutter, M., Loeb, D., Gumpert, G., O'Hara, F., & Higbie, I. (1967). Family diagnosis and therapy using videotape playback. *American Journal of Orthopsychiatry, 37,* 900–905.

Whiffen, R. (1982). The use of videotape in supervision. In R. Whiffen & J. Byng-Hall (Eds.). *Family therapy supervision: Recent developments in practice*. New York: Academic Press.

C. Group or Peer Supervision:

Allen, J. (1976). Peer group supervision in family therapy. *Child Welfare, 55,* 183–189.

Cohen, M. E., Gross, S. J., & Turner, M. B. (1976). A note on a developmental model for training family therapists through group supervision. *Journal of Marriage and Family Counseling, 2*(1), 48.

Hare, R., & Frankena, S. (1972). Peer group supervision. *American Journal of Orthopsychiatry, 42,* 527–529.

Lindsey, C., & Lloyd, J. (1982). The use of the family's relationship to the supervision groups as a therapeutic tool. In R. Whiffen & J. Byng-Hall (Eds.), *Family therapy supervision: Recent developments in practice*. New York: Grune & Stratton.

Quinn, W. H., Atkinson, B. J., & Hood, J. (1985). The stuck-case clinic as a group supervision model. *Journal of Marital and Family Therapy, 11,* 67–74.

Tucker, B., & Liddle, H. A. (1978). Intra- and interpersonal process in the group supervision of beginning family therapists. *Family Therapy 5*(1), 13–28.

Wendorf, D. J., Wendorf, R. J., & Bond, D. (1985). Growth behind the mirror: The family therapy consortium's group process. *Journal of Marriage and Family Therapy, 11,* 245–256.

D. Teams

Cade, B., Speed, B., & Seligman, P. (1986). Working in teams: The pros and cons. In F. Kaslow (Ed.), *Supervision and training: Models, dilemmas and challenges*. New York: Haworth.

Cornwell, M., & Pearson, R. (1981). Co-therapy teams and one-way screen in family therapy practice and training. *Family Process, 20,* 199–209.

Heath, A. (1982). Team family therapy training: Conceptual and pragmatic considerations. *Family Process, 21,* 187–194.

Olson, U., & Pegg, P. (1979). Direct open supervision: A team approach. *Family Process, 18,* 463–470.

Papp, P. (1980). The Greek chorus and other techniques of family therapy. *Family Process, 19*(1), 45–57.

E. Other Training and Supervision Methods

Bardill, D. (1976). The simulated family as an aid to learning family group treatment. *Child Welfare, 55*, 703–709.

Berg, B. (1978). Learning family therapy through simulation. *Psychotherapy: Theory, Research and Practice, 15*(1), 56–61.

Bockus, F. (1980). The teachable moment. In *Couple therapy* (pp. 275–314). New York: Jason Aronson.

Byng-Hall, J. (1982). The use of the earphone in supervision. In R. Whiffen, & J. Byng-Hall (Eds.), *Family therapy supervision: Recent developments in practice*. New York: Grune & Stratton.

Carter, E. (1982). Supervisory discussion in the presence of the family. In R. Whiffen & J. Byng-Hall (Eds.), *Family therapy supervision: Recent developments in practice*. New York: Grune & Stratton.

Coppersmith, E. (1978). Expanding uses of the telephone in family therapy. *Family Process, 17*, 225–230.

DeAth, E. (1979). Action models—Learning by doing. *Journal of Family Therapy, 1*(2), 231–239.

Dell, P., Scheely, M., Pulliam, G., & Goolishian, H. (1977). Family therapy process in a family therapy seminar. *Journal of Marriage and Family Counseling, 3*, 43–48.

Duhl, F. J., Kantor, D., & Duhl, B. S. (1973). Learning, space and action in family theapy: A primer of sculpture. In D. Block (Ed.), *Techniques of family psychotherapy*. New York: Grune & Stratton.

Goldenberg, I., Stier, S., & Preston, T. (1975). The use of a multiple family marathon as a teaching device. *Journal of Marriage and Family Counseling, 1*(4), 343–349.

Heath, A., McKenna, B., & Atkinson, B. (in press) Toward the identification of variables for evaluating family therapy workshops. *Journal of Marriage and Family Therapy*.

Jurasky, J. (1964). A sit-in method for training family group therapists. *Journal of Psychoanalysis in Groups, 1*, 109–114.

Kahn, M. D. (1979). Organizational consultation and the teaching of family therapy: Contrasting case histories. *Journal of Marital and Family Therapy, 5*(1), 69–80.

Kraft, I. (1966). Multiple impact therapy as a teaching device. In S. M. Cohen (Ed.), *Psychiatric research report no. 20*. [Washington, DC:] American Psychiatric Association.

Latham, T. (1982). The use of co-working (co-therapy) as a training method. *Journal of Family Therapy, 4*, 257–269.

Landau-Stanton, J., & Stanton, M. D. (1983). Aspects of supervision with the "Pick-a-Dila Circus" model. *Journal of Strategic and Systemic Therapies, 2*, 31–39.

Landau-Stanton, J., & Stanton, M. D. (1986). Family therapy and systems supervision with the "Pic-a-Dila Circus" model. In F. Kaslow (Ed.), *Supervision and training: Models, dilemmas and challenges*. New York: Haworth.

Liddle, H. A. (1980). Keeping abreast of developments in the family therapy field: The use of "concepts cards" in clinical practice. In A. Gurman (Ed.), *Questions and answers in family therapy* (Vol. 1). New York: Brunner/Mazel 1980. Also in *American Journal of Family Therapy*. 1980, 8.

Liddle, H. A. (1982). In the mind's eye: The use of imagery in training family therapists. In A. Gurman (Ed.), *Questions and answers in family therapy* (Vol. 2). 1980. New York: Brunner/Mazel. Also in *American Journal of Family Therapy, 10*(1), 68–72.

Meyerstein, I. (1979). The family behavioral snapshot: A tool for teaching family assessment. *American Journal of Family Therapy, 7*(1), 48–57.

Napier, A. Y. (1976). The consultation–demonstration interview. *Family Process, 15*(4), 419–426.

Papp, P., & Manocchio, A. (1982). In the act. In R. Whiffen & J. Byng-Hall (Eds.), *Family therapy and supervision: Recent developments in practice*. New York: Grune & Stratton.

Raasoch, J., & Lacquer, H. (1979). Learning multiple family therapy through simulated workshops. *Family Process, 18*(1), 95–98.

Schwartz, R. C. (1981). The pre-session worksheet as an adjunct to training. *American Journal of Family Therapy, 9*(3), 89–90.

Sonne, J. C. & Lincoln, G. (1964). Heterosexual co-therapy team experiences during family therapy. *Family Process, 4*(2), 177–197.

Storm, C., & Heath, A. (1982). Strategic supervision: The danger lies in the discovery. *Journal of Strategic and Systemic Therapy, 1*(4), 71.

Street, E., & Treacher, A. (1980). Microtraining and family therapy skills: Towards a possible synthesis. *Journal of Family Therapy, 2*, 243–257.

Tooley, K. (1975). The diagnostic home visit: An aid to training in case consultation. *Journal of Marriage and Family Counseling, 1*(4), 317–322.

Weingarten, K. (1979). Family awareness for nonclinicians: Participation in a simulated family as a teaching technique. *Family Process, 18*(2), 143–150.

9. TEACHING/TRAINING/SUPERVISION OF CONTENT AREAS

A. Curricula

Cooper, J., & Charnofsky, S. (1983). Curricula and program development in marriage and family counseling: Process and content. In B. F. Okun & S. T. Gladdin (Eds.), *Issues in training marriage and family therapists* (pp. 5–16). Ann Arbor, MI: ERIC/CAPS.

Freeman, D. S. (1980). A model for teaching a beginners course on family therapy. In D. S. Freeman (Ed.), *Perspectives on family therapy* (pp. 77–84). Toronto: Butterworth.

Sander, F., & Beels, C. (1970). A didactic course for family therapy trainees. *Family Process, 9,* 411–424.

Winkle, W., Piercy, F., & Hovestadt, A. (1981). A marriage and family therapy curriculum. *Journal of Marital and Family Therapy, 7,* 201–210.

B. Training Objectives

Anderson, L., Amatea, E., Munson, P., & Rudner, B. (1979). Training in family treatment: Needs and objectives. *Social Casework, 60,* 323–329.

Cleghorn, J., & Levin, S. (1973). Training family therapists by setting learning objectives. *American Journal of Orthopsychiatry, 43,* 439–446.

Falicov, C., Constantine, J., & Breunlin, D. C. (1981). Teaching family therapy: A program based on training objectives. *Journal of Marital and Family Therapy, 7,* 497–505.

Tomm, K., & Wright, L. (1979). Training in family therapy: Perceptual, conceptual and executive skills. *Family Process, 18,* 227–250.

C. Family Therapy Techniques

Constantine, J., Stone-Fish, L., & Piercy, F. (1984). A systemic procedure for teaching positive connotation. *Journal of Marital and Family Therapy, 10*(3), 313–316.

Fleuridas, C., Nelson, T., & Rosenthal, D. M. (1986). The evolution of circular questions: Training family therapists. *Journal of Marital and Family Therapy, 12*(2), 113–128.

Garrigan, J., & Bambrick, A. (1977). Introducing novice family therapists to "go-between" techniques of family therapy. *Family Process, 16*(2), 237–246.

Hoshmand, C. T. (1984). The theory-practice problem in psychotherapy training: Some proposed strategies. *Journal of Strategic and Systemic Therapies, 3*(1), 50–51.

Sherman, S. (1966). Aspects of family interviewing critical for staff training and education. *Social Service Review, 40,* 302–303.

D. Theoretical and Conceptual Ideas

Coppersmith, E. I. (1985). Teaching trainees to think in triads. *Journal of Marital and Family Therapy, 11,* 61–66.

Dell, P., Sheely, M., Pullian, G., & Goolishian, H. (1977). Family therapy in a family therapy seminar. *Journal of Marriage of Family Counseling, 3,* 43–48.

Duhl, B. (1985). Toward cognitive–behavioral integration in training systems therapists: An interactive approach to training in generic systems thinking. *Journal of Psychotherapy and the Family, 1*(4), 91–108.

Falicov, C. (1988). Learning to think culturally. In H. A. Liddle, D. C. Breunlin, & R. C. Schwartz (Eds.), *Handbook of family therapy training and supervision.* New York: Guilford Press.

Flint, A., & Rioch, M. (1963). An experiment in teaching family dynamics. *American Journal of Psychiatry, 11,* 940–944.

Liddle, H. A. (1988). Integrating developmental thinking and the family life cycle paradigm into training. In C. Falicov (Ed.), *Family transitions: Continuity and change over the life cycle.* New York: Guilford Press.

Resnikoff, R. O. (1981). Teaching family therapy: Ten key questions for understanding the family as patient. *Journal of Marital and Family Therapy, 7*(2), 135–142.

Sluzki, C. E. (1974). On training to think interactionally. *Social Science and Medicine, 8,* 483–485.

Steirlin, H., Wirsching, M., & Weber, G. (1982). How to translate dynamic perspectives into an illustrative and experimental learning process: Role play, genogram and live supervision. In R. Whiffen & J. Byng-Hall (Eds.), *Family therapy supervision: Recent developments in practice.* New York: Grune & Stratton.

E. Research

Colapinto, J. (1979). The relative value of empirical evidence. *Family Process, 18*(4), 427–441.

Reamy-Stephenson, M. (1983). The assumption of non-objective reality: A missing link in the training of strategic family therapists. *Journal of Strategic and Systemic Therapies, 2,* 51–67.

Sprenkle, D., & Piercy, F. (1984). Research in family therapy: A graduate level course. *Journal of Marital and Family Therapy, 10*(3), 225–240.

F. Gender

Caust, B., Libow, J., & Raskin, P. (1981). Challenges and promises of training women as family systems therapists. *Family Process, 20,* 439–448.

Hare-Mustin, R. (1981). Sexism in family therapy. In A. Gurman (Ed.), *Questions and answers in the practice of family therapy* (pp. 204–207). New York: Bruner/Mazel.

Libow, J. A. (1985). Training family therapists as feminists. In M. Ault-Riche (Ed.), *Women and family therapy.* Rockville, MD: Aspen.

Libow, J. A., Raskin, P. A., & Caust, B. (1982). Feminist and family systems therapy: Are they irreconcilable? *American Journal of Family Therapy, 10*(3), 3–12.

Okun, B. F. (1983). Gender issues of family systems therapists. In B. Okun & S. T. Gladdings (Eds.), *Issues in training marriage and family therapists.* Ann Arbor, MI: ERIC/CAPS.

Wheeler, D., Avis, J. M., Miller, L. A., & Chaney, S. (1985). Rethinking family therapy education and supervision: A feminist model. *Journal of Psychotherapy and the family, 1*(4), 53–72.

G. Ethics and Legal Issues

Cormier, L., & Bernard, J. (1982). Ethical and legal responsibilities of clinical supervisors. *Personnel and Guidance Journal, 60*(8), 486–490.

Margolin, G. (1982). Ethical and legal considerations in marital and family therapy. *American Psychologists, 37,* 788–801.

Piercy, F. & Sprenkle, D. (1983). Ethical, legal and professional issues in family therapy: A graduate level course. *Journal of Marital and Family Therapy, 9*(4), 393–401.

10. AAMFT ACCREDITATION ISSUES

American Association for Marriage and Family Therapy, Commission on Accreditation for Marriage and Family Therapy Education. (1979). *Marriage and family therapy: Manual on accreditation.* Upland, CA: Author.

American Association for Marriage and Family Therapy. (1986). Commission on Supervision. *Guidelines for completion of the Approved Supervisor Application.* Upland, CA: Author.

Everett, C. A. (1980). An analysis of AAMFT supervisors: Their identities, roles and resources. *Journal of Marital and Family Therapy, 6*(2), 215–226.

Mudd, E. H., & Fowler, C. R. (1976). The AAMC and the AAMFC: Nearly 40 years of form and function. In B. Ard (Ed.), *Handbook of marriage counseling* (2nd ed.). Palo Alto, CA: Science and Behavior.

Shalett, J., & Everett, C. (1981). Accreditation in family therapy education: Its history and role. *American Journal of Family Therapy, 9*(4), 82–84.

Smith, V. G., & Nichols, W. C. (1979). Accreditation in marital and family therapy. *Journal of Marital and Family Therapy, 5*(3), 95–100.

11. TRAINING AND SUPERVISION WITHIN THE FAMILY THERAPY MODELS

A. Brief Therapy, MRI

Bodin, A. M. (1981). The interactional view: Family therapy approaches of the Mental Research Institute. In A. Gurman & D. Kniskern (Eds..), *Handbook of family therapy*. New York: Brunner/Mazel.

Fisch, R. (1988). Training in the brief therapy model of the M.R.I. In H. A. Liddle, D. C. Breunlin, & R. C. Schwartz (Eds.), *Handbook of family therapy training and supervision*. New York: Guilford Press.

Watzlawick, P., Weakland, J., & Fisch, R. (1974). *Change: Principles of problem formation and resolution*. New York: Norton.

B. Strategic

Haley, J. (1980). *Leaving home: Therapy of disturbed young people*. New York: McGraw-Hill.

Haley, J., & Hoffman, L. (1967). *Techniques of family therapy*. New York: Basic Books.

Madanes, C. (1981). *Strategic family therapy*. San Francisco: Jossey-Bass.

Mazza, J. (1988). Training strategic therapists: The use of indirect techniques. In H. A. Liddle, D. C. Breunlin, & R. C. Schwartz (Eds.), *Handbook of family therapy training and supervision*. New York: Guilford Press.

Stanton, M. D. (1981). Strategic approaches to family therapy. In A. Gurman & D. Kniskern (Eds.), *Handbook of family therapy*. New York: Brunner/Mazel.

C. Structural

Aponte, H. J., & VanDeusen, J. M. (1981). Structural family therapy. In A. Gurman & D. Kniskern (Eds.), *Handbook of family therapy*. New York: Brunner/Mazel.

Colapinto, J. (1983). Beyond technique: Teaching how to think structurally. *Journal of Strategic and Systemic Therapies, 2*, 12–21.

Colapinto, J. (1988). Teaching the structural way. In H. A. Liddle, D. C. Breunlin, & R. C. Schwartz (Eds.), *Handbook of family therapy training and supervision*. New York: Guilford Press.

Hodas, G. (1985). A systems perspective in family therapy supervision. In R. L. Ziffer (Ed.), *Adjunctive techniques in family therapy*. Orlando, FL: Grune & Stratton.

Minuchin, S. (1974). *Families and family therapy*. Cambridge, MA: Harvard University Press.

Minuchin, S., & Fishman, H. C. (1981). *Family therapy techniques*. Cambridge, MA: Harvard University Press.

D. Symbolic–Experiential

Bergantino, L. (1983). I asked Carl Whitaker to teach me family therapy and this is what happened?! *American Journal of Family Therapy, 11*(2), 59–66.

Connell, G. M. (1984). An approach to supervision of symbolic–experimental psychotherapy. *Journal of Marriage and Family Therapy, 10*, 273–280.

Napier, A. Y., & Whitaker, C. (1978). *The family crucible.* New York: Harper & Row.
Whitaker, C. A., & Keith D. B. (1981). Symbolic–experiential family therapy. In A. Gurman & D. Kniskern (Eds.), *Handbook of family therapy.* New York: Brunner/Mazel.

E. Systemic (Milan)

Boscolo, L., & Cecchin, G. (1982). Training in systemic therapy at the Milan Centre. In R. Whiffin & J. Byng-Hall (Eds.), *Family therapy supervision: Recent developments in practice.* London: Academic Press.
Pirrotta, S., & Cecchin, G. (1988). The Milan training program. In H. A. Liddle, D. C. Breunlin, & R. C. Schwartz (Eds.), *Handbook of family therapy training and supervison.* New York: Guilford Press.
Selvini-Palazzoli, M., Bosocolo, L., Cecchin, G., & Prata, G. (1978). *Paradox and counterparadox: A new model for the family in schizophrenic transaction.* New York: Jason Aronson.

F. Transgenerational Models

Boszormenyi-Nagy, I. & Ulrich, D. N. (1981). Contextual family therapy. In A. Gurman & D. Kniskern (Eds.), *Handbook of family therapy.* New York: Brunner/Mazel.
Bowen, M. (1972). On the differentiation of self in one's own family. In J. Framo (Ed.), *Family interaction: A dialogue between family researchers and family therapists.* New York: Springer. [Also in M. Bowen (Ed.). (1978). *Family therapy in clinical practice.* New York: Jason Aronson.]
Framo, J. L. (1981). The integration of marital therapy with sessions with family of origin. In A. Gurman & D. Kniskern (Eds.), *Handbook of family therapy.* New York: Brunner/Mazel.
Kerr, M. E. (1981). Family systems theory and therapy. In A. Gurman & D. Kniskern (Eds.), *Handbook of family therapy.* New York: Brunner/Mazel.
Papero, D. (1988). Training in Bowen theory. In H. A. Liddle, D. C. Breunlin, & R. C. Schwartz (Eds.). *Handbook of family therapy training and supervision.* New York: Guilford Press.

G. Functional Family Therapy

Barton, C., & Alexander, J. (1977). Therapist's skills as determinants of effective systems–behavioral family therapy. *International Journal of Family Counseling, 5,* 11–20.
Barton, C., & Alexander, J. (1981). Functional family therapy: In A. Gurman & D. Kniskern (Eds.), *Handbook of family therapy.* New York: Brunner/Mazel.
Haas, T., Alexander, J., & Mas, C. H. (1988). Functional therapy: Basic concepts and training program. In H. A. Liddle, D. C. Breunlin, & R. C. Schwartz (Eds.), *Handbook of family therapy training and supervision.* New York: Guilford Press.

H. Marital Therapy

Martin, P. A. (1976). *A marital therapy manual.* New York: Brunner/Mazel.
Mezydlo, L., Wauck, L., & Foley, J. (1973). The clergy as marriage counselors: A service revisited. *Journal of Religion and Health, 22,* 278–288.
Sager, C. J. (1981). Couples therapy and marriage contracts. In A. Gurman & D. Kniskern (Eds.), *Handbook of family therapy.* New York: Brunner/Mazel.

I. Systemic Therapy

Keeney, B., & Ross, I. (1983). Learning to learn systemic therapies. *Journal of Strategic and Systemic Therapies, 2,* 22–30.
Liddle, H. A. (1980). On teaching a contextual or systemic therapy: Training content, goals and methods. *American Journal of Family Therapy, 8,* 59–69.

J. Other Models

Bargarozzi, D. (1980). Wholistic family therapy and clinical supervision: Systematic behavioral and psychoanalytic perspectives. *Family Therapy, 7,* 153–165.

Epstein, N. B., & Bishop, D. S. (1981). Problem-centered systems therapy of the family. In A. Gurman & D. Kniskern (Eds.), *Handbook of family therapy.* New York: Brunner/Mazel.

Hatcher, C. (1982). Supervision of the double axis model of therapy. In R. Whiffen & J. Byng-Hall (Eds.), *Family therapy supervision: Recent developments in practice.* New York: Grune & Stratton.

LaPerriere, K. (1979). Toward the training of broad-range family therapists. *Professional Psychology, 10,* 880–883.

Nichols, W. (1988). An integrative psychodynamic and systems approach. In H. A. Liddle, D. C. Breunlin, & R. C. Schwartz (Eds.), *Handbook of family therapy training and supervision.* New York: Guilford Press.

Rassoch, J. & Lagueur, H. P. (1979). Learning multiple family therapy through simulated workshops. *Family Process, 18*(1), 95–102.

Skynner, A. C. R. (1981). An open systems, group-analytic approach to family therapy. In A. Gurman & D. Kniskern (Eds.), *Handbook of family therapy.* New York: Brunner/Mazel.

12. CONTEXTS FOR TRAINING

A. Overviews

Bloch, D., & Weiss, H. (1981). Training facilities in marital and family therapy. *Family Process, 20,* 133–146.

Nichols, M. P. (1984). *Family therapy: Concepts and methods.* New York: Gardner Press.

Williamson, D. (1973). Training opportunities in marriage and family counseling. *Family Coordinator, 22,* 99–102.

B. Free-Standing Institutes

Andrews, E. C. (1974). Proposal for a family institute. *The emotionally disturbed family.* New York: Jason Aronson.

Berman, E., & Dixon-Murphy, T. (1979). Training in marital and family therapy at free standing institutes. *Journal of Marital and Family Therapy, 5,* 27–42.

Herz, F., & Carter, B. (1988). Born free: The life cycle of a free-standing postgraduate training institute. In H. A. Liddle, D. C. Breunlin, & R. C. Schwartz (Eds.), *Handbook of family therapy training and supervision.* New York: Guilford Press.

LaPerriere, K. (1979). Family therapy training at the Ackerman Institute: Thoughts on form and substance. *Journal of Marital and Family Therapy, 5,* 53–58.

C. Continuing Education

Matter, B. (1980). Family therapy for continuing professional education. *International Journal of Family Therapy, 2,* 39–46.

Shalett, J. S. (1979). Continuing education: An interprofessional endeavor. *Journal of Marital and Family Therapy, 5*(3), 101–105.

D. Degree-Granting Programs in Marriage and Family Therapy

Everett, C. (1979). The master's degree in marriage and family therapy. *Journal of Marital and Family Therapy, 5,* 7–14.

Garfield, R. (1979). An integrative training model for family therapists: The Hahnemann master of family therapy program. *Journal of Marital and Family Therapy, 5*(3), 15–22.

Garfield, R. (1980). Family therapy training in Hahnemann Medical College and Hospital. In M. Andolfi & I. Zwerling (Eds.), *Dimensions of family therapy*. New York: Guilford Press.

Garfield, R., & Lord, G. (1982). The Hahnemann master's of family therapy program: A design and its results. *American Journal of Family Therapy, 10,* 75–78.

Nichols, W. (1979). Doctoral programs in marital and family therapy. *Journal of Marital and Family Therapy, 5,* 23–28.

Sprenkle, D. H. (1988). Training and supervision in degree-granting programs in family therapy. In H. A. Liddle, D. C. Breunlin, & R. C. Schwartz (Eds.), *Handbook of family therapy training and supervision.* New York: Guilford Press.

Winkle, C. W., Piercy, F. P., & Hovestadt, A. J. (1981). A curriculum for graduate level marriage and family therapy education. *Journal of Marital and Family Therapy, 7*(2), 201–210.

E. Psychiatry

Combrinck-Graham, L. (1980). The role of family therapy in child psychiatry training: Why and how. In K. Flomenhaft & A. E. Christ (Eds.), *The challenge of family therapy: A dialogue for child psychiatric educators.* New York: Plenum Press.

Combrinck-Graham, L. (1988). Family therapy training in psychiatry. In H. A. Liddle, D. C. Breunlin, & R. C. Schwartz (Eds.), *Handbook of family therapy training and supervision.* New York: Guilford Press.

Erlich, F. (1973). Family therapy training in child psychiatry. *Journal of American Academy of Child Psychiatry, 12,* 461–472.

Flomenhaft, K., & Christ, A. E. (Eds.). *The challenge of family therapy: A dialogue for child psychiatric educators.* New York: Plenum Press.

Malone, C. (1974). Observations on the role of family therapy in child psychiatry training. *Journal of the American Academy of Child Psychiatry, 13,* 437–458.

Martin, P. A., & Lief, H. I. (1973). Resistance to innovation in psychiatric training as exemplified by marital therapy. In G. Usdin (Ed.), *Psychiatry: Education and image.* New York: Brunner/Mazel.

Martin, P. (1979). Training of psychiatric residents in marital therapy. *Journal of Marital and Family Therapy, 5,* 43–52.

Miyoshi, N., & Liebman, R. (1969). Training psychiatric residents in family therapy. *Family Process, 8,* 97–105.

Modlin, H. (1976). The psychiatrist and his family . . . not all understanding and insight. *Menninger Perspective, 7*(3), 12–13.

Schneiderman, C., & Pakes, E. (1976). The teaching of family therapy skills on an inpatient child psychiatry ward. *Family Therapy, 3,* 29–33.

Sugarman, S. (1981). Family therapy training in selected general psychiatric residency programs: Policy issues and alternatives. *Family Process, 20,* 147–154.

Sugarman, S. (1984). Integrating family therapy training into psychiatric residency programs: Policy issues and alternatives. *Family Process, 23,* 23–32.

Talmadge, J. (1975). Psychiatric residents, medical students and families: teaching family therapy to the uninitiated. *Family Therapy, 2,* 11–16.

Whitaker, C. A., & Abroms, G. M. (1974). New approaches to residency training in psychiatry. In G. Farwell, N. Gamsky, & P. Mathier-Couglan (Eds.), *The counselor's handbook.* New York: Intext Educational.

F. Medicine

Epstein, N., & Levin, S. (1973). Training for family therapy within a faculty of medicine. *Canadian Psychiatric Association Journal, 18,* 203–207.

Guttman, H. A., & Sigal, J. J. (1978). Teaching family psychodynamics in a family practice center—One experience. *International Journal of Psychiatry in Medicine, 8*(4), 383–392.

Messner, E., & Schmidt, D. (1974). Videotape in the training of medical students in psychiatric aspects of family medicine. *International Journal of Psychiatry in Medicine, 5*, 269–273.

Ransom, D. (1988). Family therapists teaching in family practice settings: Issues and experiences. In H. A. Liddle, D. C. Breunlin, & R. C. Schwartz (Eds.), *Handbook of family therapy training and supervision*. New York: Guilford Press.

Saunders, B. E., Roberts, J. M., & Santos, A. B. (1987). Exposure to marital and family training in medical school: A student perspective. *Journal of Marital and Family Therapy, 13*(3), 311–314.

Schopler, E., Fox, R., & Cochrane, C. (1967). Teaching family dynamics to medical students. *American Journal of Orthopsychiatry, 37*, 906–911.

Smarr, E. R., & Berkow, R. (1977). Teaching psychological medicine to family practice residents. *American Journal of Psychiatry, 134*(9), 984–986.

G. Psychology

Berger, M. (1988). Academic psychology and family training. In H. A. Liddle, D. C. Breunlin, & R. C. Schwartz (Eds.), *Handbook of family therapy training and supervision*. New York: Guilford Press.

Cooper, A., Rampage, C., & Soucy, C. (1981). Family therapy training in clinical psychology programs. *Family Process, 20*, 155–156.

Ganahl, G., Ferguson, L. R., & L'Abate, L. (1985). Training in family psychology. In L. L'Abate (Ed.), *The handbook of family psychology and therapy*. Homewood, IL: Dorsey Press.

Green, R. J., Ferguson, L. R., Framo, J. L., Shapiro, R. J., & LaPerriere, K. (1979). A symposium on family therapy training for psychologists. *Professional Psychology, 10*, 859–862.

L'Abate, L. (1983). *Family psychology: Theory, therapy and training*. Washington, DC: University Press of America.

L'Abate, L., Berger, M., Wright, L., & O'Shea, M. (1979). Training family psychologists: The Family Studies Program at Georgia State University. *Professional Psychology, 10*, 58–65.

Liddle, H., Vance, S., & Pastushak, R. (1979). Family therapy training opportunities in psychology and counselor education. *Professional Psychology, 10*, 760–765.

Solomon, J., Ott, J., & Roach, A. (1986). A survey of training opportunities for predoctoral psychology interns in marriage and family therapy. *Journal of Marital and Family Therapy, 12*(3), 269–280.

Stanton, M. (1975). Family therapy training: Academic and internship opportunities for psychologists. *Family Process, 14*, 433–439.

Stanton, M. (1975). Psychology and family therapy. *Professional Psychology, 6*, 45–49.

H. Counselor Education

Hovestadt, A., Fenell, D., & Piercy, F. (1983). Integrating marriage and family therapy within counselor education: A three-level mode. In B. Okun & S. Gladding (Eds.), *Issues in training marriage and family therapists* (pp. 31–42). Ann Arbor, MI: ERIC/CAPS.

Piercy, F., & Hovestadt, A. (1980). Marriage and family therapy within counselor education. *Counselor Education and Supervision, 20*(1), 68–74.

Thomas, M. (1983). A comparison of CACREP and AAMFT requirements for accreditation. In B. Okun & S. Gladding (Eds.), *Issues in training marriage and family therapists* (pp. 17–27). Ann Arbor, MI: ERIC/CAPS.

I. Social Work

Amatea, E. S., Munson, P. A., Anderson, L. M., & Rudner, R. A. (1980). A short-term training for caseworkers in family counseling. *Social Casework, 6*, 205–214.

Bardill, D. R. (1984). *Family therapy in schools of social work*. Unpublished survey, Florida State University.

Bardill, D. R. (1988). Marriage and family therapy and graduate social work education. In H. A. Liddle, D. C. Breunlin, & R. C. Schwartz (Eds.), *Handbook of family therapy training and supervision*. New York: Guilford Press.

Beatman, F. L. (1964). The training and preparation of workers for family group treatment. *Social Casework, 45,* 202–208.

Meltzer, R. (1973). Family treatment in the curriculum of the graduate school of social work. *Family Process, 12,* 213–216.

Reynolds, M. K., & Crymes, J. T. (1970). A survey of the use of family therapy by caseworkers. *Social Casework, 51,* 76–81.

Schulman, G. (1976). Teaching family therapy to social work students. *Social Casework, 57,* 448–457.

Siporin, M. (1980). Marriage and family therapy in social work. *Social Casework, 61*(1), 11–21.

J. Agency Settings

Bishop, D., Byles, J., & Horn, D. (1984). Family therapy training methods: Minimal contact with an agency. *Journal of Family Therapy, 6*(4), 323–334.

Coleman, S., & Stanton, M. (1978). An index for measuring agency involvement in family therapy. *Family Process, 17,* 479–484.

Flomenhaft, K., & Carter, R. (1974). Family therapy training: A statewide program for mental health centers. *Hospital and Community Psychiatry, 25*(12), 789–791.

Framo, J. I. (1976). Chronicle of a struggle to establish a family unit within a community mental health center. In P. Guerin (Ed.), *Family therapy: Theory and practice*. New York: Gardner Press.

Haley, J. (1975). Why a mental health clinic should avoid doing family therapy. *Journal of Marriage and Family Counseling, 1,* 3–12.

Meyerstein, K. (1977). Family therapy training for paraprofessionals in a community mental health center. *Family Process, 16,* 477–494.

Morrison, J. (1979). Changing a mental health team's attitudes toward family therapy. *American Journal of Family Therapy, 7*(1), 57–60.

K. Nursing

Lansky, M. R., McVey, G. G., Wendahl, N., & Keyesa, V. (1979, May). Family treatment training for psychiatric nurses: A report on serial in-service workshops. *JPN and Mental Health Services,* 19–22.

Shapiro, R. J. (1975). Some implications of training psychiatric nurses in family therapy. *Journal of Marriage and Family Counseling, 4*(1), 323–330.

Wright, L., & Leahey, M. (1988). Nursing and family therapy training. In H. A. Liddle, D. C. Breunlin, & R. C. Schwartz (Eds.), *Handbook of family therapy training and supervision*. New York: Guilford Press.

L. Other

Carpenter, J. (1984). Making training relevant—A critical review of family therapy training in the UK. *Journal of Family Therapy, 6*(3), 235–246.

Figley, C. R., Sprenkle, D. H., & Denton, W. (1976). Training marriage and family counselors in an industrial setting. *Journal of Marriage and Family Counseling, 2*(2), 167–177.

Halpern, E. (1985). Training family therapists in Israel: The necessity for indigenous models. *American Journal of Family Therapy, 13*(1), 55–60.

Van Trommell, M. J. (1982). Training in marital and family therapy in Canada and the United States. *Journal of Strategic and Systemic Therapy, 1*(3), 31–39.

Wertheimer, D. (1978). Family therapy training in Israel. *Journal of Marriage and Family Counseling, 4,* 83–90.

13. TRAINEES

A. Becoming a Family Therapist

Ferber, A. (1972). Follow the path with heart. *International Journal of Psychiatry, 10,* 6–22.

Flores, J. L. (1979). Becoming a marriage, family, and child counselor: Notes from a Chicano. *Journal of Marital and Family Therapy, 5*(4), 17–22.

Haley, J. (1972). Beginning and experienced family therapists. In A. Ferber, M. Mendelsohn, & A. Napier (Eds.), *The book of family therapy.* New York: Science House.

Haley, J. (1972). We became family therapists. In A. Ferber, M. Mendelsohn, & A. Napier (Eds.), *The book of family therapy.* Boston: Houghton Mifflin.

Haley, J. (1977). A quiz for young therapists. *Psychotherapy: Theory, research and practice, 14,* 165–168.

Haley, J. (1980). How to be a marriage therapist without knowing practically anything. *Journal of Marital and Family Therapy, 6*(4), 385–391.

Harvey, M. A. (1980). On becoming a family therapist: The first three years. *International Journal of Family Therapy, 2*(4), 263–274.

Heatherington, L. (1987). Therapists' personalities and their evaluation of three family therapy styles: An empirical investigation. *Journal of Marital and Family Therapy, 13*(2), 167–178.

Napier, A. U., & Whitaker, C. (1973). Problems of the beginning family therapist. In D. Bloch (Ed.), *Techniques of family psychotherapy: A primer* (pp. 109–122). New York: Grune & Stratton.

Sigal, J., Guttman, H., Chagoga, L., & Lasry, J. (1973). Predictability of family therapists' behavior. *Canadian Psychiatric Association Journal, 18,* 199–202.

Warburton, J., & Alexander, J. F. (1983). The family therapist: What does one do? In L. L'Abate (Ed.), *The handbook of family psychology and therapy.* Homewood, IL: Dorsey Press.

Waxenberg, B. (1973). Therapists' empathy, regard, and genuineness as factors in staying in or dropping out of short-term time limited family therapy. *Dissertation Abstracts International, 34,* 1288B.

B. Trainees' Perspectives of Training

O'Hare, C., Henrich, A., Kirschnor, N., Oberstone, A., & Ritz, M. (1975). Group training in family therapy: The student's perspective. *Journal of Marriage and Family Counseling, 1,* 157–162.

Liddle, H. A., Davidson, G., & Barrett, M. J. (1988). Outcomes of live supervision: Trainee perspectives. In H. A. Liddle, D. C. Breunlin, & R. C. Schwartz (Eds.), *Handbook of family therapy training and supervision.* New York: Guilford Press.

Stedman, J. M., & Gaines, T. (1978). Trainee response to family therapy training. *Family Therapy, 5*(1), 1–12.

C. Trainee's Family of Origin

Forman, B. (1984). Family of origin work in systemic/strategic therapy. The *Clinical Supervisor, 2,* 81–85.

Guerin, P., & Fogarty, T. (1972). The family therapist's own family. *International Journal of Psychiatry, 10*(1), 6–22.

D. Therapy for Trainees

Guldner, C. A. (1978). Family therapy for the trainee in family therapy. *Journal of Marriage and Family Counseling, 4*(1), 127–132.

Kaslow, F. W. (1984). Treatment of marital and family therapists. In F. W. Kaslow (Ed.), *Psychotherapy with psychotherapists.* New York: Haworth Press.

Nichols, W. C. (1968). Personal psychotherapy for marital therapists. *Family Coordinator, 17*, 83–88. [Also in W. C. Nichols, (Ed.), (1974), *Marriage and family therapy*. Minneapolis, MN: National Council on Family Relations.]
Ormont, L. (1974). The use of group psychotherapy in the training of marriage counselors and family life educators. In W. C. Nichols (Ed.), *Marriage and family therapy*. Minneapolis, MN: National Council on Family Relations.

E. Trainee Gender Issues

Reid, E., McDaniel, S., Donaldson, C., & Tollers, M. (1987). Taking it personally: Issues of personal authority and competence for the female in family therapy training. *Journal of Marital and Family Therapy, 13*(2), 157–166.

14. TRAINER PERSPECTIVES

Framo, J. L. (1975). Personal reflections of a family therapist. *Journal of Marriage and Family Counseling, 1*, 15–28.
Framo, J. L. (1979). A personal viewpoint on training in marital and family therapy. *Professional Psychology, 10*(6), 868–875.

15. TRAINER–TRAINEE RELATIONSHIP

Schwartz, R. C. (1988). The trainer–trainee relationship in family therapy training. In H. A. Liddle, D. C. Breunlin, & R. C. Schwartz (Eds.), *Handbook of family therapy training and supervision*. New York: Guilford Press.
Tyler, M. G., & Tyler, S. A. (1986). The sorcerer's apprenticeship: The discourse of training in family therapy. *Cultural Anthropologist, 1*(2), 238–256.

16. TRAINING TRAINERS/SUPERVISORS

Breunlin, D. C., Liddle, H. A., & Schwartz, R. C. (1988). Concurrent training of therapists and supervisors. In H. A. Liddle, D. C. Breunlin, & R. C. Schwartz (Eds.), *Handbook of family therapy training and supervision*. New York: Guilford Press.
Constantine, J., Piercy, F., & Sprenkle, D. (1984). Live supervision-of-supervision in family therapy. *Journal of Marital and Family Therapy, 10*, 95–98.
Draper, R. (1982). From trainee to trainer. In R. Whiffen & J. Byng-Hall (Eds.), *Family therapy supervision: Recent developments in practice*. New York: Grune & Stratton.
Fine, J., & Fenell, D. (1985). Supervising the supervisor-of-supervision: A supervision-of-supervision technique or an hierarchical blurring? *Journal of Strategic and Systemic Therapies, 4*(3), 55–59.
Heath, A., & Storm, C. (1983). Answering the call: A manual for beginning supervisors. *The Family Therapy Networker, 7*(2), 36–37.
Heath, A. W., & Storm, C. L. (1985). From the institute to the ivory tower: The live supervision stage approach for teaching supervision in academic settings. *American Journal of Family Therapy, 13*(3), 27–36.
Liddle, H. A., Breunlin, D. C., Schwartz, R. C., & Constantine, J. (1984). Training family therapy supervisors: Issues of content, form, and context. *Journal of Marital and Family Therapy, 10*, 139–150.
Mendelsohn, M., & Ferber, A. (1972). Is everybody watching? In A. Ferber, M. Mendelsohn, & A. Napier (Eds.), *The book of family therapy*. New York: Science House.
Wright, L., & Coppersmith, E. I. (1983). Supervision of supervision: How to be "meta" to a metaposition. *Journal of Strategic and Systemic Therapy, 2*, 40–50.

17. EVALUATION OF TRAINING

A. Overviews/Reviews

Bishop, D. S., & Epstein, N. B. (July, 1979). *Research on teaching methods*. Paper presented at the International Forum for Trainers and Family Therapists, Tavistock Clinic, London, England.

Garfield, S. L. (1977). Research on the training of professional psychotherapists. In A. Gurman & A. Razin (Eds.), *Effective psychotherapy: A handbook of research*. New York: Pergamon Press.

Kniskern, D., & Gurman, A. (1979). Research on training in marriage and family therapy: Status, issues and direction. *Journal of Marital and Family Therapy, 5*(3), 83–94.

Kniskern, D., & Gurman, A. (1988). Research. In H. A. Liddle, D. C. Breunlin, & R. C. Schwartz (Eds.), *Handbook of family therapy training and supervision*. New York: Guilford Press.

B. Instruments/Methods/Scales

Alfred, G., & Kersey, F. (1977). The AIAC, a design for systematically analyzing marriage and family counselors: A progress report. *Journal of Marriage and Family Counseling, 3*(2), 17–26.

Bartlett, W. (1982). A multidimensional framework for the analysis of supervision of counseling. *Counseling Psychologist, 11*, 9–17.

Breunlin, D. C., Schwartz, R. C., Selby, L., & Krause, M. S. (1983). Evaluating family therapy training: The development of an instrument. *Journal of Marital and Family Therapy, 9*, 37–47.

Piercy, F., Laird, R., & Mohammed, Z. (1983). A family therapist rating scale. *Journal of Marital and Family Therapy, 18*, 451–462.

Pinsof, W. (1979). The family therapist behavior scale (FTBS): Developments and evaluation of a coding system. *Family Process, 18*, 451–462.

Schumm, W. R., Bugaighis, M. R., & Jurich, A. P. (1985). Using repeated measure designs in program evaluation of family therapy. *Journal of Marriage and Family Therapy, 11*, 87–95.

C. Program Evaluation

Byles, J., Bishop, D., & Horn, D. (1983). Evaluation of a family therapy training program. *Journal of Marital and Family Therapy, 9*, 299–304.

Churven, P. (1977). Role playing, deroling, and reality in family therapy training. *Australian Social Work, 30*, 23–27.

Churven, P., & McKinnon, T. (1982). Family therapy training: An evaluation of a workshop. *Family Process, 21*, 345–352.

Dowling, E., Cade, B., Breunlin, D. C., Frude, N., & Seligman, P. (1979). A retrospective survey of students' views on a family therapy training programme. *Journal of Family Therapy, 1*(1), 61–72.

Dowling, E., & Seligman, P. (1980). Description and evaluation of a family therapy training model. *Journal of Family Therapy, 2*(2), 123–130.

Greenberg, F. Z., & Neimeyer, G. J. (1986). The impact of structural family therapy training on conceptual and executive therapy skills. *Family Process, 25*(4), 599–608.

Pulleyblank, E., & Shapiro, R. J. (1986). Evaluation of family therapy trainees: Acquisition of cognitive and therapeutic behavior skills. *Family Process, 25*(4), 591–598.

Tucker, S., & Pinsof, W. (1984). The empirical evaluation of family therapy training. *Family Process, 23*, 437–456.

West, J. D., Hosie, T. W., & Zarki, J. J. (1985). Simulation in training family therapists: Process and outcome. *International Journal of Family Therapy, 7*(1), 50–58.

D. Comparative Studies

Crane, R., Griffin, W., & Hill, R. D. (1986). Influence of therapist skills on client perceptions of marriage and family therapy outcome: Implications for supervision. *Journal of Marriage and Family Therapy, 2*, 91–96.

Fenell, D. L., Hovestadt, A. J., & Samuel, J. H. (1986). A comparison of delayed feedback and live supervision models of marriage and family therapist clinical training. *Journal of Marriage and Family Therapy, 2*, 181–186.

Fisher, B., & Embree, T. (1981). *Supervision of beginning and advanced marital and family therapists: A comparative study.* Paper presented at the Annual Meeting of the American Association for Marriage and Family Therapy, San Diego, California.

Green, R., & Kolevson, M. (1982). Three approaches to family therapy: A study of convergence and divergence. *Journal of Marital and Family Therapy, 8*, 39–50.

Haldane, D., & McCluskey, U. (1980). Working with couples and families: Experience of training, consultation and supervision. *Journal of Family Therapy, 2*(3), 163–179.

Henry, P. W., Sprenkle, D. H., & Sheehan, R. (1986). Family therapy training: Student and faculty perceptions. *Journal of Marital and Family Therapy, 12*(3), 249–258.

Kolvezon, M., & Green, R. (1983). Practice and training in family therapy: A known group study. *Family Process, 22*, 179–190.

Mead, E., & Crane, D. (1978). An empirical approach to supervision and training of relationship therapists. *Journal of Marriage and Family Counseling, 4*(4), 67–76.

Mohammed, Z., & Piercy, F. (1983). The effects of two methods of training and sequencing on structuring and relationship skills of family therapists. *American Journal of Family Therapy, 11*, 64–71.

Reilly, I., & Bayles, T. (1981). Family therapy training—Give the customer what they want. *Journal of Family Therapy, 3*(2), 167–176.

Sutton, P. M. (1985). An insider's comparison of a major family therapy doctoral program and a leading nondegree family therapy training center. *Journal of Psychotherapy and the Family, 1*(4), 41–50.

Tomm, K., & Leahy, M. (1980). Training in family assessment: A comparison of three teaching methods. *Journal of Marital and Family Therapy, 6*(4), 453–458.

18. PROBLEMS IN TRAINING

Haley, J. (1974). Fourteen ways to fail as a teacher of family therapy. *Family Therapy, 1*, 1–8.

Haley, J. (1976). Problems of training therapists. *Problem-solving therapy* (pp. 164–194). San Francisco: Jossey-Bass.

Jenkins, H. (1984). Which skills how: Options for family therapy training. *Journal of Family Therapy, 6*(1), 17–34.

Liddle, H. (1978). The emotional and political hazards of teaching and learning family therapy. *Family Therapy, 5*, 1–12.

Maguire, P. H., & Asken, M. J. (1978). Psychological problems in family practice: Implications for training. *Journal of Clinical Child Psychology, 7*(1), 13–16.

Shapiro, R. (1975). Problems in teaching family therapy. *Professional Psychology, 6*, 41–44.

Shapiro, R. (1979). The problematic position of family therapy in professional training. *Professional Psychology, 10*, 876–879.

19. BOOKS WITH SOME TRAINING CONTENT

Ackerman, N., Beatman, F. L., & Sherman, S. (Eds.). (1961). *Exploring the base for family therapy.* New York: Family Service Association of America.

Barnard, C. P., & Corrales, R. G. (1979). *The theory and technique of family therapy.* Springfield, IL: Charles C. Thomas.

Ferber, A., Mendelsohn, M., & Napier, A. (Eds.). (1972). *The book of family therapy.* New York: Science House.

Group for the Advancement of Psychiatry. (1970). *The field of family therapy.* GAP Report 78. New York: Author.

Gurman, A. S. (Ed.). (1981). *Questions and answers in the practice of family therapy.* New York: Brunner/Mazel.

Gurman, A. S., & Kniskern, D. P. (Eds.). (1981). *Handbook of family therapy.* New York: Brunner/Mazel.

Gurman, A. S., & Razin, A. M. (1977). *Effective psychotherapy: A handbook of research.* New York: Pergamon Press.

Hoffman, L. (1981). *Foundations of family therapy: A conceptual framework for systems change.* New York: Basic Books.

Kramer, C. H. (1980). *Becoming a family therapist: Developing an integrated approach to working with families.* New York: Human Sciences Press.

Luthman, S. G., & Kirchenbaum, M. (1974). *The dynamic family.* Palo Alto, CA: Science and Behavior Books.

Zuk, G. (1975). *Process and practice in family therapy.* Haverford, PA: Psychiatry and Behaviorial Science Books.

20. ARTICLES WITH SOME TRAINING CONTENT

A. Overview/Reviews of Family Therapy

Beels, C. C., & Ferber, F. (1969). Family therapy: A view. *Family Process, 8,* 280–318.

Brodkin, A. M. (1980). Family therapy: The making of a mental health movement. *American Journal of Orthopsychiatry, 50*(1), 4–17.

Green, R., & Kolevzon, M. (1982). A survey of family therapy practitioners. *Social Casework, 63,* 95–99.

Guerin, P. (1976). Family therapy: The first twenty-five years. In P. Guerin (Ed.), *Family therapy: Theory and practice* (pp. 2–22). New York: Gardner Press.

Liddle, H. A. (1985). Five factors of failure in structural–strategic family therapy. In S. Coleman (Ed.), *Failures in family therapy.* New York: Guilford Press.

Mereness, D. (1968). Family therapy: An evolving role. *Perspectives in Psychiatric Care, 6*(6), 256–259.

Olson, D. H. (1970). Marital and family therapy: Integrative review and critique. *Journal of Marriage and the Family, 32,* 501–538.

Olson, D. H., Russell, C. S., & Sprenkle, D. H. (1980). Marital and family therapy: A decade review. *Journal of Marriage and the Family, 42*(2), 973–974.

Russell, A. (1976). Contemporary concerns in family therapy. *Journal of Marriage and Family Counseling, 2,* 243–250.

Siegel, L., & Dulfano, C. (1973). Family therapy: An overview. In *Career directions* (Vol. 2). East Hanover, NJ: Sandoz Pharmaceuticals, D. J. Publications.

B. Research

Gurman, A., & Kniskern, D. (1978). Research on marital and family therapy: Progress, perspective and prospect. In S. Garfield & A. Bergin (Eds.), *Handbook of psychotherapy and behavior change: An empirical analysis* (2nd ed.). New York: Wiley.

Kniskern, D. P., & Gurman, A. S. (1980). Advances and prospects for family therapy research. In J. P. Vincent (Ed.), *Advances in family intervention, assessment and theory* (Vol. 2). Greenwich, CT: JAI Press.

Kniskern, D. P., & Gurman, A. S. (1980). Future directions for family therapy research. In D. A. Bagarrozzi (Ed.), *New perspectives in family therapy.* New York: Human Sciences Press.

Woodward, C. A., Santa-Barbara, J., Levin, S., & Epstein, N. B. (1978). The role of goal attainment scaling in evaluation of family therapy outcomes. *American Journal of Orthopsychiatry, 48,* 464–476. [Also in J. G. Howells (Ed.) (1980), *Advances in family therapy.* New York: International Universities Press.]

C. Other

Churven, P. G. (1979). Family intervention for beginners: A rationale for a brief problem-oriented approach in child and family psychiatry. *Australian and New Zealand Journal of Psychiatry, 13,* 235–239.

Coyne, J. (1983). Father of family therapy? *The Family Therapy Networker, 7*(1), 50–51.

Liddle, H. A. (1979). Some crisis points in family therapy training. *Family Therapy News.*

Liddle, H. A. (1980). Future shock in family therapy. *Family Therapy News, 11*(6).

Piercy, F. (1984). The true believer and eclectic? *The Family Therapy Networker, 8,*(1), 21.

Ritterman, M. K. (1977). Paradigmatic classification of family therapy theories. *Family Process, 16,* 29–44.

Stanton, M. D. (1981). Marital therapy from a structural–strategic viewpoint. In G. P. Sholevar (Ed.), *Handbook of marriage and marital therapy.* Jamaica, NY: Spectrum Publications.

Walter, M. (1977). On becoming a mystery. In P. Papp (Ed.), *Family therapy: Full length case studies.* New York: Gardner Press.

21. TRAINING/SUPERVISION OF PSYCHOTHERAPY (Selected Listings)

Abroms, G. M. (1977). Supervision as metatherapy. In F. Kaslow & Associates (Eds.), *Supervision, consultation and staff training in the helping profession.* San Francisco: Jossey-Bass.

Aponte, J. F., & Lyons, M. J. (1980). Supervision in community settings: Concepts, methods, and issues. In A. Hess (Ed.), *Psychotherapy Supervision* (pp. 381–406). New York: Wiley.

Appel, K. E., Goodwin, H. M., Wood, H. P., & Askren, E. (1961). Training in psychotherapy: The use of marriage counseling in a university teaching clinic. *American Journal of Psychiatry, 117,* 709–711.

Brodsky, A., & Hare-Mustin, R. (1980). *Women and psychotherapy: An assessment of research and practice.* New York: Guilford Press.

Bruch, H. (1974). *Learning psychotherapy: Rationale and ground rules.* Cambridge, MA: Harvard University Press.

Caplan, G. (1970). *The theory and practice of mental health consultation.* New York: Basic Books.

Chodoff, P. (1972). Supervision of psychotherapy with videotapes: Pros and cons. *American Journal of Psychiatry, 128,* 53–57.

Dillon, I. (1976). Teaching models for graduate training in psychotherapy. *Family Therapy, 3,* 151–162.

Ekstein, R., & Wallerstein, R. (1972). *The teaching and learning of psychotherapy* (2nd ed.). New York: International Universities Press.

Fleming, J., & Burder, T. F. (1966). *Psychoanalytic supervision.* New York: Grune & Stratton.

Ford, J. D. (1979). Research in training counselors and clinicians. *Review of Educational Research, 49,* 87–130.

Friedman, D., & Kaslow, N. (1986). The development of professional identity in psychotherapists: Six stages in the supervision process. In F. W. Kaslow (Ed.), *Supervision and training: Models, dilemmas and challenges.* New York: Haworth Press.

Gilligan, C. (1982). *In a different voice.* Cambridge, MA: Harvard University Press.

Gruenberg, P. B., Liston, E. H., & Wayne, G. T. (1969). Intensive supervision of psychotherapy with videotape recordings. *American Journal of Psychotherapy, 23,* 98–105.

Hart, G. (1982). *The process of clinical supervision.* Baltimore, MD: University Park Press.

Hendrickson, D. E., & Krause, F. H. (1972). *Counseling psychotherapy: Training and supervision.* Columbus, OH: Charles E. Merrill.

Hess, A. K. (Ed.). (1980). *Psychotherapy supervision: Theory, research and practice.* New York: Wiley.

Hess, A. K. (1986). Growth in supervision: Stages of supervisee and supervisor development. In F. W. Kaslow (Ed.), *Supervision and training: Models, dilemmas and challenges.* New York: Haworth Press.

Hess, A. K. (Ed.). (1987). Special section: Advances in psychotherapy supervision. *Professional Psychology Research and Practice, 18,* 187–259.

Hogan, R. (1964). Issues and approaches in supervision. *Psychotherapy: Theory, Research and Practice, 1*(3), 173–176.

Langs, R. (1979). *The supervisory experience.* New York: Jason Aronson.

Lewin, K. (1952). Group decision and social change. In T. Newcomb & Hartley (Eds.), *Readings in social psychology.* New York: Holt, Rinehart & Winston.

Johnson, D. (1961). *Marriage counseling: Theory and practice.* Englewood Cliffs, NJ: Prentice-Hall.

Kadushin, A. (1968). Games people play in supervision. *Social Work, 13,* 23–32.

Kadushin, A. (1974). Supervisor-supervisee: A survey. *Social Work, 19,* 288–297.

Kadushin, A. (1976). *Supervision in social work.* New York: Columbia University Press.

Kaslow, F. W. (1972). Group supervision. In F. Kaslow (Ed.), *Issues in human services: A sourcebook for supervision and staff development.* San Francisco: Jossey-Bass.

Kaslow, F. W., & Associates. (Eds.). (1977). *Supervision, consultation and staff training in the helping profession.* San Francisco: Jossey-Bass.

Kaslow, F. (Ed.). (1986). *Supervision and training: Models, dilemmas and challenges.* New York: Haworth Press.

Kutzik, A. (1977). The medical field. In F. W. Kaslow (Ed.), *Supervision, consultation, and staff training in the helping profession.* San Francisco: Jossey-Bass.

Kutzik, A. (1977). The social work field. In F. W. Kaslow (Ed.), *Supervision, consultation, and staff training in the helping profession.* San Francisco: Jossey-Bass.

Matarazzo, R. G., & Patterson, D. (1986). Research on the teaching and learning of therapeutic skills. In S. Garfield & A. Bergin (Eds.), *Handbook of psychotherapy and behavior change* (3rd ed.). New York: John Wiley.

McColley, S. H., & Baker, E. L. (1982). Training activities and styles of beginning supervisors: A survey. *Professional Psychology, 13,* 283–292.

Miars, R. D., Tracey, T. J., Roy, P. B., Cornfeld, J. L., O'Farrell, M., & Gelso, C. J. (1983). Variation in supervision process across trainee experience levels. *Journal of Counseling Psychology, 30,* 403–412.

Mueller, W., & Kell, B. (1972). *Coping with conflict: Supervising counselors and psychotherapists.* New York: Appleton-Century-Crofts.

Muslin, H., Burstein, A., Gedo, K., & Sadow, L. (1967). Research on the supervisory process: I. Supervisor's appraisal of the interview data. *Archives of General Psychiatry, 16,* 427–431.

Powell, D. J. (1980). *Clinical supervision: Skills for substance abuse counselors.* New York: Human Sciences Press.

Reiss, B. (1960). The selection and supervision of psychotherapists. In N. Dellis & H. Stone (Eds.), *The training of psychotherapists.* Baton Rouge: Louisiana State University.

Rosenblatt, A., & Mayer, J. E. (1975). Objectionable supervisory styles: Students' views. *Social Work, 20,* 184–189

Searles, H. (1955). The informational value of the supervisor's emotional experiences. In H. Searles (Ed.), *Collected papers on schizophrenia and related subjects* (pp. 157–177). New York: International Universities Press.

Searles, H. (1962). Problems of psychoanalytic supervision. In H. Searles (Ed.), *Collected papers on schizophrenia and related subjects* (pp. 584–604). New York: International Universities Press.

Stein, S. P., Karasu, T., Charles, E., & Buckley, P. (1975). Supervision of the initial interview. *Archives of General Psychiatry, 32,* 265–268.

Stoltenberg, C. (1981). Approaching supervision from a developmental perspective: The counselor complexity model. *Journal of Counseling Psychology, 28,* 58–65.

Strinhelber, J., Patterson, V., Cliffe, K., & LeGoullon, M. (1984). An investigation of some relationships between psychotherapy supervision and patient change. *Journal of Clinical Psychology, 40,* 1346–1353.

Ward, C. H. (1960). An electronic aide for teaching interviewing techniques. *Archives of General Psychiatry, 3,* 357–358.

Wright, J. C., Horlick, S., Bouchard, C., Mathieu, M., & Zeichner, A. (1977). The development of instruments to assess behavior therapy training. *Journal of Behavioral Therapy and Experimental Psychiatry, 8,* 281–286.

Index

425